CONTENTS

INTRODUCTION 9
SNACKS & APPETIZERS RECIPES 11
1. Chocolate Bacon Bites 11
2. Lemon Green Beans 11
3. Mix Nuts 11
4. Fried Mushrooms 11
5. Crust-less Meaty Pizza 11
6. Dad's Boozy Wings 11
7. Turkey Balls 11
8. Parmesan Zucchini Chips 12
9. Creamy Sausage Bites 12
10. Zucchini And Tomato Salsa 12
11. Coconut Chicken Wings 12
12. Kohlrabi Chips 12
13. Mexican-style Corn On The Cob With Bacon 12
14. Buttered Corn On The Cob 12
15. Jalapeno Cheese Dip 13
16. Old-fashioned Onion Rings 13
17. Crab Dip 13
18. Grandma's Spicy Wings 13
19. Spinach Dip 13
20. Roasted Mixed Nuts 13
21. Potato Bread Rolls 14
22. The Best Party Mix Ever 14
23. Movie Night Zucchini Fries 14
24. Cajun Cheese Sticks 14
25. Balsamic Mushroom Platter 14
26. Sugar Snap Bacon 14
27. Crispy Eggplant Slices 15
28. Mexican Cheesy Zucchini Bites 15
29. Sweet Potato Fries With Spicy Dip 15
30. Easy Carrot Dip 15
31. Broccoli And Pecorino Toscano Fat Bombs 15
32. Brussels Sprouts With Feta Cheese 15
33. Cashew Dip 16
34. Bacon Croquettes 16
35. Chili Kale Chips 16
36. Crab And Chives Balls 16
37. Paprika Bacon Shrimp 16
38. Cauliflower Bombs With Sweet & Sour Sauce ... 16
39. Portabella Pizza Treat 17
40. Sea Scallops And Bacon Skewers 17
41. Parmesan Turnip Slices 17
42. Asian Twist Chicken Wings 17
43. Coconut Celery Stalks 17
44. Tofu 17
45. Italian Dip 17
46. Air Fried Cheese Sticks 18
47. Grilled Meatball Kabobs 18
48. Roasted Parsnip 18
49. Healthy Vegetable Kabobs 18
50. Cheesy Garlic Bread 18
51. Sage Roasted Zucchini Cubes 18
52. Spicy Dip 19
53. Skinny Spinach Chips 19
54. Cheesy Bacon Bread 19
55. Garlic Chicken Meatballs 19
56. Nutty Cauliflower Poppers 19
57. Cauliflower Dip 19
58. Garlic Eggplant Chips 20
59. Romano Cheese And Broccoli Balls 20
60. Turmeric Jicama Bites 20
61. Spinach Chips With Chili Yogurt Dip 20
62. Toasted Pumpkin Seeds 20
63. Smoked Almonds 20
64. Spicy Broccoli Poppers 20
65. Hot Cheesy Dip 21
66. Crunchy Bacon Bites 21
67. Perfect Crab Dip 21
68. Roasted Parsnip Sticks With Salted Caramel 21
69. Beer Battered Vidalia Rings 21
70. Olives Fritters 21
71. Tomato Smokies 22
72. Lime Tomato Salsa 22
73. Crispy Fried Leek With Mustard 22
74. Tomato Platter 22
75. Steak Nuggets 22
76. Pizza Bites 22
77. Ranch Kale Chips 23
78. Cheese Pastries 23
79. Lemon Biscuits 23
80. Healthy Broccoli Tots 23
81. Greek-style Squash Chips 23
82. Radish Sticks 23
83. Cocktail Wieners With Spicy Sauce 24
84. Granny's Green Beans 24
85. Tasty Tofu 24
86. Sweet Potato Fries 24
87. Almond Coconut Granola 24
88. Broccoli Bites 25
89. Lemon Shrimp Bowls 25
90. Mushroom Pizza Bites 25
91. Shrimp Dip 25
92. Broccoli Cheese Nuggets 25
93. Cheesy Zucchini Sticks 25
94. Banana Peppers 25
95. Cheese Rounds 26
96. Lemon Olives Dip 26
97. Pumpkin Seeds 26
98. Potato Wedges 26
99. Party Chicken Pillows 26
100. Instant Potato Croquettes 26
101. Old-fashioned Eggplant Slices 27
102. Cucumber And Spring Onions Salsa 27
103. Teriyaki Chicken Drumettes 27
104. Turkey Sausage Patties 27
105. Chicken Jalapeno Poppers 27
106. Baby Carrots With Asian Flair 27
107. Avocado Fries With Chipotle Sauce 28
108. Thai Chili Chicken Wings 28
109. "good As Gold" Veggie Bites 28
110. Rangoon Crab Dip 28
111. Roasted Brussels Sprouts & Bacon 28
112. Lava Rice Bites 28

113. Glazed Carrot Chips With Cheese 29
114. Crunchy Spicy Chickpeas 29
115. Polenta Sticks 29
116. Greek Calamari Appetizer 29
117. Eggplant Sticks 29
118. Feta And Parsley Filo Triangles 29
119. Simple Banana Chips 30
120. Creamy Cheddar Eggs 30
121. Thyme-roasted Sweet Potatoes 30
122. Parmesan Zucchini Bites 30
123. Avocado Sticks 30
124. Brussels Sprouts 30
125. Rosemary Beans 30
126. Cheddar Cheese Lumpia Rolls 31
127. Hillbilly Cheese Surprise 31
128. Broccoli Florets 31
129. Broccoli Fries With Spicy Dip 31
130. Crunchy Roasted Chickpeas 31
131. Broccoli Coconut Dip 31
132. Pickled Fries 31
133. Sweet Corn And Bell Pepper Sandwich 32
134. Pineapple Bites 32
135. Turmeric Chicken Cubes 32
136. Mozzarella Snack 32
137. Coconut Salmon Bites 32
138. Mini Turkey And Corn Burritos 32
139. Basic Salmon Croquettes 33
140. Cocktail Cranberry Meatballs 33
141. Healthy Toasted Nuts 33
142. Kale Chips 33
143. Turmeric Cauliflower Popcorn 33
144. Chipotle Jicama Hash 33
145. Hollandaise Sauce 33
146. Cocktail Flanks 33
147. Cheese Cookies 34
148. Mexican Muffins 34
149. Italian-style Tomato-parmesan Crisps 34
150. Healthy Veggie Lasagna 34
DESSERTS RECIPES 35
151. Cinnamon Ginger Cookies 35
152. Angel Food Cake 35
153. Summer Peach Crisp 35
154. Heavenly Tasty Lava Cake 35
155. Cinnamon And Sugar Sweet Potato Fries 35
156. Poppyseed Muffins 35
157. Red Velvet Pancakes 35
158. Picnic Blackberry Muffins 36
159. Plum And Currant Tart Recipe 36
160. Apple Caramel Relish 36
161. Chocolate Biscuit Sandwich Cookies 36
162. Merengues 37
163. Orange Muffins 37
164. Mom's Orange Rolls 37
165. Raspberry-coconut Cupcake 37
166. Crusty 37
167. Lemon Mini Pies With Coconut 37
168. Chocolate Almond Cookies 38
169. Hazelnut Brownie Cups 38
170. Pumpkin Cookies 38
171. Ricotta Cheese Cake 38

172. Coconut And Berries Cream 38
173. Ninja Pop-tarts 38
174. Moon Pie 39
175. Espresso Cinnamon Cookies 39
176. Baked Plum Cream 39
177. Bread Pudding 39
178. Double Chocolate Muffins 39
179. Air Fried Doughnuts 39
180. Apple Pie In Air Fryer 40
181. Coffee Flavored Cookie Dough 40
182. Pumpkin Bars 40
183. Berry Cookies 40
184. Choco Mug Cake 40
185. Father's Day Cranberry&Whiskey Brownies .. 40
186. Almond Coconut Lemon Cake 41
187. Egg Custard 41
188. Orange Carrot Cake 41
189. Homemade Coconut Banana Treat 41
190. Pumpkin Cinnamon Pudding 41
191. Easy Fruitcake With Cranberries 41
192. Chocolate Paradise Cake 42
193. Churros 42
194. Chocolate Candies 42
195. Lemon Mousse 42
196. Ginger Vanilla Cookies 42
197. Fiesta Pastries 43
198. Avocado Cream Pudding 43
199. Easy 'n Delicious Brownies 43
200. Mouth-watering Strawberry Cobbler 43
201. Fried Pineapple Rings 43
202. Marshmallow Pastries 44
203. Dark Chocolate Cheesecake 44
204. Classic Mini Cheesecakes 44
205. Strawberry Jam 44
206. Avocado Walnut Bread 44
207. Cherry Pie 45
208. Cheesy Orange Fritters 45
209. Orange Sponge Cake 45
210. Apple Cake 45
211. Grandma's Butter Cookies 45
212. Fudge Cake With Pecans 45
213. Enchanting Coffee-apple Cake 46
214. Zucchinis Bars 46
215. Crisped 'n Chewy Chonut Holes 46
216. Baked Apples With Nuts 46
217. Blackberries Cake 46
218. Chia Chocolate Cookies 46
219. Old-fashioned Plum Dumplings 47
220. Blackberry Crisp 47
221. Birthday Chocolate Raspberry Cake 47
222. Nutty Fudge Muffins 47
223. Chocolate Molten Lava Cake 47
224. Apple-toffee Upside-down Cake 48
225. Chocolate Coffee Cake 48
226. Butter Custard 48
227. Ricotta And Lemon Cake Recipe 48
228. Chocolate Banana Pastries 48
229. Mini Almond Cakes 48
230. Coconut 'n Almond Fat Bombs 49
231. Pineapple Sticks 49

232. White Chocolate Berry Cheesecake 49
233. Strawberry Cheese Cake 49
234. Pear Fritters With Cinnamon And Ginger......... 49
235. Vanilla Soufflé.. 49
236. Easy Blueberry Muffins 49
237. Flavor-packed Clafoutis.................................... 50
238. Leche Flan Filipino Style 50
239. Strawberry Shortcake Quickie 50
240. Vanilla Bean Dream 50
241. Mock Cherry Pie 50
242. Semolina Cake 50
243. Sunday Tart With Walnuts 51
244. Chocolate Coconut Cake 51
245. Creamy Rice Pudding....................................... 51
246. Spanish-style Doughnut Tejeringos................... 51
247. Hazelnut Vinegar Cookies................................ 51
248. Raspberry Pudding Surprise.............................. 51
249. Sweet Squares Recipe 52
250. No Flour Lime Muffins 52
POULTRY RECIPES 53
251. Crispy Herbed Turkey Breast............................ 53
252. Potato Cakes & Cajun Chicken Wings 53
253. Turkey Wings With Butter Roasted Potatoes. 53
254. Classic Chicken Nuggets 53
255. Malaysian Chicken Satay With Peanut Sauce.. 53
256. Glazed Chicken Wings 54
257. Juicy & Spicy Chicken Wings 54
258. Rosemary Lemon Chicken................................ 54
259. Tasty Southwest Chicken 54
260. Chicken Breasts & Spiced Tomatoes 54
261. Awesome Sweet Turkey Bake 54
262. Creamy Chicken Breasts& Crumbled Bacon.... 55
263. Chicken & Veggie Kabobs 55
264. Indian Chicken Tenders 55
265. Tequila Glazed Chicken 55
266. Spinach 'n Bacon Egg Cups.............................. 55
267. Teriyaki Chicken 56
268. Lemon-butter Battered Thighs 56
269. Marinara Chicken 56
270. Paprika Chicken Legs With Brussels Sprouts . 56
271. Peanut Chicken And Pepper Wraps................... 56
272. Grilled Chicken Recipe From Korea................... 56
273. Grilled Sambal Chicken 57
274. Easy Turkey Kabobs 57
275. Cheesy Potato, Broccoli 'n Ham Bake.............. 57
276. Duck Breasts With Candy Onion &Coriander. 57
277. Pretzel Crusted Chicken With Spicy Mustard
Sauce 57
278. Turkey Meatloaf 58
279. Turkey Strips With Cranberry Glaze.................. 58
280. Lemon & Garlic Chicken 58
281. Basil Mascarpone Chicken Fillets 58
282. Creamy Turkey Bake.. 58
283. Eggs 'n Turkey Bake 58
284. Garlic Chicken.. 59
285. Pineapple Sauce Marinated Chicken 59
286. Dill Chicken Fritters 59
287. Sticky Greek-style Chicken Wings 59
288. Sausage Stuffed Chicken.................................. 59
289. Tomato, Eggplant 'n Chicken Skewers 59

290. Spice Lime Chicken Tenders 60
291. Old-fashioned Chicken Drumettes 60
292. Fennel Duck Legs 60
293. Country-fried Chicken Drumsticks.................... 60
294. Chicken & Pepperoni Pizza 60
295. Chives And Lemon Chicken............................. 60
296. Chicken Wonton Rolls 61
297. Garlic Rosemary Roasted Chicken..................... 61
298. The Best Pizza Chicken Ever 61
299. Dijon Turkey Drumstick 61
300. Honey-balsamic Orange Chicken 61
301. Crispy Chicken Wings...................................... 61
302. Sun-dried Tomatoes And Chicken Mix.............. 62
303. Spinach Stuffed Chicken Breasts 62
304. Almond Flour Coco-milk Battered Chicken 62
305. Peppery Turkey Sandwiches............................. 62
306. Summer Meatballs With Cheese....................... 62
307. Indian Chicken Mix 63
308. Chicken Strips... 63
309. Fried Herbed Chicken Wings 63
310. Garlic Turkey And Lemon Asparagus 63
311. Jerk Chicken, Pineapple & Veggie Kabobs 63
312. Sriracha-ginger Chicken 63
313. Crispy 'n Salted Chicken Meatballs 64
314. Kfc Like Chicken Tenders 64
315. Adobo Seasoned Chicken With Veggies 64
316. Crispy Chicken Thighs..................................... 64
317. Ham & Cheese Chicken................................... 64
318. Chicken With Asparagus And Zucchini 65
319. Chicken Wings And Vinegar Sauce 65
320. Green Curry Hot Chicken Drumsticks............... 65
321. Chicken Fajita Casserole.................................. 65
322. Buffalo Chicken Wings 65
323. Italian-style Chicken With Roma Tomatoes 65
324. Saucy Chicken With Leeks 66
325. Paprika Turkey And Shallot Sauce 66
326. Duck And Walnut Rice..................................... 66
327. Bacon Wrapped Chicken Breasts 66
328. Chicken Pockets.. 66
329. Pizza Stuffed Chicken...................................... 66
330. Oregano-thyme Rubbed Thighs........................ 67
331. Chicken And Chickpeas Mix 67
332. Beastly Bbq Drumsticks 67
333. Duck With Peppers And Pine Nuts Sauce 67
334. Chicken With Veggies & Rice........................... 67
335. Sweet Curried Chicken Cutlets......................... 68
336. Pepper-salt Egg 'n Spinach Casserole 68
337. Breaded Chicken Cutlets.................................. 68
338. Oregano Duck Spread...................................... 68
339. Garlic Paprika Rubbed Chicken Breasts 68
340. Air Fried Southern Drumsticks.......................... 68
341. Air Fried Chicken With Honey & Lemon 69
342. Easy Chicken Fried Rice................................... 69
343. Simple Chicken Wings..................................... 69
344. Lemon Grilled Chicken Breasts......................... 69
345. Parmesan Chicken Cutlets................................ 69
346. Creamy Chicken-veggie Pasta.......................... 69
347. Delicious Chicken Burgers 70
348. Bacon Chicken Mix... 70
349. Peppery Lemon-chicken Breast......................... 70

350. Ginger And Coconut Chicken 70
351. Italian Seasoned Chicken Tenders 70
352. Basil-garlic Breaded Chicken Bake 70
353. Chicken With Golden Roasted Cauliflower 71
354. Cauliflower Stuffed Chicken 71
355. Chicken With Veggies 71
356. Grilled Hawaiian Chicken 71
357. Mixed Vegetable Breakfast Frittata 72
358. Chicken, Rice & Vegetables 72
359. Shaking Tarragon Chicken Tenders 72
360. Chicken Wrapped In Bacon 72
361. Chicken Stuffed With Sage And Garlic 72
362. Parmesan Chicken Nuggets 72
363. Tasty Caribbean Chicken 73
364. Chinese-style Sticky Turkey Thighs 73
365. Graceful Mango Chicken 73
366. Chicken Bbq Recipe From Peru 73
367. Quick 'n Easy Brekky Eggs 'n Cream 73
368. Sweet & Sour Chicken Thighs 74
369. Sweet And Sour Grilled Chicken 74
370. Chicken And Ghee Mix 74
371. Simple Turkey Breasts 74
372. Air Fried Cheese Chicken 74
373. Duck Breast With Fig Sauce Recipe 74
374. Chinese Chili Chicken 75
375. Chili And Paprika Chicken Wings 75
376. Crusted Chicken 75
377. Greek Chicken Meatballs 75
378. Buffalo Chicken 75
379. Bacon-wrapped Turkey With Cheese 75
380. Creamy Scrambled Eggs With Broccoli 76
381. Sweet Chili Chicken Wings 76
382. Chicken Pizza Crusts 76
383. Nacho-fried Chicken Burgers 76
384. Holiday Colby Turkey Meatloaf 76
385. Bacon 'n Egg-substitute Bake 76
386. Flavorful Cornish Hen 77
387. Chicken Bbq On Kale Salad 77
388. Tomato, Cheese 'n Broccoli Quiche 77
389. Creamy Onion Chicken 77
390. Sweet Turmeric Chicken Wings 77
391. Mouthwatering Turkey Roll 77
392. Chinese Chicken Drumsticks 78
393. Bbq Turkey Meatballs With Cranberry Sauce 78
394. Sriracha-vinegar Marinated Chicken 78
395. Chicken Gruyere 78
396. Easy How-to Hard Boil Egg In Air Fryer 78
397. Chicken Popcorn 78
398. Vermouth Bacon And Turkey Burgers 79
399. Coconut Chicken Bake 79
400. Thyme And Sage Turkey Breasts 79
BEEF,PORK & LAMB RECIPES 80
401. Asian-style Round Steak.. 80
402. Rich Meatball And Mushroom Cassoulet 80
403. Cinnamon Lamb Meatloaf.. 80
404. Spiced Lamb Steaks 80
405. Top Chuck With Mustard And Herbs 80
406. Paprika Burgers With Blue Cheese 81
407. Pork Belly Marinated 81
408. Herbed Crumbed Filet Mignon.............................. 81

409. Beef & Kale Omelet 81
410. Bolognese Sauce With A Twist 81
411. Ginger And Turmeric Lamb 81
412. Crispy Roast Garlic-salt Pork 82
413. Beef And Broccoli 82
414. Meaty Pasta Bake From The Southwest 82
415. Spicy Pork With Herbs And Candy Onions......82
416. Pork Chops Marinate In Honey-mustard 82
417. Tamales 82
418. Flatiron Steak Grill On Parsley Salad..................83
419. Beef Roast In Worcestershire-rosemary...........83
420. Champagne-vinegar Marinated Skirt Steak.....83
421. Hickory Smoked Beef Jerky 83
422. Beef, Pearl Onions And Cauliflower 83
423. Pork Tenderloin With Bacon & Veggies..............84
424. Air Fryer Beef Casserole 84
425. Saucy Beef With Cotija Cheese 84
426. Korean Beef Bulgogi Burgers..................................84
427. Beefy Bell Pepper'n Egg Scramble........................84
428. Ground Beef On Deep Dish Pizza 84
429. Spicy Mexican Beef With Cotija Cheese 85
430. Spicy And Saucy Pork Sirloin 85
431. Cheesy Sausage'n Grits Bake 85
432. Garlic Burgers...85
433. Sweet & Sour Pork Chops 85
434. Gourmet Meatloaf..86
435. Almond Flour 'n Egg Crusted Beef........................86
436. Cajun Pork And Peppers Mix..................................86
437. Bbq Skirt Steak...86
438. Moist Stuffed Pork Roll 86
439. Top Loin Beef Strips With Blue Cheese..............87
440. Beef And Garlic Onions Sauce 87
441. Garlic Pork And Bok Choy 87
442. Pork Tenderloin With Bell Peppers 87
443. Herbed Beef Roast 87
444. Garlic Fillets...87
445. Simple New York Strip Steak 87
446. Spicy Buttered Steaks 88
447. Mustard Beef And Garlic Spinach........................88
448. Marinated Flank Steak 88
449. Coffee Flavored Steaks Recipe...............................88
450. Saffron Spiced Rack Of Lamb 88
451. Balsamic London Broil With Garlic......................88
452. Teriyaki Steak With Fresh Herbs..........................89
453. Italian Beef Meatballs 89
454. Easy Beef Medallions With Parsley &Peppers 89
455. Stuffed Pork Steaks Recipe.....................................89
456. Cumin-paprika Rubbed Beef Brisket....................89
457. Saucy Lemony Beef Steaks 90
458. Bacon With Shallot And Greens 90
459. Marjoram Lamb 90
460. Steak Rolls..90
461. Italian Pork 90
462. Favorite Beef Stroganoff..90
463. Spicy Pork...91
464. Scrumptious Lamb Chops..91
465. Easy Cheeseburger Meatballs................................91
466. Spicy Meatloaf With Peppers 91
467. Cardamom Lamb Mix 91
468. Sausage 'n Cauliflower Frittata 92

469. Sriracha-hoisin Glazed Grilled Beef......................92
470. Tomato Stuffed Pork Roll.................................92
471. Coriander, Mustard 'n Cumin Rubbed Flank Steak...92
472. Fat Burger Bombs...92
473. Cilantro Steak..93
474. Orange Carne Asada..93
475. Beef Schnitzel...93
476. Classic Skirt Steak Strips With Veggies.............93
477. Sloppy Joes With A Twist................................93
478. Buttered Filet Mignon....................................94
479. Beef And Thyme Cabbage Mix...............................94
480. Easy Corn Dog Bites......................................94
481. Bjorn's Beef Steak.......................................94
482. Max's Meatloaf...94
483. Bacon Stuffing...94
484. Curry Pork Roast In Coconut Sauce.......................95
485. Mexican Beef Mix Recipe..................................95
486. Cheesy Mini Meatloaves...................................95
487. Herbed Pork Chops..95
488. Fried Sausage And Mushrooms Recipe..................96
489. Beef Sausage And Vegetable Medley......................96
490. Pork Butt With Herb-garlic Sauce.......................96
491. Classic Keto Cheeseburgers..............................96
492. Grilled Steak On Tomato-olive Salad....................96
493. Italian Fennel Lamb......................................96
494. Beef Bulgogi...97
495. Beef Recipe Texas-rodeo Style...........................97
496. Lamb And Vinaigrette.....................................97
497. Caraway, Sichuan 'n Cumin Lamb Kebabs........97
498. Pork With Padrón Peppers And Green Olives 97
499. Italian Peperonata With A Twist.........................97
500. Lamb Racks And Fennel Mix Recipe....................98
FISH & SEAFOOD RECIPES....................99
501. Crumbed Cod..99
502. Fish Packets..99
503. Cod And Shallot Frittata................................99
504. Butterflied Prawns With Garlic-sriracha 99
505. Lobster Tails With Olives And Butter................99
506. Butter Flounder Fillets.................................99
507. Fried Anchovies..100
508. Rich Crab Croquettes...................................100
509. Baked Scallops With Garlic Aioli 100
510. Italian Sardinas Fritas................................100
511. Butter Mussels...100
512. Swordfish With Roasted Peppers........................101
513. Crispy Tilapia Fillets.................................101
514. English-style Flounder Fillets........................101
515. Monkfish With Sautéed Vegetables 101
516. Crispy Mustardy Fish Fingers..........................101
517. Miso Sauce Over Grilled Salmon........................102
518. Creamy Salmon..102
519. Mahi Mahi With Green Beans............................102
520. Buttered Baked Cod With Wine..........................102
521. Salmon With Asparagus..................................102
522. Cod Nuggets..102
523. Simple Salmon Patties..................................103
524. Tartar Sauce 'n Crispy Cod Nuggets 103
525. Shrimp Scampi Linguine.................................103
526. Cayenne Salmon...103

527. Soy Sauce Glazed Cod...................................103
528. Chili Salmon Recipe....................................103
529. Paprika And Cumin Shrimp..............................104
530. Delicious Prawns And Sweet Potatoes...........104
531. Coconut Calamari.......................................104
532. Cajun Seasoned Salmon Filet...........................104
533. Butter Crab Muffins....................................104
534. Smoked And Creamed White Fish.....................104
535. Lime Cod...105
536. Salmon Cakes..105
537. Cod Fillets With Lemon And Mustard.............105
538. Wrapped Scallops.......................................105
539. Creamy Tuna Cakes......................................105
540. Fried Haddock Fillets..................................105
541. Crispy Cod Sticks......................................106
542. Lemon Garlic Shrimp....................................106
543. Paprika Tilapia..106
544. Beer Battered Cod Filet...............................106
545. Creamy Shrimp..106
546. Louisiana-style Shrimp................................106
547. Crispy Fish Fingers With Lemon Herbs 107
548. Garlic Shrimp Mix......................................107
549. Spicy Cod..107
550. Crab Stuffed Flounder..................................107
551. Summer Fish Packets....................................107
552. Thyme Catfish..107
553. Creole Crab..108
554. Sunday Fish With Sticky Sauce.....................108
555. Best Cod Ever..108
556. Stevia Cod...108
557. Chili Sea Bass Mix.....................................108
558. Cajun Fish Cakes With Cheese......................108
559. Grilled Shrimp With Chipotle-orange Seasoning 109
560. Grilled Salmon Fillets.................................109
561. Tuna Steaks With Pearl Onions.........................109
562. Shrimp Magic...109
563. Mediterranean Salad....................................109
564. Old Bay Calamari.......................................109
565. Breaded Scallops.......................................110
566. Lemony-sage On Grilled Swordfish 110
567. Tuna Cake Burgers With Beer Cheese Sauce 110
568. Sesame Prawns With Firecracker Sauce 110
569. Cheesy Crab Dip..110
570. Full Baked Trout En Papillote With Herbs 111
571. Leamony-parsley Linguine&Grilled Tuna......111
572. Paprika Cod And Endives...............................111
573. Herbed Calamari Rings..................................111
574. Crispy Coconut Covered Shrimps 111
575. Citrusy Branzini On The Grill........................111
576. Salmon And Blackberry Sauce..........................111
577. Coconut Shrimp With Orange Sauce.............112
578. Salmon Patties...112
579. Snapper Fillets And Veggies Recipe...............112
580. Perfect Salmon Fillets.................................112
581. Filipino Bistek..112
582. Wild Alaskan Salmon With Parsley Sauce 113
583. Grilled Shellfish With Vegetables................113
584. Parmesan And Garlic Trout.............................113
585. Honey-ginger Soy Sauce Over Grilled Tuna ..113

586. Shrimp Scampi Dip With Cheese...................... 113
587. Pistachio Crusted Salmon............................... 114
588. Cajun Fish Fritters... 114
589. Celery Leaves 'n Garlic-oil Grilled Turbot...... 114
590. Delicious Snapper En Papillote...................... 114
591. Char-grilled 'n Herbed Sea Scallops................ 114
592. Favorite Shrimp Fritatta............................... 114
593. Minty Trout And Pine Nuts............................ 114
594. Coriander Cod And Green Beans..................... 115
595. Salad Niçoise With Peppery Halibut................ 115
596. Lemon And Oregano Tilapia Mix.................... 115
597. Drunken Skewered Shrimp, Tomatoes............ 115
598. Cheese Crust Salmon.................................... 115
599. Creamed Trout Salad..................................... 116
600. Lime, Oil 'n Leeks On Grilled Swordfish......... 116
VEGAN & VEGETARIAN RECIPES 117
601. Crispy Shawarma Broccoli............................. 117
602. Hearty Celery Croquettes With Chive Mayo. 117
603. Radish And Mozzarella Salad.......................... 117
604. Easy Vegan "chicken".................................... 117
605. Baked Potato Topped With Cream Cheese.... 117
606. Easy Roast Winter Vegetable Delight............. 117
607. Cauliflower, Broccoli And Chickpea Salad..... 118
608. Keto Cauliflower Hash Browns....................... 118
609. Corn Cakes... 118
610. Sesame Seeds Bok Choy(2)............................ 118
611. Parsnip & Potato Bake.................................. 118
612. Black Bean Burger With Garlic-chipotle......... 119
613. Hearty Carrots... 119
614. Open-faced Vegan Flatbread-wich.................. 119
615. Eggplant Cheeseburger................................. 119
616. Eggplant Gratin With Mozzarella Crust.......... 119
617. Crispy Green Beans With Pecorino Romano 119
618. Vegetable Kabobs With Peanut Sauce............. 120
619. Ultra-crispy Tofu... 120
620. Broccoli With Olives..................................... 120
621. Herby Zucchini 'n Eggplant Bake................... 120
622. Baked Polenta With Chili-cheese................... 120
623. Shallots 'n Almonds On French Green Beans 121
624. Oatmeal Stuffed Bell Peppers........................ 121
625. Vegetable Spring Rolls.................................. 121
626. Air-fried Falafel... 121
627. Salted Beet Chips... 121
628. Air-fried Veggie Sushi................................... 121
629. Surprising Quinoa Eggplant Rolls.................. 122
630. Polenta Fries... 122
631. Garlic Broccoli... 122
632. Tomato Sandwiches With Feta And Pesto..... 122
633. Garlic-roasted Brussels Sprouts.................... 122
634. Banana Pepper Stuffed With Tofu 'n Spices . 122
635. Cheesy Muffins.. 123
636. Vegetable Tortilla Pizza................................ 123
637. Vegetable Bake With Cheese And Olives........ 123
638. Baked Zucchini Recipe From Mexico............. 123
639. Crispy Brussels Sprout Chips........................ 123
640. Baby Portabellas With Romano Cheese.......... 123
641. Zoodles With Cheese.................................... 124
642. Spicy Tofu... 124
643. Broccoli With Cauliflower.............................. 124
644. Tofu With Peanut Butter Sauce 124

645. Three Veg Bake.. 124
646. Tofu With Veggies... 125
647. Barbecue Tofu With Green Beans................... 125
648. Grilled 'n Glazed Strawberries....................... 125
649. Crispy Vegie Tempura Style........................... 125
650. Air Fried Vegetables With Garlic.................... 125
651. Sautéed Bacon With Spinach.......................... 126
652. Cinnamon Pear Chips.................................... 126
653. Easy Fry Portobello Mushroom...................... 126
654. Mushrooms With Tahini Sauce....................... 126
655. Prawn Toast... 126
656. Rice & Beans Stuffed Bell Peppers................. 126
657. Delightful Mushrooms.................................. 126
658. Jalapeno Stuffed With Bacon 'n Cheeses........ 127
659. Rosemary Olive-oil Over Shrooms.................. 127
660. Rainbow Roasted Vegetables......................... 127
661. Classic Vegan Chili....................................... 127
662. Pesto Tomatoes... 127
663. The Best Avocado Fries Ever 128
664. Tender Butternut Squash Fry......................... 128
665. Quinoa & Veggie Stuffed Peppers.................. 128
666. Greek-style Roasted Vegetables..................... 128
667. Caramelized Carrots..................................... 129
668. The Best Falafel Ever.................................... 129
669. Rich Asparagus And Mushroom Patties.......... 129
670. Vegetable Skewers With Peanut Sauce........... 129
671. Dad's Roasted Pepper Salad.......................... 129
672. Healthy Apple-licious Chips........................... 130
673. Warm Farro Salad With Roasted Tomatoes. 130
674. Grilled 'n Spiced Tomatoes On Garden Salad 130
675. Traditional Indian Bhaji............................... 130
676. Cottage Cheese And Potatoes........................ 130
677. Refreshingly Zesty Broccoli........................... 131
678. Spiced Soy Curls.. 131
679. Fried Broccoli Recipe From India................... 131
680. Almond Asparagus.. 131
681. Curly Vegan Fries... 131
682. Curried Cauliflower Florets........................... 131
683. Eggplant Salad... 132
684. Ricotta Cauliflower Fritters........................... 132
685. Easy Glazed Carrots...................................... 132
686. Herbed Potatoes.. 132
687. Tofu With Capers Sauce................................ 132
688. Crispy Bacon-wrapped Asparagus Bundles.. 132
689. Radish Salad.. 133
690. Your Traditional Mac 'n Cheese..................... 133
691. Two-cheese Vegetable Frittata 133
692. Kurkuri Bhindi (indian Fried Okra)................ 133
693. Sweet & Spicy Parsnips................................. 134
694. Lemony Green Beans..................................... 134
695. Air Fried Halloumi With Veggies.................... 134
696. Avocado Rolls.. 134
697. Classic Baked Banana................................... 134
698. Mediterranean-style Potato Chips With Dip 134
699. Baked Spicy Tortilla Chips............................. 135
700. Mozzarella Cabbage With Blue Cheese 135
OTHER AIR FRYER RECIPES 136
701. Spring Chocolate Doughnuts........................ 136
702. Frittata With Porcini Mushrooms................... 136
703. Zesty Broccoli Bites With Hot Sauce.............. 136

704. Wine-braised Turkey Breasts...............................136
705. Homemade Pork Scratchings............................136
706. Baked Apples With Crisp Topping 137
707. Cornbread With Pulled Pork..............................137
708. Double Cheese Mushroom Balls.......................137
709. Rosemary Roasted Mixed Nuts 137
710. Creamed Asparagus And Egg Salad 137
711. Delicious Hot Fruit Bake 138
712. Gorgonzola Stuffed Mushrooms With Mayo. 138
713. Scrambled Egg Muffins With Cheese...............138
714. French Toast With Blueberries And Honey.. 138
715. Vegetarian Tofu Scramble.................................138
716. Breakfast Eggs With Swiss Chard And Ham. 138
717. Baked Eggs With Linguica Sausage.................139
718. Steak Fingers With Mushrooms &Cheese......139
719. Japanese Fried Rice With Eggs.........................139
720. Eggs Florentine With Spinach 139
721. Party Pancake Kabobs.......................................139
722. Savory Italian Crespelle.....................................140
723. Country-style Pork Meatloaf 140
724. Easy Fried Button Mushrooms.........................140
725. Cheese Sticks With Ketchup..............................140
726. Oatmeal Pizza Cups...140
727. Keto Rolls With Halibut And Eggs 141
728. Easy Roasted Hot Dogs 141
729. Hearty Southwestern Cheeseburger Frittata141
730. Sweet Mini Monkey Rolls..................................141
731. Potato And Kale Croquettes 141
732. Easiest Vegan Burrito Ever 141
733. Hanukkah Latkes..142
734. Mozzarella Stick Nachos...................................142
735. Rum Roasted Cherries.......................................142
736. The Best Sweet Potato Fries Ever....................142
737. Super Easy Sage And Lime Wings....................142
738. Egg Salad With Asparagus And Spinach.........143
739. Traditional Onion Bhaji.....................................143
740. Dijon And Curry Turkey Cutlets 143
741. Snapper With Gruyere Cheese 143
742. Fingerling Potatoes With Cashew Sauce 143
743. Mother's Day Pudding..144
744. Scrambled Eggs With Sausage...........................144
745. Quinoa With Baked Eggs And Bacon.................144
746. Italian Creamy Frittata With Kale.....................144
747. Roasted Turkey Sausage With Potatoes.........144
748. Red Currant Cupcakes..145
749. Sweet Corn And Kernel Fritters 145
750. Italian Sausage And Veggie Bake 145
751. Easy Frittata With Chicken Sausage.................145
752. Bourbon Glazed Mango With Walnuts............145
753. Onion Rings With Mayo Dip.................................146
754. Chive, Feta And Chicken Frittata......................146
755. Crispy Wontons With Asian Dipping Sauce.. 146
756. Roasted Green Bean Salad With Cheese.........146
757. Creamy Lemon Turkey.......................................147
758. Easy Cheesy Broccoli 147
759. Greek-style Roasted Figs....................................147
760. Celery And Bacon Cakes.....................................147
761. Cheesy Pasilla Turkey..147
762. Cheesy Cauliflower Balls....................................147
763. Cheese Balls With Spinach 148
764. Grilled Chicken Tikka Masala............................148
765. Stuffed Mushrooms With Cheese......................148
766. Easy Frittata With Mozzarella And Kale.........148
767. Cheese And Chive Stuffed Chicken Rolls 149
768. Two Cheese And Shrimp Dip..............................149
769. Peanut Butter And Chicken Bites......................149
770. Easiest Pork Chops Ever....................................149
771. Keto Brioche With Caciocavallo.........................149
772. Creamed Cajun Chicken.....................................150
773. Double Cheese Crêpes...150
774. Tangy Paprika Chicken.......................................150
775. Parmesan Broccoli Fritters 150
776. Baked Eggs With Beef And Tomato 151
777. Award Winning Breaded Chicken.....................151
778. Baked Eggs With Cheese And Cauli Rice 151
779. Scrambled Eggs With Spinach And Tomato.. 151
780. Dinner Turkey Sandwiches...............................151
781. Parmesan-crusted Fish Fingers.........................152
782. Philadelphia Mushroom Omelet........................152
783. Turkey With Cheese And Pasilla Peppers......152
784. Muffins With Brown Mushrooms.......................152
785. Easy Greek Revithokeftedes...............................152
786. Chicken Drumsticks With Sauce........................153
787. Western Eggs With Ham And Cheese 153
788. Greek Omelet With Halloumi Cheese...............153
789. Winter Baked Eggs With Italian Sausage......153
790. Spicy Eggs With Sausage And Swiss Cheese.153
791. Masala-style Baked Eggs 154
792. Super-easy Chicken With Tomato Sauce........154
793. Cheddar Cheese And Pastrami Casserole 154
794. Dinner Avocado Chicken Sliders 154
795. Easy Zucchini Chips..154
796. Double Cheese Asparagus Casserole................155
797. Baked Eggs Florentine..155
798. Omelet With Mushrooms And Peppers..........155
799. Italian-style Broccoli Balls With Cheese.........155
800. Za'atar Eggs With Chicken.................................155

INTRODUCTION

Air fryers use a circulation of hot air to cook food that would otherwise be submerged in oil. The air fryer's cooking chamber radiates heat from a heating element near the food, and a fan circulates hot air. There is an air inlet on the top and an exhaust at the back that controls the temperature by releasing any excess hot air. The temperatures can go up to 230 °C (445 °F) depending on the model. Oil cannot be used inside the air fryer, as it could burn. Cooking times in the air fryer are typically reduced by 20% in comparison with traditional ovens, depending on the model, and the particular food. The taste and consistency of foods cooked using traditional fried methods compared with air fried techniques are not identical, because the larger quantity of oil used in traditional frying penetrates the foods (or the coating batter, if it is used) and adds its own flavor. With air fryers, if food is coated only in a wet batter without an external barrier of a dry coating like breadcrumbs that are pressed firmly to ensure adhesion, the air fryer's fan can blow the batter off the food. We can use the TOWER air Fryer to cook Meat, vegetables, poultry, fruit, fish and a wide variety of desserts. It is possible to prepare your entire meals, starting from appetizers to main courses as well as desserts. Not to mention, TOWER air fryer also allows home made preserves or even delicious sweets and cakes.

Advantages Of Air Fryer
1. Easy To Clean

An air fryer is easy to clean up since it has dishwasher-safe parts. These parts are the basket, the tray and the pan which are washed similar to how you do to other dishes: with soap and hot water.   Apart from this, you may need to use a comfortable bristle brush to keep your air fryer sparkling all the time. You can also choose to use the best dishwasher in India. Yet, you will first have to check the instruction manual of your model for safety purposes. Then proceed by drying each part completely before assembling the air fryer again. Furthermore, since air fryers do not use a lot of oil, the process of cleaning is made simpler. In most cases, one only needs to use hot water, washing soap and some elbow grease to get the job done. Apart from As compared to deep fat fryers which get extremely messy when cooking thus making the cooking process more complicated since one uses a lot of oil, air fryers are very easy to clean.

2. Safer To Use

As compared to other cooking devices, air fryers are safer since they are self-contained cooking appliances that ensure that the user is protected from the heating element and any form of oil that may splatter when cooking. As compared to the customary deep fryers which splatter and burn anything in their immediate vicinity, air fryers ensure that the immediate space is safe and no one gets burned. Considering that they use hot oil that is more than three hundred degrees Fahrenheit, this is very good. feature to consider when investing in a cooking appliance. Moreover, apart from mitigating the risk of personal injury, air fryers have little chance of starting fires which can lead to damage of property and sometimes even death. The main reason for their safety is that they come with auto-shutdown safety features so that when the timer is done, they immediately turn off. This ensures that the food does not get burnt or dried out but also that when the timer hits, the air fryer will turn off. This is a huge plus as compared to convection ovens and grills which do not have such a safety feature.

3. Air Fryers Are Economical To Use

Cooking oil is an expensive commodity especially in the instance when you need to use a gallon or more to cook either for a friend, guests or even colleagues from work. To cook food with a countertop deep fryer, you will need to purchase a gallon or so of cooking oils which can be a tad bit expensive and this is where an air fryer comes in since it uses a very little amount of oil. Sure, some of you might argue that cooking oil is reusable but you can only use it for a couple of times before it goes rancid. Once this happens, you will have no option but to get rid of it and buy new cooking oil for your deep fryer. Another point to consider on the economic front is the amount of power used. Deep fryers need a significant amount of power so that they can operate. Contrastingly, air fryers are economical since they do not take a long time to get the heated meaning that they will require less power to operate. All in all, air fryers are inexpensive and more convenient to use as compared to other kitchen appliances used for cooking.

4. Use Less Oil For Cooking

As established earlier, traditional deep fryers can utilize up to a gallon of cooking oil when operating at full capacity. Contrastingly, air fryers can use even as little oil as a tablespoon depending on the food you are cooking or the recipe you are using. The advantages of using less oil are numerous. First and foremost, it is economical and cheap meaning that you will not have to spend large sums of money purchasing cooking oil. Secondly, it makes the job of cleaning the air fryer much easy. Too much oil makes deep fryers messier and thus very difficult to clean. Thirdly, cooking with less oil means that you will eat fewer calories which makes it all the healthier to cook using an air fryer. However, it is advisable to use an oil sprayer or mister when cooking using an air fryer so that you can coat the food with oil properly.

5. Food Cooked With An Air Fryer Has Fewer Calories And Fats

When cooking with an air fryer, you will need to factor in that one tablespoon of commonly used cooking oil only has about one twenty calories and ten to fourteen grams of fat. Depending on the type of oil you are using, this translates to fewer calories when using an air fryer. When cooking with an air fryer, you only need to use a tablespoon or so of cooking oil. We can then safely say that one's intake of calories will be lower when using an air fryer are compared to food prepared using a deep fryer. It also means that you will get fried, tasty, textured and crunchy food all without having to intake large amounts of calories. When cooking using a deep fryer, the food is fully submerged in cooking oil which means that it will absorb a lot of oil, which approximately adds up to two hundred and forty calories or twenty-five grams of fat. This extra fat may make the food tastier but it comes at a huge cost to your overall health.

6. They Do Not Take Up Much Space In Your Kitchen

Typical air fryers are 1 foot cubed which is a relatively small size for a cooking appliance in your kitchen. To put this into perspective, they are only a little bit bigger than a typical coffee maker but in essence smaller than a toaster oven. Their small sizes come with several advantages. For one, they are small enough to be tucked away in a pantry when they are not in use and if you decide to leave it at the countertop, they will not take up much space. The main difference with a countertop deep fryer is that it has a basket for cooking that sticks out at the front. This takes away their aesthetic features and so most people prefer to always keep their deep fryers in the pantry every time they are not in use.

SNACKS & APPETIZERS RECIPES

1. Chocolate Bacon Bites

Servings: 4   Cooking Time: 10 Minutes

Ingredients:

4 bacon slices, halved
A pinch of pink salt

1 cup dark chocolate, melted

Directions:

Dip each bacon slice in some chocolate, sprinkle pink salt over them, put them in your air fryer's basket and cook at 350 degrees F for 10 minutes. Serve as a snack.

2. Lemon Green Beans

Servings: 4   Cooking Time: 20 Minutes

Ingredients:

1 lb. green beans, washed and destemmed
¼ tsp. extra virgin olive oil

1 lemon, juiced
Sea salt to taste
Black pepper to taste

Directions:

Pre-heat the Air Fryer to 400°F.   Put the green beans in your Air Fryer basket and drizzle the lemon juice over them.   Sprinkle on the pepper and salt. Pour in the oil, and toss to coat the green beans well. Cook for 10 – 12 minutes and serve warm.

3. Mix Nuts

Servings: 8   Cooking Time: 15 Minutes

Ingredients:

2 cup mixed nuts
1 tsp. chipotle chili powder
1 tsp. ground cumin

1 tbsp. butter, melted
1 tsp. pepper
1 tsp. salt

Directions:

In a bowl, combine all of the ingredients, coating the nuts well.   Set your Air Fryer to 350°F and allow to heat for 5 minutes.   Place the mixed nuts in the fryer basket and roast for 4 minutes, shaking the basket halfway through the cooking time.

4. Fried Mushrooms

Servings: 4   Cooking Time: 40 Minutes

Ingredients:

2 lb. button mushrooms
3 tbsp. white or French vermouth [optional]

1 tbsp. coconut oil
2 tsp. herbs of your choice
½ tsp. garlic powder

Directions:

1 Wash and dry the mushrooms. Slice them into quarters.   2 Pre-heat your Air Fryer at 320°F and add the coconut oil, garlic powder, and herbs to the basket.   3 Briefly cook the ingredients for 2 minutes and give them a stir. Put the mushrooms in the air fryer and cook for 25 minutes, stirring occasionally throughout.   4 Pour in the white vermouth and mix. Cook for an additional 5 minutes. 5 Serve hot.

5. Crust-less Meaty Pizza

Servings: 1   Cooking Time: 15 Minutes

Ingredients:

½ cup mozzarella cheese, shredded
2 slices sugar-free bacon, cooked and crumbled

¼ cup ground sausage, cooked
7 slices pepperoni
1 tbsp. parmesan cheese, grated

Directions:

Spread the mozzarella across the bottom of a six-inch cake pan. Throw on the bacon, sausage, and pepperoni, then add a sprinkle of the parmesan cheese on top. Place the pan inside your air fryer. Cook at 400°F for five minutes. The cheese is ready once brown in color and bubbly. Take care when removing the pan from the fryer and serve.

6. Dad's Boozy Wings

Servings: 4   Cooking Time: 1 Hour 15 Minutes

Ingredients:

2 teaspoons coriander seeds
1 ½ tablespoons soy sauce
3/4 pound chicken wings
1 ½ tablespoons each fish sauce

1/3 cup vermouth
2 tablespoons melted butter
1 teaspoon seasoned salt
Freshly ground black pepper, to taste

Directions:

Rub the chicken wings with the black pepper and seasoned salt; now, add the other ingredients. Next, soak the chicken wings in this mixture for 55 minutes in the refrigerator.   Air-fry the chicken wings at 365 degrees F for 16 minutes or until warmed through. Bon appétit!

7. Turkey Balls

Servings: 8   Cooking Time: 20 Minutes

Ingredients:

2 cups mozzarella, grated
1 pound turkey breast, skinless, boneless and ground
½ cup almond meal
3 tablespoons ghee, melted

½ cup coconut milk
1 tablespoon Italian seasoning
1 teaspoon garlic powder
½ cup parmesan, grated
Cooking spray

Directions:

In a bowl, mix all the ingredients except the parmesan and the cooking spray and stir well. Shape medium balls out of this mix, coat each in the parmesan, and arrange them in your air fryer.

Grease the balls with cooking spray and cook at 380 degrees F for 20 minutes. Serve as an appetizer.

8.   Parmesan Zucchini Chips

Servings: 1   Cooking Time: 10 Minutes
Ingredients:

2 medium zucchini	½ cup parmesan cheese, grated
1 oz. pork rinds, finely ground	1 egg

Directions:
Cut the zucchini into slices about a quarter-inch thick. Lay on a paper towel to dry.   In a bowl, combine the ground pork rinds and the grated parmesan.   In a separate bowl, beat the egg with a fork.   Take a zucchini slice and dip it into the egg, then into the pork rind-parmesan mixture, making sure to coat it evenly. Repeat with the rest of the slices. Lay them in the basket of your fryer, taking care not to overlap. This step may need to be completed in more than one batch.   Cook at 320°F for five minutes. Turn the chips over and allow to cook for another five minutes.   Allow to cool to achieve a crispier texture or serve warm. Enjoy!

9.   Creamy Sausage Bites

Servings: 6   Cooking Time: 9 Minutes
Ingredients:

1 cup ground pork sausages	1 egg, beaten
¼ cup almond flour	½ teaspoon dried dill
¼ teaspoon baking powder	2 tablespoons heavy cream
¼ teaspoon salt	1 teaspoon sunflower oil
1 teaspoon flax meal	

Directions:
In the bowl mix up ground pork sausages, almond flour, baking powder, salt, flax meal, egg, dried dill, and heavy cream. Make the small balls from the mixture. Preheat the air fryer to 400F. Place the sausage balls in the air fryer in one layer and cook them for 9 minutes. Flip the balls on another side after 5 minutes of cooking.

10.   Zucchini And Tomato Salsa

Servings: 6   Cooking Time: 15 Minutes
Ingredients:

1 and ½ pounds zucchinis, roughly cubed	2 tomatoes, cubed
	Salt and black pepper to the taste
2 spring onions, chopped	1 tablespoon balsamic vinegar

Directions:
In a pan that fits your air fryer, mix all the ingredients, toss, introduce the pan in the fryer and cook at 360 degrees F for 15 minutes. Divide the salsa into cups and serve cold.

11.   Coconut Chicken Wings

Servings: 4   Cooking Time: 10 Minutes
Ingredients:

1 teaspoon keto tomato sauce	4 chicken wings
2 tablespoons coconut cream	1 teaspoon nut oil
	¼ teaspoon salt

Directions:
Sprinkle the chicken wings with tomato sauce, nut oil, coconut cream, and salt. Massage the chicken wings with the help of the fingertips and put in the air fryer. Cook the chicken at 400f for 6 minutes. Then flip the wings on another side and cook for 4 minutes more.

12.   Kohlrabi Chips

Servings: 10   Cooking Time: 20 Minutes
Ingredients:

1 lb kohlrabi, peel and slice thinly	1 tbsp olive oil
1 tsp paprika	1 tsp salt

Directions:
Preheat the air fryer to 320 F.   Add all ingredients into the bowl and toss to coat.   Transfer kohlrabi into the air fryer basket and cook for 20 minutes. Toss halfway through.   Serve and enjoy.

13.   Mexican-style Corn On The Cob With Bacon

Servings: 4   Cooking Time: 20 Minutes
Ingredients:

4 ears fresh corn, shucked and cut into halves	2 slices bacon
	2 garlic cloves
1 avocado, pitted, peeled and mashed	2 tablespoons cilantro, chopped
1 teaspoon ancho chili powder	1 teaspoon lime juice
	Salt and black pepper, to taste

Directions:
Start by preheating your Air Fryer to 400 degrees F. Cook the bacon for 6 to 7 minutes; chop into small chunks and reserve.   Spritz the corn with cooking spray. Cook at 395 degrees F for 8 minutes, turning them over halfway through the cooking time.   Mix the reserved bacon with the remaining ingredients. Spoon the bacon mixture over the corn on the cob and serve immediately. Bon appétit!

14.   Buttered Corn On The Cob

Servings: 2   Cooking Time: 20 Minutes
Ingredients:

2 corn on the cob	Salt and black pepper, to taste
2 tablespoons butter, softened and divided	

Directions:
Preheat the Air fryer to 320F and grease an Air fryer basket.   Season the cobs evenly with salt and black pepper and rub with 1 tablespoon butter.   Wrap the cobs in foil paper and arrange in the Air fryer

basket. Cook for about 20 minutes and top with remaining butter. Dish out and serve warm.

15. Jalapeno Cheese Dip

Servings: 6   Cooking Time: 16 Minutes

Ingredients:

1 1/2 cup Monterey jack cheese, shredded	1/3 cup mayonnaise
1 1/2 cup cheddar cheese, shredded	8 oz cream cheese, softened
2 jalapeno pepper, minced	8 bacon slices, cooked and crumbled
1 tsp garlic powder	Pepper
1/3 cup sour cream	Salt

Directions:

Preheat the air fryer to 325 F.   Add all ingredients into the bowl and mix until combined.   Transfer bowl mixture into the air fryer baking dish and place in the air fryer and cook for 16 minutes.   Serve and enjoy.

16. Old-fashioned Onion Rings

Servings: 4   Cooking Time: 10 Minutes

Ingredients:

1 large onion, cut into rings	1 egg
1¼ cups all-purpose flour	¾ cup dry bread crumbs
1 cup milk	Salt, to taste

Directions:

Preheat the Air fryer to 360F and grease the Air fryer basket.   Mix together flour and salt in a dish. Whisk egg with milk in a second dish until well mixed.   Place the breadcrumbs in a third dish. Coat the onion rings with the flour mixture and dip into the egg mixture.   Lastly dredge in the breadcrumbs and transfer the onion rings in the Air fryer basket.   Cook for about 10 minutes and dish out to serve warm.

17. Crab Dip

Servings: 4   Cooking Time: 20 Minutes

Ingredients:

8 ounces cream cheese, soft	1 pound artichoke hearts, drained and chopped
1 tablespoon lemon juice	12 ounces jumbo crab meat
1 cup coconut cream	
1 tablespoon lemon juice	A pinch of salt and black pepper
1 bunch green onions, minced	1 and ½ cups mozzarella, shredded

Directions:

In a bowl, combine all the ingredients except half of the cheese and whisk them really well. Transfer this to a pan that fits your air fryer, introduce in the machine and cook at 400 degrees F for 15 minutes. Sprinkle the rest of the mozzarella on top and cook

for 5 minutes more. Divide the mix into bowls and serve as a party dip.

18. Grandma's Spicy Wings

Servings: 4   Cooking Time: 40 Minutes + Chilling Time

Ingredients:

2 cloves garlic, smashed	3 tablespoons melted butter
Ground black pepper and fine sea salt, to taste	8 chicken wings
	A few dashes of hot sauce

Directions:

First of all, steam chicken wings for 8 minutes; pat them dry and place in the refrigerator for about 55 minutes.   Now, bake in the preheated Air Fryer at 335 degrees F for 28 minutes, turning halfway through. While the chicken wings are cooking, combine the other ingredients to make the sauce. To finish, toss air fried chicken wings with the sauce and serve immediately.

19. Spinach Dip

Servings: 8   Cooking Time: 40 Minutes

Ingredients:

8 oz cream cheese, softened	1 cup mayonnaise
1/4 tsp garlic powder	1 cup parmesan cheese, grated
1/2 cup onion, minced	1 cup frozen spinach, thawed and squeeze out all liquid
1/3 cup water chestnuts, drained and chopped	1/2 tsp pepper

Directions:

Spray air fryer baking dish with cooking spray. Add all ingredients into the bowl and mix until well combined.   Transfer bowl mixture into the prepared baking dish and place dish in air fryer basket.   Cook at 300 F for 35-40 minutes. After 20 minutes of cooking stir dip.   Serve and enjoy.

20. Roasted Mixed Nuts

Servings: 6   Cooking Time: 20 Minutes

Ingredients:

½ cup walnuts	1 packet stevia
½ cup pecans	½ tablespoon ground cinnamon
½ cup almonds	
2 tablespoons egg white	A pinch of cayenne pepper

Directions:

Set the temperature of Air Fryer to 320 degrees F. Take a bowl and mix together all the listed ingredients.   Place the nuts in an Air Fryer basket in a single layer. (you can lay a piece of grease-proof baking paper)   Air Fry for about 20 minutes, stirring once halfway through.   Once done, transfer the hot nuts in a glass or steel bowl and serve.

21. Potato Bread Rolls

Servings: 8   Cooking Time: 13 Minutes

Ingredients:

5 large potatoes, boiled and mashed
2 small onions, chopped finely
2 green chilies, seeded and chopped
8 bread slices, trimmed
2 curry leaves
2 tablespoons vegetable oil, divided
½ teaspoon ground turmeric
Salt, to taste

Directions:
Preheat the Air fryer to 390F and grease an Air fryer basket.   Heat 1 teaspoon of vegetable oil in a skillet on medium heat and add onions.   Sauté for about 5 minutes and add green chilies, curry leaves and turmeric.   Sauté for about 1 minute and add mashed potatoes and salt.   Stir well until combined and remove from heat.   Make 8 equal sized oval shaped patties from the mixture.   Wet the bread slices completely with water and press the bread slices to drain completely.   Put a patty in a bread slice and roll it in a spindle shape.   Seal the edges to secure the filling and coat with vegetable oil. Repeat with the remaining bread slices, filling mixture and vegetable oil.   Place the potato rolls in the Air fryer basket and cook for about 13 minutes. Remove from the Air fryer and serve warm.

22. The Best Party Mix Ever

Servings: 10   Cooking Time: 15 Minutes

Ingredients:

2 cups mini pretzels
1 cup mini crackers
1 tablespoon Creole seasoning
1 cup peanuts
2 tablespoons butter, melted

Directions:
Toss all ingredients in the Air Fryer basket.   Cook in the preheated Air Fryer at 360 degrees F approximately 9 minutes until lightly toasted. Shake the basket periodically. Enjoy!

23. Movie Night Zucchini Fries

Servings: 4   Cooking Time: 26 Minutes

Ingredients:

2 zucchinis, slice into sticks
2 teaspoons shallot powder
1/4 teaspoon dried dill weed
2 teaspoons garlic powder
1/3 teaspoon cayenne pepper
1/2 cup Parmesan cheese, preferably freshly grated
3 egg whites
1/3 cup almond meal
Cooking spray
Salt and ground black pepper, to your liking

Directions:
Pat the zucchini sticks dry using a kitchen towel. Grab a mixing bowl and beat the egg whites until pale; then, add all the seasonings in the order listed above and beat again   Take another mixing bowl and mix together almond meal and the Parmesan cheese.   Then, coat the zucchini sticks with the seasoned egg mixture; then, roll them over the parmesan cheese mixture.   Lay the breaded zucchini sticks in a single layer on the tray that is coated lightly with cooking spray.   Bake at 375 degrees F for about 20 minutes until the sticks are golden brown. Serve with your favorite sauce for dipping.

24. Cajun Cheese Sticks

Servings: 4   Cooking Time: 15 Minutes

Ingredients:

1/2 cup all-purpose flour
2 eggs
1/2 cup parmesan cheese, grated
1 tablespoon Cajun seasonings
8 cheese sticks, kid-friendly
1/4 cup ketchup

Directions:
To begin, set up your breading station. Place the all-purpose flour in a shallow dish. In a separate dish, whisk the eggs.   Finally, mix the parmesan cheese and Cajun seasoning in a third dish.   Start by dredging the cheese sticks in the flour; then, dip them into the egg. Press the cheese sticks into the parmesan mixture, coating evenly.   Place the breaded cheese sticks in the lightly greased Air Fryer basket. Cook at 380 degrees F for 6 minutes. Serve with ketchup and enjoy!

25. Balsamic Mushroom Platter

Servings: 4   Cooking Time: 12 Minutes

Ingredients:

2 tablespoons balsamic vinegar
2 tablespoons olive oil
½ teaspoon basil, dried
½ teaspoon tarragon, dried
½ teaspoon rosemary, dried
½ teaspoon thyme, dried
A pinch of salt and black pepper
12 ounces Portobello mushrooms, sliced

Directions:
In a bowl, mix all the ingredients and toss well. Arrange the mushroom slices in your air fryer's basket and cook at 380 degrees F for 12 minutes. Arrange the mushroom slices on a platter and serve.

26. Sugar Snap Bacon

Servings: 4   Cooking Time: 10 Minutes

Ingredients:

3 cups sugar snap peas
½ tbsp lemon juice
2 tbsp bacon fat
2 tsp garlic
½ tsp red pepper flakes

Directions:
In a skillet, cook the bacon fat until it begins to smoke.   Add the garlic and cook for 2 minutes. Add the sugar peas and lemon juice.   Cook for 2-3

minutes.   Remove and sprinkle with red pepper flakes and lemon zest.   Serve!

27. Crispy Eggplant Slices

Servings: 4   Cooking Time: 16 Minutes

Ingredients:

1 medium eggplant, peeled and cut into ½-inch round slices	Salt, as required
	2 eggs, beaten
½ cup all-purpose flour	1 cup Italian-style breadcrumbs
	¼ cup olive oil

Directions:

In a colander, add the eggplant slices and sprinkle with salt.   Set aside for about 45 minutes and pat dry the eggplant slices.   Add the flour in a shallow dish.   Crack the eggs in a second dish and beat well.   In a third dish, mix together the oil, and breadcrumbs.   Coat each eggplant slice with flour, then dip into beaten eggs and finally, evenly coat with the breadcrumbs mixture.   Set the temperature of Air Fryer to 390 degrees F. Arrange the eggplant slices in an Air Fryer basket in a single layer in 2 batches.   Air Fry for about 8 minutes.   Serve.

28. Mexican Cheesy Zucchini Bites

Servings: 4   Cooking Time: 25 Minutes

Ingredients:

1 large-sized zucchini, thinly sliced	1/2 cup tortilla chips, crushed
1/2 cup flour	1/2 cup Queso Añejo, grated
1/4 cup yellow cornmeal	Salt and cracked pepper, to taste
1 egg, whisked	

Directions:

Pat dry the zucchini slices with a kitchen towel. Mix the remaining ingredients in a shallow bowl; mix until everything is well combined. Dip each zucchini slice in the prepared batter.   Cook in the preheated Air Fryer at 400 degrees F for 12 minutes, shaking the basket halfway through the cooking time.   Work in batches until the zucchini slices are crispy and golden brown. Enjoy!

29. Sweet Potato Fries With Spicy Dip

Servings: 3   Cooking Time: 50 Minutes

Ingredients:

3 medium sweet potatoes, cut into 1/3-inch sticks	Spicy Dip:
	1/4 cup mayonnaise
2 tablespoons olive oil	1/4 cup Greek yogurt
	1/4 teaspoon Dijon mustard
1 teaspoon kosher salt	1 teaspoon hot sauce

Directions:

Soak the sweet potato in icy cold water for 30 minutes. Drain the sweet potatoes and pat them dry with paper towels.   Toss the sweet potatoes with olive oil and salt.   Place in the lightly greased cooking basket. Cook in the preheated Air Fryer at 360 degrees F for 14 minutes. Wok in batches. While the sweet potatoes are cooking, make the spicy dip by whisking the remaining ingredients. Place in the refrigerator until ready to serve. Enjoy!

30. Easy Carrot Dip

Servings: 6   Cooking Time: 15 Minutes

Ingredients:

2 cups carrots, grated	1 tbsp chives, chopped
1/4 tsp cayenne pepper	Pepper
4 tbsp butter, melted	Salt

Directions:

Add all ingredients into the air fryer baking dish and stir until well combined.   Place dish in the air fryer and cook at 380 F for 15 minutes.   Transfer cook carrot mixture into the blender and blend until smooth.   Serve and enjoy.

31. Broccoli And Pecorino Toscano Fat Bombs

Servings: 6   Cooking Time: 20 Minutes

Ingredients:

1 large-sized head of broccoli, broken into small florets	1/2 teaspoon sea salt
	1 teaspoon groundnut oil
1/4 teaspoon ground black pepper, or more to taste	1 cup bacon bits
	1 cup Pecorino Toscano, freshly grated
1 tablespoon Shoyu sauce	Paprika, to taste

Directions:

Add the broccoli florets to boiling water; boil approximately 4 minutes; drain well.   Season with salt and pepper; drizzle with Shoyu sauce and groundnut oil. Mash with a potato masher.   Add the bacon and cheese to the mixture; shape the mixture into bite-sized balls.   Air-fry at 390 degrees F for 10 minutes; shake the Air Fryer basket, push the power button again, and continue to cook for 5 minutes more.   Toss the fried keto bombs with paprika. Bon appétit!

32. Brussels Sprouts With Feta Cheese

Servings: 4   Cooking Time: 20 Minutes

Ingredients:

1 teaspoon kosher salt	3/4 pound Brussels sprouts, trimmed and cut off the ends
1 tablespoon lemon zest	
	1 cup feta cheese, cubed
Non-stick cooking spray	

Directions:

Firstly, peel the Brussels sprouts using a small paring knife. Toss the leaves with salt and lemon zest; spritz them with a cooking spray, coating all sides. Bake at 380 degrees for 8 minutes; shake the cooking basket halfway through the cooking time and cook for 7 more minutes.   Make sure to work in batches so everything can cook evenly. Taste and adjust the seasonings. Serve with feta cheese. Bon appétit!

33. Cashew Dip

Servings: 6   Cooking Time: 8 Minutes

Ingredients:

½ cup cashews, soaked in water for 4 hours and drained	2 garlic cloves, minced
3 tablespoons cilantro, chopped	A pinch of salt and black pepper
1 teaspoon lime juice	2 tablespoons coconut milk

Directions:

In a blender, combine all the ingredients, pulse well and transfer to a ramekin. Put the ramekin in your air fryer's basket and cook at 350 degrees F for 8 minutes. Serve as a party dip.

34. Bacon Croquettes

Servings: 6   Cooking Time: 8 Minutes

Ingredients:

1 pound thin bacon slices	1 cup all-purpose flour
1 pound sharp cheddar cheese block, cut into 1-inch rectangular pieces	3 eggs
	1 cup breadcrumbs
	Salt, as required
	¼ cup olive oil

Directions:

Wrap 2 bacon slices around 1 piece of cheddar cheese, covering completely.   Repeat with the remaining bacon and cheese pieces.   Arrange the croquettes in a baking dish and freeze for about 5 minutes.   Add the flour in a shallow dish.   In a second dish, crack the eggs and beat well.   In a third dish, mix together the breadcrumbs, salt, and oil.   Coat the croquettes with flour, then dip into beaten eggs and finally, evenly coat with the breadcrumbs mixture.   Set the temperature of Air Fryer to 390 degrees F.   Arrange the croquettes in an Air Fryer basket in a single layer.   Air Fry for about 7-8 minutes.   Serve hot.

35. Chili Kale Chips

Servings: 4   Cooking Time: 5 Minutes

Ingredients:

1 teaspoon nutritional yeast	½ teaspoon chili flakes
1 teaspoon salt	1 teaspoon sesame oil
2 cups kale, chopped	

Directions:

Mix up kale leaves with nutritional yeast, salt, chili flakes, and sesame oil. Shake the greens well. Preheat the air fryer to 400F and put the kale leaves in the air fryer basket. Cook them for 3 minutes and then give a good shake. Cook the kale leaves for 2 minutes more.

36. Crab And Chives Balls

Servings: 8   Cooking Time: 20 Minutes

Ingredients:

½ cup coconut cream	16 ounces lump crabmeat, chopped
2 tablespoons chives, mined	2/3 cup almond meal
1 egg, whisked	A pinch of salt and black pepper
1 teaspoon mustard	Cooking spray
1 teaspoon lemon juice	

Directions:

In a bowl, mix all the ingredients except the cooking spray and stir well. Shape medium balls out of this mix, place them in the fryer and cook at 390 degrees F for 20 minutes. Serve as an appetizer.

37. Paprika Bacon Shrimp

Servings: 10   Cooking Time: 45 Minutes

Ingredients:

1 ¼ pounds shrimp, peeled and deveined	1 teaspoon chili powder
1 teaspoon paprika	1 tablespoon shallot powder
1/2 teaspoon ground black pepper	1/4 teaspoon cumin powder
1/2 teaspoon red pepper flakes, crushed	1 ¼ pounds thin bacon slices
1 tablespoon salt	

Directions:

Toss the shrimps with all the seasoning until they are coated well.   Next, wrap a slice of bacon around the shrimps, securing with a toothpick; repeat with the remaining ingredients; chill for 30 minutes.   Air-fry them at 360 degrees F for 7 to 8 minutes, working in batches. Serve with cocktail sticks if desired. Enjoy!

38. Cauliflower Bombs With Sweet & Sour Sauce

Servings: 4   Cooking Time: 25 Minutes

Ingredients:

Cauliflower Bombs:	1 clove garlic, minced
1/2 pound cauliflower	1 teaspoon sherry vinegar
2 ounces Ricotta cheese	1 tablespoon tomato puree
1/3 cup Swiss cheese	2 tablespoons olive oil
1 egg	
1 tablespoon Italian seasoning mix	Salt and black pepper, to taste
Sweet & Sour Sauce:	
1 red bell pepper, jarred	

Directions:

Blanch the cauliflower in salted boiling water about 3 to 4 minutes until al dente. Drain well and pulse in a food processor.   Add the remaining ingredients for the cauliflower bombs; mix to combine well. Bake in the preheated Air Fryer at 375 degrees F for 16 minutes, shaking halfway through the cooking time.   In the meantime, pulse all ingredients for the sauce in your food processor until combined. Season to taste. Serve the cauliflower bombs with the Sweet & Sour Sauce on the side. Bon appétit!

39. Portabella Pizza Treat

Servings: 2   Cooking Time: 6 Minutes

Ingredients:

2 Portabella caps, stemmed	2 tablespoons canned tomatoes with basil
2 tablespoons mozzarella cheese, shredded	2 tablespoon olive oil
	1/8 teaspoon dried Italian seasonings
4 pepperoni slices	Salt, to taste
2 tablespoons Parmesan cheese, grated freshly	1 teaspoon red pepper flakes, crushed

Directions:
Preheat the Air fryer to 320F and grease an Air fryer basket.   Drizzle olive oil on both sides of portabella cap and season salt, red pepper flakes and Italian seasonings.   Top canned tomatoes on the mushrooms, followed by mozzarella cheese. Place portabella caps in the Air fryer basket and cook for about 2 minutes.   Top with pepperoni slices and cook for about 4 minutes.   Sprinkle with Parmesan cheese and dish out to serve warm.

40. Sea Scallops And Bacon Skewers

Servings: 6   Cooking Time: 50 Minutes

Ingredients:

1/2 pound sea scallops	1 tablespoon vermouth
1/2 cup coconut milk	1/2 pound bacon, diced
6 ounces orange juice	1 shallot, diced
Sea salt and ground black pepper, to taste	1 teaspoon garlic powder
	1 teaspoon paprika

Directions:
In a ceramic bowl, place the sea scallops, coconut milk, orange juice, vermouth, salt, and black pepper; let it marinate for 30 minutes.   Assemble the skewers alternating the scallops, bacon, and shallots. Sprinkle garlic powder and paprika all over the skewers.   Bake in the preheated air Fryer at 400 degrees F for 6 minutes. Serve warm and enjoy!

41. Parmesan Turnip Slices

Servings: 8   Cooking Time: 10 Minutes

Ingredients:

1 lb turnip, peel and cut into slices	1 tbsp olive oil
3 oz parmesan cheese, shredded	1 tsp garlic powder
	1 tsp salt

Directions:
Preheat the air fryer to 360 F.   Add all ingredients into the mixing bowl and toss to coat.   Transfer turnip slices into the air fryer basket and cook for 10 minutes.   Serve and enjoy.

42. Asian Twist Chicken Wings

Servings: 6   Cooking Time: 20 Minutes

Ingredients:

1 ½ pounds chicken wings	Kosher salt and ground black pepper, to taste
2 teaspoons sesame oil	
2 tablespoons tamari sauce	2 garlic clove, minced
	2 tablespoons honey
1 tablespoon rice vinegar	2 sun-dried tomatoes, minced

Directions:
Toss the chicken wings with the sesame oil, salt, and pepper. Add chicken wings to a lightly greased baking pan.   Roast the chicken wings in the preheated Air Fryer at 390 degrees F for 7 minutes. Turn them over once or twice to ensure even cooking. In a mixing dish, thoroughly combine the tamari sauce, vinegar, garlic, honey, and sun-dried tomatoes.   Pour the sauce all over the chicken wings; bake an additional 5 minutes. Bon appétit!

43. Coconut Celery Stalks

Servings: 4   Cooking Time: 4 Minutes

Ingredients:

4 celery stalks	1 egg, beaten
1 teaspoon flax meal	1 teaspoon sunflower oil
1 teaspoon coconut flour	

Directions:
In the bowl mix up flax meal and coconut flour. Then dip the celery stalks in the egg and coat in the flax meal mixture. Sprinkle the celery stalks with sunflower oil and place in the air fryer basket. Cook for 4 minutes at 400F.

44. Tofu

Servings: 4   Cooking Time: 20 Minutes

Ingredients:

15 oz. extra firm tofu, drained and cut into cubes	¾ cup cornstarch
	¼ cup cornmeal
1 tsp. chili flakes	Pepper to taste
	Salt to taste

Directions:
In a bowl, combine the cornmeal, cornstarch, chili flakes, pepper, and salt.   Coat the tofu cubes completely with the mixture.   Pre-heat your Air Fryer at 350°F.   Spritz the basket with cooking spray.   Transfer the coated tofu to the basket and air fry for 8 minutes, shaking the basket at the 4-minute mark.

45. Italian Dip

Servings: 8   Cooking Time: 12 Minutes

Ingredients:

8 oz cream cheese, softened	1/2 cup roasted red peppers
1 cup mozzarella	

cheese, shredded
1/3 cup basil pesto

1/4 cup parmesan
cheese, grated

Directions:
Add parmesan cheese and cream cheese into the food processor and process until smooth. Transfer cheese mixture into the air fryer pan and spread evenly.   Pour basil pesto on top of cheese layer.   Sprinkle roasted pepper on top of basil pesto layer.   Sprinkle mozzarella cheese on top of pepper layer and place dish in air fryer basket. Cook dip at 250 F for 12 minutes.   Serve and enjoy.

46. Air Fried Cheese Sticks

Servings: 4 Minutes   Cooking Time: 8 Minutes

Ingredients:

6 mozzarella cheese
sticks
1/4 tsp garlic powder
1 tsp Italian
seasoning
1/3 cup almond flour

1/2 cup parmesan
cheese, grated
1 large egg, lightly
beaten
1/4 tsp sea salt

Directions:
In a small bowl, whisk the egg.   In a shallow bowl, mix together almond flour, parmesan cheese, Italian seasoning, garlic powder, and salt. Dip mozzarella cheese stick in egg then coat with almond flour mixture and place on a plate. Place in refrigerator for 1 hour.   Spray air fryer basket with cooking spray.   Place prepared mozzarella cheese sticks into the air fryer basket and cook at 375 F for 8 minutes.   Serve and enjoy.

47. Grilled Meatball Kabobs

Servings: 6   Cooking Time: 20 Minutes

Ingredients:

1/2 pound ground
pork
1/2 pound ground
beef
1 teaspoon dried
onion flakes
1 teaspoon fresh
garlic, minced
1 teaspoon dried
parsley flakes

Salt and black
pepper, to taste
1 red pepper, 1-inch
pieces
1 cup pearl onions
1/2 cup barbecue
sauce, no sugar
added

Directions:
Mix the ground meat with the onion flakes, garlic, parsley flakes, salt, and black pepper. Shape the mixture into 1-inch balls.   Thread the meatballs, pearl onions, and peppers alternately onto skewers. Place the skewers on the Air Fryer grill pan. Microwave the barbecue sauce for 10 seconds. Cook in the preheated Air Fryer at 380 degrees for 5 minutes. Turn the skewers over halfway through the cooking time. Brush with the sauce and cook for a further 5 minutes. Work in batches.   Serve with the remaining barbecue sauce and enjoy!

48. Roasted Parsnip

Servings: 5   Cooking Time: 55 Minutes

Ingredients:

2 lb. parsnips [about
6 large parsnips]
2 tbsp. maple syrup

1 tbsp. coconut oil
1 tbsp. parsley, dried
flakes

Directions:
1 Melt the duck fat or coconut oil in your Air Fryer for 2 minutes at 320°F.   2 Rinse the parsnips to clean them and dry them. Chop into 1-inch cubes. Transfer to the fryer.   3 Cook the parsnip cubes in the fat/oil for 35 minutes, tossing them regularly. 4 Season the parsnips with parsley and maple syrup and allow to cook for another 5 minutes or longer to achieve a soft texture throughout.   Serve straightaway.

49. Healthy Vegetable Kabobs

Servings: 4   Cooking Time: 10 Minutes

Ingredients:

1/2 onion
1 zucchini
1 eggplant

2 bell peppers
Pepper
Salt

Directions:
Cut all vegetables into 1-inch pieces.   Thread vegetables onto the soaked wooden skewers and season with pepper and salt.   Place skewers into the air fryer basket and cook for 10 minutes at 390 F. Turn halfway through.   Serve and enjoy.

50. Cheesy Garlic Bread

Servings: 2   Cooking Time: 20 Minutes

Ingredients:

1 friendly baguette
4 tsp. butter, melted
3 chopped garlic
cloves

5 tsp. sundried
tomato pesto
1 cup mozzarella
cheese, grated

Directions:
1 Cut your baguette into 5 thick round slices.   2 Add the garlic cloves to the melted butter and brush onto each slice of bread.   3 Spread a teaspoon of sun dried tomato pesto onto each slice.   4 Top each slice with the grated mozzarella.   5 Transfer the bread slices to the Air Fryer and cook them at 180°F for 6 – 8 minutes.   6 Top with some freshly chopped basil leaves, chili flakes and oregano if desired.

51. Sage Roasted Zucchini Cubes

Servings: 6   Cooking Time: 20 Minutes

Ingredients:

1 ½ pounds zucchini,
peeled and cut into
1/2-inch chunks
2 tablespoons melted
coconut oil
A pinch of coarse salt

A pinch of pepper
2 tablespoons sage,
finely chopped
Zest of 1 small-sized
lemon
1/8 teaspoon ground
allspice

Directions:
Toss the squash chunks with the other items. Roast in the Air Fryer cooking basket at 350 degrees F for 10 minutes.   Pause the machine, and turn the

temperature to 400 degrees F; stir and roast for additional 8 minutes. Bon appétit!

52. Spicy Dip

Servings: 6   Cooking Time: 5 Minutes
Ingredients:

12 oz hot peppers, chopped	1 1/2 cups apple cider vinegar
Pepper	Salt

Directions:
Add all ingredients into the air fryer baking dish and stir well.   Place dish in the air fryer and cook at 380 F for 5 minutes.   Transfer pepper mixture into the blender and blend until smooth.   Serve and enjoy.

53. Skinny Spinach Chips

Servings: 3   Cooking Time: 20 Minutes
Ingredients:

3 cups fresh spinach leaves	1 teaspoon garlic powder
1 tablespoon extra-virgin olive oil	Chili Yogurt Dip: 1/4 cup yogurt
1 teaspoon sea salt	2 tablespoons mayonnaise
1/2 teaspoon cayenne pepper	1/2 teaspoon chili powder

Directions:
Toss the spinach leaves with the olive oil and seasonings.   Bake in the preheated Air Fryer at 350 degrees F for 10 minutes, shaking the cooking basket occasionally.   Bake until the edges brown, working in batches.   In the meantime, make the sauce by whisking all ingredients in a mixing dish. Serve immediately.

54. Cheesy Bacon Bread

Servings: 2   Cooking Time: 25 Minutes
Ingredients:

4 slices sugar-free bacon, cooked and chopped	2 eggs
1/4 cup pickled jalapenos, chopped	1/4 cup parmesan cheese, grated
	2 cups mozzarella cheese, shredded

Directions:
Add all of the ingredients together in a bowl and mix together.   Cut out a piece of parchment paper that will fit the base of your fryer's basket. Place it inside the fryer   With slightly wet hands, roll the mixture into a circle. You may have to form two circles to cook in separate batches, depending on the size of your fryer.   Place the circle on top of the parchment paper inside your fryer. Cook at 320°F for ten minutes.   Turn the bread over and cook for another five minutes.   The bread is ready when it is golden and cooked all the way through. Slice and serve warm.

55. Garlic Chicken Meatballs

Servings: 12   Cooking Time: 20 Minutes
Ingredients:

A pinch of salt and black pepper	2 pound chicken breast, skinless, boneless and ground
2 garlic cloves, minced	6 tablespoons keto hot sauce
2 spring onions, chopped	3/4 cup almond meal
2 tablespoons ghee, melted	Cooking spray

Directions:
In a bowl, mix all the ingredients except the cooking spray, stir well and shape medium meatballs out of this mix. Arrange the meatballs in your air fryer's basket, grease them with cooking spray and cook at 360 degrees F for 20 minutes. Serve as an appetizer.

56. Nutty Cauliflower Poppers

Servings: 4   Cooking Time: 12 Minutes
Ingredients:

1/4 cup golden raisins	1 cup boiling water
1/4 cup toasted pine nuts	1/2 cup olive oil, divided
1 head of cauliflower, cut into small florets	1 tablespoon curry powder
	1/4 teaspoon salt

Directions:
Preheat the Air fryer to 390F and grease an Air fryer basket.   Put raisins in boiling water in a bowl and keep aside.   Drizzle 1 teaspoon olive oil on the pine nuts in another bowl.   Place the pine nuts in an Air fryer basket and cook for about 2 minutes. Remove the pine nuts from the Air fryer and keep aside.   Mix together cauliflower, salt, curry powder and remaining olive oil in a large bowl. Transfer this mixture into the Air fryer basket and cook for about 12 minutes   Dish out the cauliflower in a serving bowl and stir in the pine nuts. Drain raisins and add to the serving bowl.

57. Cauliflower Dip

Servings: 10   Cooking Time: 40 Minutes
Ingredients:

1 cauliflower head, cut into florets	1 tsp Worcestershire sauce
1 1/2 cups parmesan cheese, shredded	1/2 cup sour cream
2 tbsp green onions, chopped	3/4 cup mayonnaise
2 garlic clove	8 oz cream cheese, softened
	2 tbsp olive oil

Directions:
Toss cauliflower florets with olive oil.   Add cauliflower florets into the air fryer basket and cook at 390 F for 20-25 minutes. Shake basket halfway through.   Add cooked cauliflower, 1 cup parmesan cheese, green onion, garlic, Worcestershire sauce, sour cream, mayonnaise, and cream cheese into the food processor and process until smooth.

Transfer cauliflower mixture into the 7-inch dish and top with remaining parmesan cheese. Place dish in air fryer basket and cook at 360 F for 10-15 minutes. Serve and enjoy.

58. Garlic Eggplant Chips

Servings: 4   Cooking Time: 25 Minutes
Ingredients:

1 eggplant, sliced	1 tablespoon olive oil
1 teaspoon garlic powder	

Directions:
Mix up olive oil and garlic powder. Then brush every eggplant slice with a garlic powder mixture. Preheat the air fryer to 400F. Place the eggplant slices in the air fryer basket in one layer and cook them for 15 minutes. Then flip the eggplant slices on another side and cook for 10 minutes.

59. Romano Cheese And Broccoli Balls

Servings: 4   Cooking Time: 25 Minutes
Ingredients:

1/2 pound broccoli	4 eggs, beaten
1/2 cup Romano cheese, grated	1/2 teaspoon paprika
2 garlic cloves, minced	1/4 teaspoon dried basil
1 shallot, chopped	Sea salt and ground black pepper, to taste
2 tablespoons butter, at room temperature	

Directions:
Add the broccoli to your food processor and pulse until the consistency resembles rice. Stir in the remaining ingredients; mix until everything is well combined. Shape the mixture into bite-sized balls and transfer them to the lightly greased cooking basket. Cook in the preheated Air Fryer at 375 degrees F for 16 minutes, shaking halfway through the cooking time. Serve with cocktail sticks and tomato ketchup on the side.

60. Turmeric Jicama Bites

Servings: 4   Cooking Time: 3 Minutes
Ingredients:

8 oz Jicama, peeled	1/4 teaspoon dried dill
1/2 teaspoon ground turmeric	1 tablespoon avocado oil

Directions:
Cut the Jicama on the wedges and sprinkle them with turmeric and dried dill. Then sprinkle the vegetables with avocado oil. Preheat the air fryer to 400F. Place the Jicama wedges in the air fryer basket in one layer and cook them for 3 minutes.

61. Spinach Chips With Chili Yogurt Dip

Servings: 3   Cooking Time: 20 Minutes
Ingredients:

3 cups fresh spinach leaves	1 teaspoon garlic powder
1 tablespoon extra-virgin olive oil	Chili Yogurt Dip:
1 teaspoon sea salt	1/4 cup yogurt
1/2 teaspoon cayenne pepper	2 tablespoons mayonnaise
	1/2 teaspoon chili powder

Directions:
Toss the spinach leaves with the olive oil and seasonings. Bake in the preheated Air Fryer at 350 degrees F for 10 minutes, shaking the cooking basket occasionally. Bake until the edges brown, working in batches. In the meantime, make the sauce by whisking all ingredients in a mixing dish. Serve immediately.

62. Toasted Pumpkin Seeds

Servings: 4   Cooking Time: 25 Minutes
Ingredients:

1 1/2 cups pumpkin seeds [cut a whole pumpkin & scrape out the insides	using a large spoon, separating the seeds from the flesh]
1 tsp. smoked paprika	1 1/2 tsp. salt
	Olive oil

Directions:
1 Run the pumpkin seeds under some cold water. 2 Over a medium heat, boil two quarts of salted water in a pot. 3 Add in the pumpkin seeds and cook in the water for 8 to 10 minutes. 4 Dump the contents of the pot into a sieve to drain the seeds. Place them on paper towels and allow them to dry for at least 20 minutes. 5 Pre-heat your Air Fryer to 350°F. 6 In a medium bowl coat the pumpkin seeds with olive oil, smoked paprika and salt. 7 Put them in the fryer's basket and air fry for at least 30 minutes until slightly browned and crispy. Shake the basket a few times during the cooking time. 8 Allow the seeds to cool. Serve with a salad or keep in an airtight container for snacking.

63. Smoked Almonds

Servings: 6   Cooking Time: 6 Minutes
Ingredients:

1 cup almonds	1/4 tsp smoked paprika
1/4 tsp cumin	
1 tsp chili powder	2 tsp olive oil

Directions:
Add almond into the bowl and remaining ingredients and toss to coat. Transfer almonds into the air fryer basket and cook at 320 F for 6 minutes. Shake halfway through. Serve and enjoy.

64. Spicy Broccoli Poppers

Servings: 4   Cooking Time: 10 Minutes
Ingredients:

2 tablespoons plain yogurt
1 pound broccoli, cut into small florets
2 tablespoons chickpea flour
Salt, to taste
½ teaspoon red chili powder
¼ teaspoon ground cumin
¼ teaspoon ground turmeric

Directions:
Preheat the Air fryer to 400F and grease an Air fryer basket. Mix together the yogurt, red chili powder, cumin, turmeric and salt in a bowl until well combined. Stir in the broccoli and generously coat with marinade. Refrigerate for about 30 minutes and sprinkle the broccoli florets with chickpea flour. Arrange the broccoli florets in the Air fryer basket and cook for about 10 minutes, flipping once in between. Dish out and serve warm.

65. Hot Cheesy Dip

Servings: 6   Cooking Time: 12 Minutes
Ingredients:

12 ounces coconut cream
2 teaspoons keto hot sauce
8 ounces cheddar cheese, grated

Directions:
In ramekin, mix the cream with hot sauce and cheese and whisk. Put the ramekin in the fryer and cook at 390 degrees F for 12 minutes. Whisk, divide into bowls and serve as a dip.

66. Crunchy Bacon Bites

Servings: 4   Cooking Time: 10 Minutes
Ingredients:

4 bacon strips, cut into small pieces
1/4 cup hot sauce
1/2 cup pork rinds, crushed

Directions:
Add bacon pieces in a bowl. Add hot sauce and toss well. Add crushed pork rinds and toss until bacon pieces are well coated. Transfer bacon pieces in air fryer basket and cook at 350 F for 10 minutes. Serve and enjoy.

67. Perfect Crab Dip

Servings: 4   Cooking Time: 7 Minutes
Ingredients:

1 cup crabmeat
2 tbsp parsley, chopped
2 tbsp fresh lemon juice
2 tbsp hot sauce
1/2 cup green onion, sliced
2 cups cheese, grated
1/4 cup mayonnaise
1/4 tsp pepper
1/2 tsp salt

Directions:
In a 6-inch dish, mix together crabmeat, hot sauce, cheese, mayo, pepper, and salt. Place dish in air fryer basket and cook dip at 400 F for 7 minutes. Remove dish from air fryer. Drizzle dip with lemon juice and garnish with parsley. Serve and enjoy.

68. Roasted Parsnip Sticks With Salted Caramel

Servings: 4   Cooking Time: 25 Minutes
Ingredients:

1 pound parsnip, trimmed, scrubbed, cut into sticks
2 tablespoon avocado oil
2 tablespoons butter
2 tablespoons granulated sugar
1/4 teaspoon ground allspice
1/2 teaspoon coarse salt

Directions:
Toss the parsnip with the avocado oil; bake in the preheated Air Fryer at 380 degrees F for 15 minutes, shaking the cooking basket occasionally to ensure even cooking. Then, heat the sugar and 1 tablespoon of water in a small pan over medium heat. Cook until the sugar has dissolved; bring to a boil. Keep swirling the pan around until the sugar reaches a rich caramel color. Pour in 2 tablespoons of cold water. Now, add the butter, allspice, and salt. The mixture should be runny. Afterwards, drizzle the salted caramel over the roasted parsnip sticks and enjoy!

69. Beer Battered Vidalia Rings

Servings: 4   Cooking Time: 30 Minutes
Ingredients:

1/2 pound Vidalia onions, sliced into rings
1/2 cup all-purpose flour
1/2 teaspoon baking powder
Sea salt and freshly cracked black pepper, to taste
1/4 cup cornmeal
1/4 teaspoon garlic powder
2 eggs, beaten
1/2 cup lager-style beer
1 cup plain breadcrumbs
2 tablespoons peanut oil

Directions:
Place the onion rings in the bowl with icy cold water; let them soak approximately 20 minutes; drain the onion rings and pat them dry. In a shallow bowl, mix the flour, cornmeal, baking powder, salt, and black pepper. Add the garlic powder, eggs and beer; mix well to combine. In another shallow bowl, mix the breadcrumbs with the peanut oil. Dip the onion rings in the flour/egg mixture; then, dredge in the breadcrumb mixture. Roll to coat them evenly. Spritz the Air Fryer basket with cooking spray; arrange the breaded onion rings in the basket. Cook in the preheated Air Fryer at 400 degrees F for 4 to 5 minutes, turning them over halfway through the cooking time. Bon appétit!

70. Olives Fritters

Servings: 6   Cooking Time: 12 Minutes
Ingredients:

Cooking spray
½ cup parsley, chopped
1 egg
½ cup almond flour
Salt and black pepper to the taste

3 spring onions, chopped
½ cup kalamata olives, pitted and minced
3 zucchinis, grated

Directions:
In a bowl, mix all the ingredients except the cooking spray, stir well and shape medium fritters out of this mixture. Place the fritters in your air fryer's basket, grease them with cooking spray and cook at 380 degrees F for 6 minutes on each side. Serve them as an appetizer.

71. Tomato Smokies

Servings: 10   Cooking Time: 10 Minutes
Ingredients:
12 oz pork and beef smokies
3 oz bacon, sliced
1 teaspoon keto tomato sauce

1 teaspoon Erythritol
1 teaspoon avocado oil
½ teaspoon cayenne pepper

Directions:
Sprinkle the smokies with cayenne pepper and tomato sauce. Then sprinkle them with Erythritol and olive oil. After this, wrap every smokie in the bacon and secure it with the toothpick. Preheat the air fryer to 400F. Place the bacon smokies in the air fryer and cook them for 10 minutes. Shake them gently during cooking to avoid burning.

72. Lime Tomato Salsa

Servings: 4   Cooking Time: 8 Minutes
Ingredients:
4 tomatoes, cubed
3 chili peppers, minced
2 spring onions, chopped
1 garlic clove, minced

2 tablespoons lime juice
2 teaspoons cilantro, chopped
2 teaspoons parsley, chopped
Cooking spray

Directions:
Grease a pan that fits your air fryer with the cooking spray, and mix all the ingredients inside. Introduce the pan in the machine and cook at 360 degrees F for 8 minutes. Divide into bowls and serve as an appetizer.

73. Crispy Fried Leek With Mustard

Servings: 4   Cooking Time: 15 Minutes
Ingredients:
1 large-sized leek, cut into 1/2-inch wide rings
Salt and pepper, to taste
1 teaspoon mustard
1 cup milk

1 egg
1/2 cup almond flour
1/2 teaspoon baking powder
1/2 cup pork rinds, crushed

Directions:
Toss your leeks with salt and pepper.   In a mixing bowl, whisk the mustard, milk and egg until frothy and pale.   Now, combine almond flour and baking powder in another mixing bowl. In the third bowl, place the pork rinds.   Coat the leek slices with the almond meal mixture. Dredge the floured leek slices into the milk/egg mixture, coating well. Finally, roll them over the pork rinds.   Air-fry for approximately 10 minutes at 370 degrees F. Bon appétit!

74. Tomato Platter

Servings: 6   Cooking Time: 20 Minutes
Ingredients:
6 tomatoes, halved
3 teaspoons sugar-free apricot jam
2 ounces watercress
2 teaspoons oregano, dried

1 tablespoon olive oil
A pinch of salt and black pepper
3 ounces cheddar cheese, grated

Directions:
Spread the jam on each tomato half, sprinkle oregano, salt and pepper, and drizzle the oil all over them Introduce them in the fryer's basket, sprinkle the cheese on top and cook at 360 degrees F for 20 minutes. Arrange the tomatoes on a platter, top each half with some watercress and serve as an appetizer.

75. Steak Nuggets

Servings: 4   Cooking Time: 15 Minutes
Ingredients:
1 lb beef steak, cut into chunks
1 large egg, lightly beaten
1/2 tsp salt

1/2 cup pork rind, crushed
1/2 cup parmesan cheese, grated

Directions:
Add egg in a small bowl.   In a shallow bowl, mix together pork rind, cheese, and salt.   Dip each steak chunk in egg then coat with pork rind mixture and place on a plate. Place in refrigerator for 30 minutes.   Spray air fryer basket with cooking spray.   Preheat the air fryer to 400 F.   Place steak nuggets in air fryer basket and cook for 15-18 minutes or until cooked. Shake after every 4 minutes. Serve and enjoy.

76. Pizza Bites

Servings: 10   Cooking Time: 3 Minutes
Ingredients:
10 Mozzarella cheese slices

10 pepperoni slices

Directions:
Preheat the air fryer to 400F. Line the air fryer pan with baking paper and put Mozzarella in it in one layer. After this, place the pan in the air fryer basket and cook the cheese for 3 minutes or until it is melted. After this, remove the cheese from the air fryer and cool it to room temperature. Then remove

the melted cheese from the baking paper and put the pepperoni slices on it. Fold the cheese in the shape of turnovers.

77. Ranch Kale Chips

Servings: 4   Cooking Time: 5 Minutes
Ingredients:

4 cups kale, stemmed	2 tsp ranch seasoning
1 tbsp nutritional yeast flakes	2 tbsp olive oil
	1/4 tsp salt

Directions:
Add all ingredients into the large mixing bowl and toss well.   Spray air fryer basket with cooking spray.   Add kale in air fryer basket and cook for 4-5 minutes at 370 F. Shake halfway through.   Serve and enjoy.

78. Cheese Pastries

Servings: 6   Cooking Time: 5 Minutes
Ingredients:

4 ounces feta cheese, crumbled	1 egg yolk
1 scallion, finely chopped	Salt and ground black pepper, as needed
2 tablespoons fresh parsley, finely chopped	2 frozen filo pastry sheets, thawed
	2 tablespoons olive oil

Directions:
In a large bowl, add the egg yolk, and beat well. Add in the feta cheese, scallion, parsley, salt, and black pepper. Mix well.   Cut each filo pastry sheet in three strips.   Add about 1 teaspoon of feta mixture on the underside of a strip.   Fold the tip of sheet over the filling in a zigzag manner to form a triangle.   Repeat with the remaining strips and fillings.   Set the temperature of Air Fryer to 390 degrees F.   Coat each pastry evenly with oil. Place the pastries in an Air Fryer basket in a single layer.   Air Fry for about 3 minutes, then air fryer for about 2 minutes on 360 degrees F.   Serve.

79. Lemon Biscuits

Servings: 10   Cooking Time: 5 Minutes
Ingredients:

8½ ounces self-rising flour	3½ ounces cold butter
3½ ounces caster sugar	1 small egg
1 teaspoon fresh lemon zest, finely grated	2 tablespoons fresh lemon juice
	1 teaspoon vanilla extract

Directions:
In a bowl, mix together the flour, and sugar. Using two forks, cut in the butter until coarse crumb forms.   Add in the egg, vanilla extract, lemon juice, and zest. Mix until a soft dough forms.   Then, take out the dough from bowl and put onto a floured surface.   Now, roll it into an even thickness. (½ inch)   Cut the dough into medium-sized biscuits

using a cookie cutter.   Set the temperature of Air Fryer to 355 degrees F.   Place the biscuits in a baking sheet in a single layer.   Put the baking sheet in an Air Fryer basket.   Air Fry for about 5 minutes or until golden brown.   Enjoy!

80. Healthy Broccoli Tots

Servings: 4   Cooking Time: 25 Minutes
Ingredients:

1 lb broccoli, chopped	1/2 cup almond flour
1/4 cup ground flaxseed	1/2 tsp garlic powder
	1 tsp salt

Directions:
Add broccoli into the microwave-safe bowl and microwave for 3 minutes.   Transfer steamed broccoli into the food processor and process until it looks like rice.   Transfer broccoli to a large mixing bowl.   Add remaining ingredients into the bowl and mix until well combined.   Spray air fryer basket with cooking spray.   Make small tots from broccoli mixture and place into the air fryer basket. Cook broccoli tots for 12 minutes at 375 F.   Serve and enjoy.

81. Greek-style Squash Chips

Servings: 4   Cooking Time: 25 Minutes
Ingredients:

1/2 cup seasoned breadcrumbs	1/4 teaspoon oregano
1/2 cup Parmesan cheese, grated	Sauce:
	1/2 cup Greek-style yogurt
Sea salt and ground black pepper, to taste	1 tablespoon fresh cilantro, chopped
2 yellow squash, cut into slices	1 garlic clove, minced
2 tablespoons grapeseed oil	Freshly ground black pepper, to your liking

Directions:
In a shallow bowl, thoroughly combine the seasoned breadcrumbs, Parmesan, salt, black pepper, and oregano.   Dip the yellow squash slices in the prepared batter, pressing to adhere.   Brush with the grapeseed oil and cook in the preheated Air Fryer at 400 degrees F for 12 minutes. Shake the Air Fryer basket periodically to ensure even cooking. Work in batches.   While the chips are baking, whisk the sauce ingredients; place in your refrigerator until ready to serve. Enjoy!

82. Radish Sticks

Servings: 2   Cooking Time: 12 Minutes
Ingredients:

1 large radish, peeled and cut into sticks	1 tablespoon olive oil
1 tablespoon fresh rosemary, finely chopped	¼ teaspoon cayenne pepper
2 teaspoons sugar	Salt and black pepper, as needed

Directions:

Preheat the Air fryer to 390F and grease an Air fryer basket.   Mix radish with all other ingredients in a bowl until well combined.   Arrange the radish sticks in the Air fryer basket and cook for about 12 minutes.   Dish out and serve warm.

83. Cocktail Wieners With Spicy Sauce

Servings: 4   Cooking Time: 20 Minutes
Ingredients:

1 pound pork cocktail sausages	1 teaspoon balsamic vinegar
For the Sauce:	1 garlic clove, finely minced
1/4 cup mayonnaise	1 teaspoon chili powder
1/4 cup cream cheese	
1 whole grain mustard	

Directions:
Take your sausages, give them a few pricks using a fork and place them on the Air Fryer grill pan.   Set the timer for 15 minutes; after 8 minutes, pause the Air Fryer, turn the sausages over and cook for further 7 minutes.   Check for doneness and take the sausages out of the machine.   In the meantime, thoroughly combine all the ingredients for the sauce. Serve with warm sausages and enjoy!

84. Granny's Green Beans

Servings: 4   Cooking Time: 10 Minutes
Ingredients:

1 lb green beans, trimmed	1 cup butter
2 cloves garlic, minced	1 cup toasted pine nuts

Directions:
Boil a pot of water.   Add the green beans and cook until tender for 5 minutes.   Heat the butter in a large skillet over a high heat. Add the garlic and pine nuts and sauté for 2 minutes or until the pine nuts are lightly browned.   Transfer the green beans to the skillet and turn until coated.   Serve!

85. Tasty Tofu

Servings: 4   Cooking Time: 35 Minutes
Ingredients:

1x 12 oz. package low-fat and extra firm tofu	1 tbsp. coriander paste
2 tbsp. low-sodium soy sauce	1 tsp. sesame oil
2 tbsp. fish sauce	1 tsp. duck fat or coconut oil
	1 tsp. Maggi sauce

Directions:
1 Remove the liquid from the package of tofu and chop the tofu into 1-inch cubes. Line a plate with paper towels and spread the tofu out on top in one layer. Place another paper towel on top, followed by another plate, weighting it down with a heavier object if necessary. This is to dry the tofu out completely. Leave for a minimum of 30 minutes or a maximum of 24 hours, replacing the paper towels once or twice throughout the duration.   2 In a medium bowl, mix together the sesame oil, Maggi sauce, coriander paste, fish sauce, and soy sauce. Stir to combine fully.   3 Coat the tofu cubes with this mixture and allow to marinate for at least a half-hour, tossing the cubes a few times throughout to ensure even coating. Add another few drops of fish sauce or soy sauce to thin out the marinade if necessary.   4 Melt the duck fat/coconut oil in your Air Fryer at 350°F for about 2 minutes. Place the tofu cubes in the basket and cook for about 20 minutes or longer to achieve a crispier texture. Flip the tofu over or shake the basket every 10 minutes. 5 Serve hot with the dipping sauce of your choosing.

86. Sweet Potato Fries

Servings: 5   Cooking Time: 35 Minutes
Ingredients:

2 large sweet potatoes	1 tbsp. extra virgin olive oil

Directions:
1 Wash the sweet potatoes. Dry and peel them before chopping them into shoestring fries. In a bowl, toss the fries with the olive oil to coat well.   2 Set your Air Fryer to 320°F and briefly allow to warm. Put the sweet potatoes in the Air Fryer basket and fry for 15 minutes, stirring them at the halfway point.   3 Once done, toss again to make sure no fries are sticking to each other.   4 Turn the heat to 350°F and cook for a further 10 minutes, again giving them a good stir halfway through the cooking time.   5 Serve your fries straightaway.

87. Almond Coconut Granola

Servings: 4   Cooking Time: 12 Minutes
Ingredients:

1 teaspoon monk fruit	½ teaspoon pumpkin pie spices
1 teaspoon almond butter	2 tablespoons coconut flakes
1 teaspoon coconut oil	2 tablespoons pumpkin seeds, crushed
2 tablespoons almonds, chopped	1 teaspoon hemp seeds
1 teaspoon pumpkin puree	1 teaspoon flax seeds
	Cooking spray

Directions:
In the big bowl mix up almond butter and coconut oil. Microwave the mixture until it is melted. After this, in the separated bowl mix up monk fruit, pumpkin spices, coconut flakes, pumpkin seeds, hemp seeds, and flax seeds. Add the melted coconut oil and pumpkin puree. Then stir the mixture until it is homogenous. Preheat the air fryer to 350F. Then put the pumpkin mixture on the baking paper and make the shape of the square. After this, cut the square on the serving bars and transfer in the preheated air fryer. Cook the pumpkin granola for 12 minutes.

88. Broccoli Bites

Servings: 10   Cooking Time: 12 Minutes
Ingredients:

2 cups broccoli florets	2 eggs, beaten
1¼ cups cheddar cheese, grated	1¼ cups panko breadcrumbs
¼ cup Parmesan cheese, grated	Salt and black pepper, to taste

Directions:
Preheat the Air fryer to 350F and grease an Air fryer basket.   Mix broccoli with rest of the ingredients and mix until well combined.   Make small equal-sized balls from mixture and arrange these balls on a baking sheet.   Refrigerate for about half an hour and then transfer into the Air fryer basket.   Cook for about 12 minutes and dish out to serve warm.

89. Lemon Shrimp Bowls

Servings: 4   Cooking Time: 10 Minutes
Ingredients:

1 pound shrimp, peeled and deveined	Juice of ½ lemon
3 garlic cloves, minced	A pinch of salt and black pepper
¼ cup olive oil	¼ teaspoon cayenne pepper

Directions:
In a pan that fits your air fryer, mix all the ingredients, toss, introduce in the fryer and cook at 370 degrees F for 10 minutes. Serve as a snack.

90. Mushroom Pizza Bites

Servings: 6   Cooking Time: 7 Minutes
Ingredients:

6 cremini mushroom caps	½ tomato, chopped
3 oz Parmesan, grated	½ teaspoon dried basil
1 tablespoon olive oil	1 teaspoon ricotta cheese

Directions:
Preheat the air fryer to 400F. Sprinkle the mushroom caps with olive oil and put in the air fryer basket in one layer. Cook them for 3 minutes. After this, mix up tomato and ricotta cheese. Fill the mushroom caps with tomato mixture. Then top them with parmesan and sprinkle with dried basil. Cook the mushroom pizzas for 4 minutes at 400F.

91. Shrimp Dip

Servings: 4   Cooking Time: 20 Minutes
Ingredients:

2 tablespoons ghee, melted	1 pound shrimp, peeled, deveined and minced
¼ pound mushrooms, minced	1 tablespoon parsley, chopped
½ cup mozzarella, shredded	Salt and black pepper to the taste

4 garlic cloves, minced
Directions:
In a bowl, mix all the ingredients, stir well, divide into small ramekins and place them in your air fryer's basket. Cook at 360 degrees F for 20 minutes and serve as a party dip.

92. Broccoli Cheese Nuggets

Servings: 4   Cooking Time: 15 Minutes
Ingredients:

1/4 cup almond flour	1 cup cheddar cheese, shredded
2 cups broccoli florets, cooked until soft	2 egg whites
	1/8 tsp salt

Directions:
Preheat the air fryer to 325 F.   Spray air fryer basket with cooking spray.   Add cooked broccoli into the bowl and using masher mash broccoli into the small pieces.   Add remaining ingredients to the bowl and mix well to combine.   Make small nuggets from broccoli mixture and place into the air fryer basket.   Cook broccoli nuggets for 15 minutes. Turn halfway through.   Serve and enjoy.

93. Cheesy Zucchini Sticks

Servings: 2   Cooking Time: 20 Minutes
Ingredients:

1 zucchini, slice into strips	Sea salt and black pepper, to your liking
2 tablespoons mayonnaise	1 tablespoon garlic powder
1/4 cup tortilla chips, crushed	1/2 teaspoon red pepper flakes
1/4 cup Romano cheese, shredded	

Directions:
Coat the zucchini with mayonnaise.   Mix the crushed tortilla chips, cheese and spices in a shallow dish.   Then, coat the zucchini sticks with the cheese/chips mixture.   Cook in the preheated Air Fryer at 400 degrees F for 12 minutes, shaking the basket halfway through the cooking time.   Work in batches until the sticks are crispy and golden brown. Bon appétit!

94. Banana Peppers

Servings: 8   Cooking Time: 20 Minutes
Ingredients:

1 cup full-fat cream cheese	16 slices salami
Cooking spray	Salt and pepper to taste
16 avocado slices	16 banana peppers

Directions:
1 Pre-heat the Air Fryer to 400°F.   2 Spritz a baking tray with cooking spray.   3 Remove the stems from the banana peppers with a knife.   4 Cut a slit into one side of each banana pepper.   5 Season the cream cheese with the salt and pepper and combine well.   6 Fill each pepper with one

spoonful of the cream cheese, followed by one slice of avocado.   7 Wrap the banana peppers in the slices of salami and secure with a toothpick.   8 Place the banana peppers in the baking tray and transfer it to the Air Fryer. Bake for roughly 8 - 10 minutes.

95. Cheese Rounds

Servings: 4   Cooking Time: 6 Minutes
Ingredients:
1 cup Cheddar cheese, shredded
Directions:
Preheat the air fryer to 400F. Then line the air fryer basket with baking paper. Sprinkle the cheese on the baking paper in the shape of small rounds. Cook them for 6 minutes or until the cheese is melted and starts to be crispy.

96. Lemon Olives Dip

Servings: 6   Cooking Time: 5 Minutes
Ingredients:
1 cup black olives, pitted and chopped
¼ cup capers
3 tablespoons lemon juice
2 garlic cloves, minced
½ cup olive oil
2 teaspoon apple cider vinegar
1 cup parsley leaves
1 cup basil leaves
A pinch of salt and black pepper
Directions:
In a blender, combine all the ingredients, pulse well and transfer to a ramekin. Place the ramekin in your air fryer's basket and cook at 350 degrees F for 5 minutes. Serve as a snack.

97. Pumpkin Seeds

Servings: 1 ½ Cups   Cooking Time: 55 Minutes
Ingredients:
1 ½ cups pumpkin seeds from a large whole pumpkin
Olive oil
1 ½ tsp. salt
1 tsp. smoked paprika
Directions:
1 Boil two quarts of well-salted water in a pot. Cook the pumpkin seeds in the boiling water for 10 minutes.   2 Dump the content of the pot into a sieve and dry the seeds on paper towels for at least 20 minutes.   3 Pre-heat the Air Fryer to 350°F. 4 Cover the seeds with olive oil, salt and smoked paprika, before placing them in the Air Fryer basket. 5 Air fry for 35 minutes. Give the basket a good shake several times throughout the cooking process to ensure the pumpkin seeds are crispy and lightly browned.   6 Let the seeds cool before serving. Alternatively, you can keep them in an air-tight container or bag for snacking or for use as a yogurt topping.

98. Potato Wedges

Servings: 4   Cooking Time: 30 Minutes
Ingredients:
4 medium potatoes, cut into wedges
1 tbsp. Cajun spice
1 tbsp. olive oil
Pepper to taste
Salt to taste
Directions:
Place the potato wedges in the Air Fryer basket and pour in the olive oil.   Cook wedges at 370°F for 25 minutes, shaking the basket twice throughout the cooking time.   Put the cooked wedges in a bowl and coat them with the Cajun spice, pepper, and salt. Serve warm.

99. Party Chicken Pillows

Servings: 4   Cooking Time: 20 Minutes
Ingredients:
1 teaspoon olive oil
1 cup ground chicken
1 (8-ounces) can Pillsbury Crescent Roll dough
Sea salt and ground black pepper, to taste
1 teaspoon onion powder
1/2 teaspoon garlic powder
4 tablespoons tomato paste
4 ounces cream cheese, at room temperature
2 tablespoons butter, melted
Directions:
Heat the olive oil in a pan over medium-high heat. Then, cook the ground chicken until browned or about 4 minutes.   Unroll the crescent dough. Roll out the dough using a rolling pin; cut into 8 pieces. Place the browned chicken, salt, black pepper, onion powder, garlic powder, tomato paste, and cheese in the center of each piece.   Fold each corner over the filling using wet hands. Press together to cover the filling entirely and seal the edges.   Now, spritz the bottom of the Air Fryer basket with cooking oil. Lay the chicken pillows in a single layer in the cooking basket. Drizzle the melted butter all over chicken pillows.   Bake at 370 degrees F for 6 minutes or until golden brown. Work in batches. Bon appétit!

100.   Instant Potato Croquettes

Servings: 4   Cooking Time: 8 Minutes
Ingredients:
2 medium Russet potatoes, boiled, peeled and mashed
2 tablespoons all-purpose flour
½ cup Parmesan cheese, grated
3 eggs
½ cup breadcrumbs
2 tablespoons vegetable oil
Pinch of ground nutmeg
Salt and black pepper, to taste
Directions:
Mix together potatoes with egg yolk, Parmesan, nutmeg, salt and black pepper.   Make equal sized small balls from this mixture and keep aside. Whisk the eggs in a shallow dish.   Mix together oil and breadcrumbs in another shallow dish.   Dip the croquettes evenly in the eggs and dredge in the

breadcrumb mixture.   Place the croquettes in an Air fryer basket and cook for about 8 minutes and dish out to serve warm.

101. Old-fashioned Eggplant Slices

Servings: 2   Cooking Time: 26 Minutes

Ingredients:

1 medium eggplant, peeled and cut into ½-inch round slices	1 cup Italian-style breadcrumbs
½ cup all-purpose flour	2 tablespoons milk
2 eggs, beaten	Salt, to taste
	¼ cup olive oil

Directions:

Preheat the Air fryer to 390F and grease in an Air fryer basket.   Season the eggplant slices with salt and keep aside for 1 hour.   Place flour in a shallow dish.   Whisk the eggs with milk in a second dish. Mix together oil and breadcrumbs in a third shallow dish.   Coat the eggplant slices evenly with flour, then dip in the egg mixture and finally coat with breadcrumb mixture.   Transfer the eggplant slices in the Air fryer basket and cook for about 8 minutes. Dish out and serve warm.

102. Cucumber And Spring Onions Salsa

Servings: 4   Cooking Time: 5 Minutes

Ingredients:

1 and ½ pounds cucumbers, sliced	2 tablespoons ginger, grated
2 spring onions, chopped	1 tablespoon balsamic vinegar
2 tomatoes cubed	A drizzle of olive oil
2 red chili peppers, chopped	

Directions:

In a pan that fits your air fryer, mix all the ingredients, toss, introduce in the fryer and cook at 340 degrees F for 5 minutes. Divide into bowls and serve cold as an appetizer.

103. Teriyaki Chicken Drumettes

Servings: 6   Cooking Time: 40 Minutes

Ingredients:

1 ½ pounds chicken drumettes	1/4 cup honey
Sea salt and cracked black pepper, to taste	1/2 teaspoon Five-spice powder
2 tablespoons fresh chives, roughly chopped	2 tablespoons rice wine vinegar
Teriyaki Sauce:	1/2 teaspoon fresh ginger, grated
1 tablespoon sesame oil	2 cloves garlic, crushed
1/4 cup soy sauce	1 tablespoon corn starch dissolved in 3
1/2 cup water	tablespoons of water

Directions:

Start by preheating your Air Fryer to 380 degrees F. Rub the chicken drumettes with salt and cracked black pepper.   Cook in the preheated Air Fryer approximately 15 minutes. Turn them over and cook an additional 7 minutes.   While the chicken drumettes are roasting, combine the sesame oil, soy sauce, water, honey, Five-spice powder, vinegar, ginger, and garlic in a pan over medium heat. Cook for 5 minutes, stirring occasionally.   Add the cornstarch slurry, reduce the heat, and let it simmer until the glaze thickens.   After that, brush the glaze all over the chicken drumettes. Air-fry for a further 6 minutes or until the surface is crispy. Serve topped with the remaining glaze and garnished with fresh chives. Bon appétit!

104. Turkey Sausage Patties

Servings: 6   Cooking Time: 20 Minutes

Ingredients:

1 lb. lean ground turkey	3⁄4 tsp. paprika
1 tsp. olive oil	Kosher salt and pepper to taste
1 tbsp. chopped chives	Pinch of raw sugar
1 small onion, diced	1 tbsp. vinegar
1 large garlic clove, chopped	1 tsp. fennel seed
	Pinch of nutmeg

Directions:

1 Pre-heat the Air Fryer to 375°F.   2 Add a half-teaspoon of the oil to the fryer, along with the onion and garlic. Air fry for 30 seconds before adding in the fennel. Place everything on a plate.   3 In a bowl, combine the ground turkey with the sugar, paprika, nutmeg, vinegar, chives and the onion mixture. Divide into equal portions and shape each one into a patty.   4 Add another teaspoon of oil to the fryer. Put the patties in the fryer and cook for roughly 3 minutes.   5 Serve with salad or on hamburger buns.

105. Chicken Jalapeno Poppers

Servings: 12   Cooking Time: 20 Minutes

Ingredients:

1/2 cup chicken, cooked and shredded	1/4 cup Monterey jack cheese, shredded
6 jalapenos, halved and seed removed	4 oz cream cheese
1/4 cup green onion, sliced	1/4 tsp dried oregano
1/4 tsp garlic powder	1/4 tsp dried basil
	1/4 tsp salt

Directions:

Preheat the air fryer to 370 F.   Spray air fryer basket with cooking spray.   Mix all ingredients in a bowl except jalapenos.   Spoon 1 tablespoon mixture into each jalapeno halved and place into the air fryer basket.   Cook jalapeno for 20 minutes. Serve and enjoy.

106. Baby Carrots With Asian Flair

Servings: 3   Cooking Time: 20 Minutes

Ingredients:

1 pound baby carrots	1 tablespoon honey
2 tablespoons sesame oil	1 large garlic clove, crushed
1/2 teaspoon Szechuan pepper	1 (1-inch) piece fresh ginger root, peeled
1 teaspoon Wuxiang powder (Five-spice powder)	and grated
	2 tablespoons tamari sauce

Directions:
Start by preheating your Air Fryer to 380 degrees F. Toss all ingredients together and place them in the Air Fryer basket. Cook for 15 minutes, shaking the basket halfway through the cooking time. Enjoy!

107. Avocado Fries With Chipotle Sauce

Servings: 3   Cooking Time: 20 Minutes

Ingredients:

2 tablespoons fresh lime juice	1 egg
	1/2 cup breadcrumbs
1 avocado, pitted, peeled, and sliced	1 chipotle chili in adobo sauce
Pink Himalayan salt and ground white pepper, to taste	1/4 cup light mayonnaise
1/4 cup flour	1/4 cup plain Greek yogurt

Directions:
Drizzle lime juice all over the avocado slices and set aside. Then, set up your breading station. Mix the salt, pepper, and all-purpose flour in a shallow dish. In a separate dish, whisk the egg. Finally, place your breadcrumbs in a third dish. Start by dredging the avocado slices in the flour mixture; then, dip them into the egg. Press the avocado slices into the breadcrumbs, coating evenly. Cook in the preheating Air Fryer at 380 degrees F for 11 minutes, shaking the cooking basket halfway through the cooking time. Meanwhile, blend the chipotle chili, mayo, and Greek yogurt in your food processor until the sauce is creamy and uniform. Serve the warm avocado slices with the sauce on the side. Enjoy!

108. Thai Chili Chicken Wings

Servings: 6   Cooking Time: 16 Minutes

Ingredients:

1/2 lb chicken wings	2 tsp ginger powder
1 tsp paprika	2 1/2 tbsp dry sherry
1/3 cup Thai chili sauce	Pepper
2 tsp garlic powder	Salt

Directions:
Toss chicken wings with dry sherry, paprika, garlic powder, ginger, powder, pepper, and salt. Add chicken wings into the air fryer basket and cook at 365 F for 16 minutes. Serve with Thai chili sauce and enjoy.

109. "good As Gold" Veggie Bites

Servings: 10   Cooking Time: 10 Minutes

Ingredients:

1½ pound fresh spinach, blanched, drained and chopped	2 bread slices, toasted and processed into breadcrumbs
½ of onion, chopped	1 garlic clove, minced
1 carrot, peeled and chopped	1 teaspoon red chili flakes
2 American cheese slices, cut into tiny pieces	Salt, to taste

Directions:
Preheat the Air fryer to 395F and grease an Air fryer basket. Mix all the ingredients in a bowl except breadcrumbs until well combined. Make small equal-sized balls from mixture and arrange these balls on a baking sheet. Refrigerate for about half an hour. Place the bread crumbs in a shallow dish and coat the balls evenly in bread crumbs. Transfer the balls into the Air fryer basket and cook for about 10 minutes. Dish out and serve warm.

110. Rangoon Crab Dip

Servings: 8   Cooking Time: 16 Minutes

Ingredients:

2 cups crab meat	2 tsp coconut amino
1 cup mozzarella cheese, shredded	2 tsp mayonnaise
	8 oz cream cheese, softened
1/2 tsp garlic powder	
1/4 cup pimentos, drained and diced	1 tbsp green onion
	1/4 tsp pepper
1/4 tsp stevia	Salt
1/2 lemon juice	

Directions:
Preheat the air fryer to 325 F. Add all ingredients except half mozzarella cheese into the large bowl and mix until well combined. Transfer bowl mixture into the air fryer baking dish and sprinkle with remaining mozzarella cheese. Place into the air fryer and cook for 16 minutes. Serve and enjoy.

111. Roasted Brussels Sprouts & Bacon

Servings: 2   Cooking Time: 45 Minutes

Ingredients:

24 oz brussels sprouts	¼ cup bacon grease
¼ cup fish sauce	6 strips bacon
	Pepper to taste

Directions:
De-stem and quarter the brussels sprouts. Mix them with the bacon grease and fish sauce. Slice the bacon into small strips and cook. Add the bacon and pepper to the sprouts. Spread onto a greased pan and cook at 450°F/230°C for 35 minutes. Stir every 5 minute or so. Broil for a few more minutes and serve.

112. Lava Rice Bites

Servings: 4   Cooking Time: 20 Minutes

Ingredients:

3 cups cooked risotto
1/3 cup Parmesan cheese, grated
3-ounce mozzarella cheese, cubed

1 egg, beaten
¾ cup bread crumbs
1 tablespoon olive oil

Directions:
Preheat the Air fryer to 390F and grease an Air fryer basket. Mix risotto, olive oil, Parmesan cheese and egg in a bowl until well combined. Make small equal-sized balls from mixture and put a mozzarella cube in the center of each ball. Smooth the risotto mixture with your finger to cover the cheese. Place the bread crumbs in a shallow dish and coat the balls evenly in bread crumbs. Transfer the balls into the Air fryer basket and cook for about 10 minutes. Dish out and serve warm.

113. Glazed Carrot Chips With Cheese

Servings: 3   Cooking Time: 20 Minutes
Ingredients:
3 carrots, sliced into sticks
1 tablespoon coconut oil
2 teaspoons granulated garlic

1/3 cup Romano cheese, preferably freshly grated
Sea salt and ground black pepper, to taste

Directions:
Toss all ingredients in a mixing bowl until the carrots are coated on all sides. Cook at 380 degrees F for 15 minutes, shaking the basket halfway through the cooking time. Serve with your favorite dipping sauce. Bon appétit!

114. Crunchy Spicy Chickpeas

Servings: 4   Cooking Time: 20 Minutes
Ingredients:
1 tablespoon olive oil
½ teaspoon ground cumin
½ teaspoon cayenne pepper

1 (15-ounce) can chickpeas, rinsed and drained
½ teaspoon smoked paprika
Salt, taste

Directions:
Preheat the Air fryer to 390F and grease an Air fryer basket. Mix together all the ingredients in a bowl and toss to coat well. Place half of the chickpeas in the Air fryer basket and cook for about 10 minutes. Repeat with the remaining chickpeas and dish out to serve warm.

115. Polenta Sticks

Servings: 4   Cooking Time: 6 Minutes
Ingredients:
2½ cups cooked polenta
Salt, as required

¼ cup Parmesan cheese, shredded

Directions:
Add the polenta evenly into a greased baking dish and with the back of a spoon, smooth the top surface.

Cover the baking dish and refrigerate for about 1 hour or until set. Remove from the refrigerator and cut down the polenta into the desired size slices. Set the temperature of Air Fryer to 350 degrees F. Grease a baking dish. Arrange the polenta sticks into the prepared baking dish in a single layer and sprinkle with salt. Place the baking dish into an Air Fryer basket. Air Fry for about 5-6 minutes. Top with the cheese and serve.

116. Greek Calamari Appetizer

Servings: 6   Cooking Time: 20 Minutes
Ingredients:
1 ½ pounds calamari tubes, cleaned, cut into rings
Sea salt and ground black pepper, to taste

2 tablespoons lemon juice
1/2 cup almond meal
2 eggs, whisked
1/4 cup buttermilk

Directions:
Preheat your Air Fryer to 390 degrees F. Rinse the calamari and pat it dry. Season with salt and black pepper. Drizzle lemon juice all over the calamari. Now, combine the almond meal, eggs, and buttermilk. Dredge the calamari in the batter. Arrange them in the Air Fryer cooking basket. Spritz with cooking oil and cook for 9 to 12 minutes, shaking the basket occasionally. Work in batches. Serve with toothpicks. Bon appétit!

117. Eggplant Sticks

Servings: 3   Cooking Time: 8 Minutes
Ingredients:
6 oz eggplant, trimmed
½ teaspoon dried oregano
½ teaspoon dried cilantro
½ teaspoon dried thyme

½ teaspoon ground cumin
½ teaspoon salt
1 tablespoon olive oil
¼ teaspoon garlic powder

Directions:
Cut the eggplant into the fries and sprinkle with dried oregano, cilantro, thyme, cumin, salt, and garlic powder. Then sprinkle the eggplant fries with olive oil and shake well. Preheat the air fryer to 400F. Place the eggplant fries in the air fryer and cook them for 4 minutes from each side.

118. Feta And Parsley Filo Triangles

Servings: 6   Cooking Time: 5 Minutes
Ingredients:
1 egg yolk
4-ounce feta cheese, crumbled
1 scallion, chopped finely
2 tablespoons fresh parsley, chopped finely

2 frozen filo pastry sheets, thawed and cut into three strips
2 tablespoons olive oil
Salt and black pepper, to taste

Directions:

Preheat the Air fryer to 390F and grease an Air fryer basket. Whisk egg yolk in a large bowl and beat well. Stir in feta cheese, scallion, parsley, salt and black pepper. Brush pastry with olive oil and put a tablespoon of feta mixture over one corner of filo strip. Fold diagonally to create a triangle and keep folding until filling is completely wrapped. Repeat with the remaining strips and filling and coat the triangles with olive oil. Place the triangles in the Air fryer basket and cook for about 3 minutes. Now, set the Air fryer to 360 degrees F and cook for another 2 minutes. Dish out and serve warm.

119. Simple Banana Chips

Servings: 8   Cooking Time: 10 Minutes
Ingredients:

2 raw bananas, peeled and sliced	Salt and black pepper, to taste
2 tablespoons olive oil	

Directions:
Preheat the Air fryer to 355F and grease an Air fryer basket. Drizzle banana slices evenly with olive oil and arrange in the Air fryer basket. Cook for about 10 minutes and season with salt and black pepper. Dish out and serve warm.

120. Creamy Cheddar Eggs

Servings: 8   Cooking Time: 16 Minutes
Ingredients:

4 eggs	1 tablespoon heavy cream
2 oz pork rinds	1 teaspoon fresh dill, chopped
¼ cup Cheddar cheese, shredded	

Directions:
Place the eggs in the air fryer and cook them at 255F for 16 minutes. Then cool the eggs in the cold water and peel. Cut every egg into the halves and remove the egg yolks. Transfer the egg yolks in the mixing bowl. Add shredded cheese, heavy cream, and fresh dill. Stir the mixture with the help of the fork until smooth and add pork rinds. Mix it up. Fill the egg whites with the egg yolk mixture.

121. Thyme-roasted Sweet Potatoes

Servings: 3   Cooking Time: 35 Minutes
Ingredients:

1 pound sweet potatoes, peeled, cut into bite-sized pieces	1 teaspoon sea salt
	1/4 teaspoon freshly ground black pepper
2 tablespoons olive oil	1/2 teaspoon cayenne pepper
	2 fresh thyme sprigs

Directions:
Arrange the potato slices in a single layer in the lightly greased cooking basket. Add the olive oil, salt, black pepper, and cayenne pepper; toss to coat. Bake at 380 degrees F for 30 minutes, shaking the cooking basket occasionally. Bake until tender

and slightly browned, working in batches. Serve warm, garnished with thyme sprigs. Bon appétit!

122. Parmesan Zucchini Bites

Servings: 6   Cooking Time: 10 Minutes
Ingredients:

4 zucchinis, grated and squeeze out all liquid	1 egg, lightly beaten
	1 tsp Italian seasoning
1 cup shredded coconut	1/2 cup parmesan cheese, grated

Directions:
Add all ingredients into the bowl and mix until well combined. Spray air fryer basket with cooking spray. Make small balls from zucchini mixture and place into the air fryer basket and cook at 400 F for 10 minutes. Serve and enjoy.

123. Avocado Sticks

Servings: 2   Cooking Time: 10 Minutes
Ingredients:

2 avocados	Salt and pepper
4 egg yolks	1 cup flour
1 ½ tbsp. water	1 cup herbed butter

Directions:
Halve the avocados, twist to open, and take out the pits. Cut each half into three equal slices. In a bowl, combine the egg yolks and water. Season with salt and pepper to taste and whisk together. Pour the flour into a shallow bowl. Coat each slice of avocado in the flour, then in the egg, before dipping it in the flour again. Ensure the flour coats the avocado well and firmly. Pre-heat the fryer at 400°F. When it is warm, put the avocados inside and cook for eight minutes. Take care when removing the avocados from the fryer and enjoy with a side of the herbed butter.

124. Brussels Sprouts

Servings: 2   Cooking Time: 15 Minutes
Ingredients:

2 cups Brussels sprouts, sliced in half	1 tbsp. balsamic vinegar
1 tbsp. olive oil	¼ tsp. salt

Directions:
Toss all of the ingredients together in a bowl, coating the Brussels sprouts well. Place the sprouts in the Air Fryer basket and air fry at 400°F for 10 minutes, shaking the basket at the halfway point.

125. Rosemary Beans

Servings: 2   Cooking Time: 5 Minutes
Ingredients:

1 cup green beans, chopped	2 tbsp rosemary, chopped
2 garlic cloves, minced	1 tbsp butter, melted
	1/2 tsp salt

Directions:

Preheat the air fryer to 390 F. Add all ingredients into the bowl and toss well. Transfer green beans into the air fryer basket and cook for 5 minutes. Serve and enjoy.

126. Cheddar Cheese Lumpia Rolls

Servings: 5   Cooking Time: 20 Minutes

Ingredients:

- 15 pieces spring roll lumpia wrappers
- 2 tablespoons sesame oil
- 5 ounces mature cheddar cheese, cut into 15 sticks

Directions:

Wrap the cheese sticks in the lumpia wrappers. Transfer to the Air Fryer basket. Brush with sesame oil. Bake in the preheated Air Fryer at 395 degrees for 10 minutes or until the lumpia wrappers turn golden brown. Work in batches. Shake the Air Fryer basket occasionally to ensure even cooking. Bon appétit!

127. Hillbilly Cheese Surprise

Servings: 6   Cooking Time: 40 Minutes

Ingredients:

- 4 cups broccoli florets
- ¼ cup ranch dressing
- ½ cup sharp cheddar cheese, shredded
- ¼ cup heavy whipping cream
- Kosher salt and pepper to taste

Directions:

Preheat your fryer to 375°F/190°C. In a bowl, combine all of the ingredients until the broccoli is well-covered. In a casserole dish, spread out the broccoli mixture. Bake for 30 minutes. Take out of your fryer and mix. If the florets are not tender, bake for another 5 minutes until tender. Serve!

128. Broccoli Florets

Servings: 4   Cooking Time: 20 Minutes

Ingredients:

- 1 lb. broccoli, cut into florets
- 1 tbsp. lemon juice
- 1 tbsp. olive oil
- 1 tbsp. sesame seeds
- 3 garlic cloves, minced

Directions:

In a bowl, combine all of the ingredients, coating the broccoli well. Transfer to the Air Fryer basket and air fry at 400°F for 13 minutes.

129. Broccoli Fries With Spicy Dip

Servings: 4   Cooking Time: 15 Minutes

Ingredients:

- 3/4 pound broccoli florets
- 1/2 teaspoon onion powder
- 1 teaspoon granulated garlic
- 1/2 teaspoon cayenne
- Sea salt and ground black pepper, to taste
- 2 tablespoons sesame oil
- Spicy Dip:
- 1/4 cup mayonnaise
- 1/4 cup Greek yogurt
- pepper
- 4 tablespoons parmesan cheese, preferably freshly grated
- 1/4 teaspoon Dijon mustard
- 1 teaspoon hot sauce

Directions:

Start by preheating the Air Fryer to 400 degrees F. Blanch the broccoli in salted boiling water until al dente, about 3 to 4 minutes. Drain well and transfer to the lightly greased Air Fryer basket. Add the onion powder, garlic, cayenne pepper, salt, black pepper, sesame oil, and parmesan cheese. Cook for 6 minutes, tossing halfway through the cooking time. Meanwhile, mix all of the spicy dip ingredients. Serve broccoli fries with chilled dipping sauce. Bon appétit!

130. Crunchy Roasted Chickpeas

Servings: 4   Cooking Time: 25 Minutes

Ingredients:

- 1 (15-ounce) can chickpeas, drained and patted dry
- 1 tablespoon sesame oil
- 1/8 cup Romano cheese, grated
- 1/4 teaspoon mustard powder
- 1/2 teaspoon shallot powder
- 1/2 teaspoon garlic powder
- 1 teaspoon coriander, minced
- 1/2 teaspoon red pepper flakes, crushed
- Coarse sea salt and ground black pepper, to taste

Directions:

Toss all ingredients in a mixing bowl. Roast in the preheated Air Fryer at 380 degrees F for 10 minutes, shaking the basket halfway through the cooking time. Work in batches. Bon appétit!

131. Broccoli Coconut Dip

Servings: 4   Cooking Time: 15 Minutes

Ingredients:

- 1 and ½ cups veggie stock
- 3 cups broccoli florets
- 2 garlic cloves, minced
- 1/3 cup coconut milk
- Salt and black pepper to the taste
- 1 tablespoon balsamic vinegar
- 1 tablespoon olive oil

Directions:

In a pan that fits your air fryer, mix all the ingredients, toss, introduce in the fryer and cook at 390 degrees F for 15 minutes. Divide into bowls and serve.

132. Pickled Fries

Servings: 4   Cooking Time: 8 Minutes

Ingredients:

- 2 pickles, sliced
- 1 tablespoon dried dill
- 1 egg, beaten
- 2 tablespoons flax meal

Directions:

Dip the sliced pickles in the egg and then sprinkle with dried ill and flax meal. Place them in the air fryer basket in one layer and cook at 400F for 8 minutes.

133. Sweet Corn And Bell Pepper Sandwich With Barbecue Sauce

Servings: 2   Cooking Time: 23 Minutes
Ingredients:

2 tablespoons butter, softened
4 bread slices, trimmed and cut horizontally

1 cup sweet corn kernels
1 roasted green bell pepper, chopped
¼ cup barbecue sauce

Directions:
Preheat the Air fryer to 355F and grease an Air fryer basket.   Heat butter in a skillet on medium heat and add corn.   Sauté for about 2 minutes and dish out in a bowl.   Add bell pepper and barbecue sauce to the corn.   Spread corn mixture on one side of 2 bread slices and top with remaining slices. Dish out and serve warm.

134. Pineapple Bites

Servings: 4   Cooking Time: 10 Minutes
Ingredients:

For Pineapple Sticks:
½ of pineapple
¼ cup desiccated coconut

For Yogurt Dip:
1 tablespoon fresh mint leaves, minced
1 cup vanilla yogurt

Directions:
With a sharp knife, remove the outer peel of pineapple and then, cut into 1-2 inch thick sticks lengthwise.   Add the desiccated coconut in a shallow dish.   Coat the pineapple sticks evenly with coconut.   Set the temperature of Air Fryer to 390 degrees F.   Add the pineapple sticks in an Air Fryer basket in a single layer.   Air Fry for about 10 minutes.   For dip: in a bowl, mix together the mint, and yogurt.   Serve the pineapple sticks with yogurt dip.

135. Turmeric Chicken Cubes

Servings: 6   Cooking Time: 12 Minutes
Ingredients:

8 oz chicken fillet
½ teaspoon ground black pepper
½ teaspoon ground turmeric
¼ teaspoon ground coriander

½ teaspoon ground paprika
3 egg whites, whisked
4 tablespoons almond flour
Cooking spray

Directions:
In the shallow bowl mix up ground black pepper, turmeric, coriander, and paprika. Then chop the chicken fillet on the small cubes and sprinkle them with spice mixture. Stir well and ad egg white. Mix up the chicken and egg whites well. After this, coat every chicken cube in the almond flour. Preheat the air fryer to 375F. Put the chicken cubes in the air fryer basket in one layer and gently spray with cooking spray. Cook the chicken popcorn for 7 minutes. Then shake the chicken popcorn well and cook it for 5 minutes more.

136. Mozzarella Snack

Servings: 8   Cooking Time: 5 Minutes
Ingredients:

2 cups mozzarella, shredded
2 teaspoons psyllium husk powder

¾ cup almond flour
¼ teaspoon sweet paprika

Directions:
Put the mozzarella in a bowl, melt it in the microwave for 2 minutes, add all the other ingredients quickly and stir really until you obtain a dough. Divide the dough into 2 balls, roll them on 2 baking sheets and cut into triangles. Arrange the tortillas in your air fryer's basket and bake at 370 degrees F for 5 minutes. Transfer to bowls and serve as a snack.

137. Coconut Salmon Bites

Servings: 12   Cooking Time: 10 Minutes
Ingredients:

2 avocados, peeled, pitted and mashed
4 ounces smoked salmon, skinless, boneless and chopped
2 tablespoons coconut cream

1 teaspoon avocado oil
1 teaspoon dill, chopped
A pinch of salt and black pepper

Directions:
In a bowl, mix all the ingredients, stir well and shape medium balls out of this mix. Place them in your air fryer's basket and cook at 350 degrees F for 10 minutes. Serve as an appetizer.

138. Mini Turkey And Corn Burritos

Servings: 6   Cooking Time: 25 Minutes
Ingredients:

1 tablespoon olive oil
1/2 pound ground turkey
2 tablespoons shallot, minced
1 garlic clove, smashed
1 red bell pepper, seeded and chopped
Sea salt and freshly ground black pepper, to taste

1 ancho chili pepper, seeded and minced
1/2 teaspoon ground cumin
1/3 cup salsa
6 ounces sweet corn kernels
12 (8-inch) tortilla shells
1 tablespoon butter, melted
1/2 cup sour cream, for serving

Directions:
Heat the olive oil in a sauté pan over medium-high heat. Cook the ground meat and shallots for 3 to 4 minutes.   Add the garlic and peppers and cook an additional 3 minutes or until fragrant. After that, add the spices, salsa, and corn. Stir until everything is well combined.   Place about 2 tablespoons of the meat mixture in the center of each tortilla. Roll your tortillas to seal the edges and make the burritos. Brush each burrito with melted butter and place them in the lightly greased cooking basket. Bake at

395 degrees F for 10 minutes, turning them over halfway through the cooking time. Garnish each burrito with a dollop of sour cream and serve.

139. Basic Salmon Croquettes

Servings: 16   Cooking Time: 14 Minutes

Ingredients:

1 large can red salmon, drained	1 cup breadcrumbs
2 eggs, lightly beaten	2 tablespoons milk
2 tablespoons fresh parsley, chopped	Salt and black pepper, to taste
	1/3 cup vegetable oil

Directions:
Preheat the Air fryer to 390F and grease an Air fryer basket. Mash the salmon completely in a bowl and stir in eggs, parsley, breadcrumbs, milk, salt and black pepper. Mix until well combined and make 16 equal-sized croquettes from the mixture. Mix together oil and breadcrumbs in a shallow dish and coat the croquettes in this mixture. Place half of the croquettes in the Air fryer basket and cook for about 7 minutes. Repeat with the remaining croquettes and serve warm.

140. Cocktail Cranberry Meatballs

Servings: 5   Cooking Time: 15 Minutes

Ingredients:

1/2 pound ground beef	Sea salt and ground black pepper, to taste
1/2 pound ground turkey	1 teaspoon red pepper flakes, crushed
1/4 cup Parmesan cheese, grated	1 tablespoon soy sauce
1/4 cup breadcrumbs	1 (8-ounce can jellied cranberry sauce
1 small shallot, chopped	6 ounces tomato-based chili sauce
2 eggs, whisked	
1/2 teaspoon garlic powder	
1/2 teaspoon porcini powder	

Directions:
In a mixing bowl, combine the ground meat together with the cheese, breadcrumbs, shallot, eggs, and spices. Shape the mixture into 1-inch balls. Cook the meatballs in the preheated Air Fryer at 380 degrees for 5 minutes. Shake halfway through the cooking time. Work in batches. Whisk the soy sauce, cranberry sauce, and chili sauce in a mixing bowl. Pour the sauce over the meatballs and bake an additional 2 minutes. Serve with cocktail sticks. Bon appétit!

141. Healthy Toasted Nuts

Servings: 4   Cooking Time: 9 Minutes

Ingredients:

1/2 cup macadamia nuts	1/4 cup walnuts
1/2 cup pecans	1/4 cup hazelnuts
1 tbsp olive oil	1 tsp salt

Directions:
Preheat the air fryer to 320 F. Add all nuts into the air fryer basket and cook for 8 minutes. Shake halfway through. Drizzle nuts with olive oil and season with salt and toss well. Cook nuts for 1 minute more. Serve and enjoy.

142. Kale Chips

Servings: 2   Cooking Time: 15 Minutes

Ingredients:

1 head kale	1 tsp. soy sauce
1 tbsp. olive oil	

Directions:
De-stem the head of kale and shred each leaf into a 1 ½" piece. Wash and dry well. Toss the kale with the olive oil and soy sauce to coat it completely. Transfer to the Air Fryer and cook at 390°F for 2 to 3 minutes, giving the leaves a good toss at the halfway mark.

143. Turmeric Cauliflower Popcorn

Servings: 4   Cooking Time: 11 Minutes

Ingredients:

1 cup cauliflower florets	2 tablespoons almond flour
1 teaspoon ground turmeric	1 teaspoon salt
2 eggs, beaten	Cooking spray

Directions:
Cut the cauliflower florets into small pieces and sprinkle with ground turmeric and salt. Then dip the vegetables in the eggs and coat in the almond flour. Preheat the air fryer to 400F. Place the cauliflower popcorn in the air fryer in one layer and cook for 7 minutes. Give a good shake to the vegetables and cook them for 4 minutes more.

144. Chipotle Jicama Hash

Servings: 2   Cooking Time: 15 Minutes

Ingredients:

4 slices bacon, chopped	1 oz green bell pepper (or poblano), seeded and chopped
12 oz jicama, peeled and diced	4 tbsp Chipotle mayonnaise
4 oz purple onion, chopped	

Directions:
Using a skillet, brown the bacon on a high heat. Remove and place on a towel to drain the grease. Use the remaining grease to fry the onions and jicama until brown. When ready, add the bell pepper and cook the hash until tender. Transfer the hash onto two plates and serve each plate with 4 tablespoons of Chipotle mayonnaise.

145. Hollandaise Sauce

Servings: 8   Cooking Time: 2 Minutes

Ingredients:

8 large egg yolks	½ tsp salt
2 tbsp fresh lemon juice	1 cup unsalted butter

Directions:
Combine the egg yolks, salt, and lemon juice in a blender until smooth. Put the butter in your microwave for around 60 seconds, until melted and hot. Turn the blender on a low speed and slowly pour in the butter until the sauce begins to thicken. Serve!

146. Cocktail Flanks

Servings: 4   Cooking Time: 45 Minutes

Ingredients:

1x 12-oz. package cocktail franks	1x 8-oz. can crescent rolls

Directions:
1 Drain the cocktail franks and dry with paper towels. 2 Unroll the crescent rolls and slice the dough into rectangular strips, roughly 1" by 1.5". 3 Wrap the franks in the strips with the ends poking out. Leave in the freezer for 5 minutes. 4 Pre-heat the Air Fryer to 330°F. 5 Take the franks out of the freezer and put them in the cooking basket. Cook for 6 – 8 minutes. 6 Reduce the heat to 390°F and cook for another 3 minutes or until a golden-brown color is achieved.

147. Cheese Cookies

Servings: 10   Cooking Time: 12 Minutes

Ingredients:

For Dough:	Salt, as required
3.38 fluid ounces cream	½ teaspoon baking powder
5.30 ounces margarine	For Topping:
6.35 ounces Gruyere cheese, grated	1 tablespoon milk
1 teaspoon paprika	2 egg yolks, beaten
5.30 ounces flour, sifted	2 tablespoons poppy seeds

Directions:
For cookies: in a bowl, mix together the cream, margarine, cheese, paprika, and salt.   Place the flour, and baking powder onto a smooth surface. Mix them well.   Using your hands, create a well in the center of flour.   Add the cheese mixture and knead until a soft dough forms.   Roll the dough into 1-1½-inch thickness.   Cut the cookies using a cookie cutter.   In another bowl, mix together the milk, and egg yolks.   Coat the cookies with milk mixture and then, sprinkle with poppy seeds.   Set the temperature of Air Fryer to 340 degrees F. Place cookies onto the grill pan of an Air Fryer in a single layer.   Air Fry for about 12 minutes. Serve.

148. Mexican Muffins

Servings: 4   Cooking Time: 15 Minutes

Ingredients:

1 teaspoon taco seasonings	1 cup ground beef
2 oz Mexican blend cheese, shredded	1 teaspoon keto tomato sauce
	Cooking spray

Directions:
Preheat the air fryer to 375F. Meanwhile, in the mixing bowl mix up ground beef and taco seasonings. Spray the muffin molds with cooking spray. Then transfer the ground beef mixture in the muffin molds and top them with cheese and tomato sauce. Transfer the muffin molds in the preheated air fryer and cook them for 15 minutes.

149. Italian-style Tomato-parmesan Crisps

Servings: 4   Cooking Time: 20 Minutes

Ingredients:

4 Roma tomatoes, sliced	1 teaspoon Italian seasoning mix
2 tablespoons olive oil	4 tablespoons Parmesan cheese, grated
Sea salt and white pepper, to taste	

Directions:
Start by preheating your Air Fryer to 350 degrees F. Generously grease the Air Fryer basket with nonstick cooking oil.   Toss the sliced tomatoes with the remaining ingredients. Transfer them to the cooking basket without overlapping.   Cook in the preheated Air Fryer for 5 minutes. Shake the cooking basket and cook an additional 5 minutes. Work in batches.   Serve with Mediterranean aioli for dipping, if desired. Bon appétit!

150. Healthy Veggie Lasagna

Servings: 4   Cooking Time: 1 Hour

Ingredients:

1½ pounds pumpkin, peeled and chopped finely	½ pound fresh lasagna sheets
¾ pound tomatoes, cubed	¼ cup Parmesan cheese, grated
1 pound cooked beets, sliced thinly	2 tablespoons sunflower oil

Directions:
Preheat the Air fryer to 300F and lightly grease a baking dish.   Put pumpkin and 1 tablespoon sunflower oil in a skillet and cook for about 10 minutes.   Put the pumpkin mixture and tomatoes in a blender and pulse until smooth.   Return to the skillet and cook on low heat for about 5 minutes.   Transfer the pumpkin puree into the baking dish and layer with lasagna sheets.   Top with the beet slices and cheese and place in the Air fryer.   Cook for about 45 minutes and dish out to serve warm.

Desserts Recipes

151. Cinnamon Ginger Cookies

Servings: 8   Cooking Time: 12 Minutes

Ingredients:

1 egg	1 1/2 cups almond
1/2 tsp vanilla	flour
1/8 tsp ground cloves	1/4 tsp ground
1 tsp baking powder	nutmeg
3/4 cup erythritol	1/4 tsp ground
2/4 cup butter,	cinnamon
melted	1/2 tsp ground ginger
	Pinch of salt

Directions:

In a large bowl, mix together all dry ingredients. In a separate bowl, mix together all wet ingredients. Add dry ingredients to the wet ingredients and mix until dough is formed. Cover and place in the fridge for 30 minutes.   Preheat the air fryer to 325 F. Make cookies from dough and place into the air fryer and cook for 12 minutes.   Serve and enjoy.

152.   Angel Food Cake

Servings: 12   Cooking Time: 30 Minutes

Ingredients:

¼ cup butter, melted	12 egg whites
1 cup powdered	2 teaspoons cream of
erythritol	tartar
1 teaspoon strawberry	A pinch of salt
extract	

Directions:

Preheat the air fryer for 5 minutes.   Mix the egg whites and cream of tartar.   Use a hand mixer and whisk until white and fluffy.   Add the rest of the ingredients except for the butter and whisk for another minute.   Pour into a baking dish.   Place in the air fryer basket and cook for 30 minutes at 400F or if a toothpick inserted in the middle comes out clean.   Drizzle with melted butter once cooled.

153.   Summer Peach Crisp

Servings: 4   Cooking Time: 40 Minutes

Ingredients:

2 cups fresh peaches,	1/2 teaspoon ground
pitted and sliced	cinnamon
1/4 cup cornmeal	A pinch of fine sea
1/4 cup brown sugar	salt
1 teaspoon pure	1 stick cold butter
vanilla extract	1/2 cup rolled oats

Directions:

Toss the sliced peaches with the cornmeal, brown sugar, vanilla extract, cinnamon, and sea salt. Place in a baking pan coated with cooking spray.   In a mixing dish, thoroughly combine the cold butter and rolled oats. Sprinkle the mixture over each peach. Bake in the preheated Air Fryer at 330 degrees F for 35 minutes. Bon appétit!

154.   Heavenly Tasty Lava Cake

Servings: 6   Cooking Time: 3 Minutes

Ingredients:

2/3 cup unsalted	2 eggs
butter	1/3 cup fresh
2/3 cup all-purpose	raspberries
flour	5 tablespoons sugar
1 cup chocolate chips,	Salt, to taste
melted	

Directions:

Preheat the Air fryer to 355F and grease 6 ramekins lightly.   Mix sugar, butter, eggs, chocolate mixture, flour and salt in a bowl until well combined.   Fold in the melted chocolate chips and divide this mixture into the prepared ramekins.   Transfer into the Air fryer basket and cook for about 3 minutes.   Garnish with raspberries and serve immediately.

155. Cinnamon And Sugar Sweet Potato Fries

Servings: 2   Cooking Time: 30 Minutes

Ingredients:

1 large sweet potato,	1/4 teaspoon ground
peeled and sliced into	cardamom
sticks	1/4 cup sugar
1 teaspoon ghee	1 tablespoon ground
1 tablespoon	cinnamon
cornstarch	

Directions:

Toss the sweet potato sticks with the melted ghee and cornstarch.   Cook in the preheated Air Fryer at 380 degrees F for 20 minutes, shaking the basket halfway through the cooking time.   Sprinkle the cardamom, sugar, and cinnamon all over the sweet potato fries and serve. Bon appétit!

156.   Poppyseed Muffins

Servings: 12   Cooking Time: 14 Minutes

Ingredients:

3 eggs	1 tsp baking powder
4 true lemon packets	1 cup almond flour
2 tbsp poppy seeds	1 tsp lemon extract
1/4 cup coconut oil	1/4 cup heavy
1/4 cup ricotta cheese	whipping cream
	1/3 cup swerve

Directions:

Add all ingredients into the large bowl and beat using a hand mixer until fluffy.   Pour batter into the silicone muffin molds and place in the air fryer. In batches.   Cook at 320 F for 14 minutes. Serve and enjoy.

157. Red Velvet Pancakes

Servings: 3   Cooking Time: 35 Minutes

Ingredients:

1/2 cup flour	1/2 cup milk
1 teaspoon baking powder	1 teaspoon vanilla
1/4 teaspoon salt	Topping:
2 tablespoons white sugar	2 ounces cream cheese, softened
1/2 teaspoon cinnamon	2 tablespoons butter, softened
1 teaspoon red paste food color	3/4 cup powdered sugar
1 egg	

Directions:
Mix the flour, baking powder, salt, sugar, cinnamon, red paste food color in a large bowl. Gradually add the egg and milk, whisking continuously, until well combined. Let it stand for 20 minutes. Spritz the Air Fryer baking pan with cooking spray. Pour the batter into the pan using a measuring cup. Cook at 230 degrees F for 4 to 5 minutes or until golden brown. Repeat with the remaining batter. Meanwhile, make your topping by mixing the ingredients until creamy and fluffy. Decorate your pancakes with topping. Bon appétit!

---

158.   Picnic Blackberry Muffins

Servings: 8   Cooking Time: 20 Minutes

Ingredients:

1 ½ cups almond flour	2 eggs, whisked
1/2 teaspoon baking soda	1/2 cup milk
1 teaspoon baking powder	1/4 cup coconut oil, melted
1/4 teaspoon kosher salt	1/2 teaspoon vanilla paste
1/2 cup swerve	1/2 cup fresh blackberries

Directions:
In a mixing bowl, combine the almond flour, baking soda, baking powder, swerve, and salt. Whisk to combine well. In another mixing bowl, mix the eggs, milk, coconut oil, and vanilla. Now, add the wet egg mixture to dry the flour mixture. Then, carefully fold in the fresh blackberries; gently stir to combine. Scrape the batter mixture into the muffin cups. Bake your muffins at 350 degrees F for 12 minutes or until the tops are golden brown. Sprinkle some extra icing sugar over the top of each muffin if desired. Serve and enjoy!

---

159.   Plum And Currant Tart Recipe

Servings: 6   Cooking Time: 65 Minutes

Ingredients:

For the crumble:	1 cup white currants
1/4 cup almond flour	2 tbsp. cornstarch
1/4 cup millet flour	3 tbsp. sugar
1 cup brown rice flour	1/2 tsp. vanilla extract
1/2 cup cane sugar	1/2 tsp. cinnamon
10 tbsp. butter; soft	

3 tbsp. milk	powder
For the filling:	1/4 tsp. ginger powder
1 lb. small plums; pitted and halved	1 tsp. lime juice

Directions:
In a bowl; mix brown rice flour with 1/2 cup sugar, millet flour, almond flour, butter and milk and stir until you obtain a sand like dough Reserve 1/4 of the dough, press the rest of the dough into a tart pan that fits your air fryer and keep in the fridge for 30 minutes. Meanwhile; in a bowl, mix plums with currants, 3 tbsp. sugar, cornstarch, vanilla extract, cinnamon, ginger and lime juice and stir well Pour this over tart crust, crumble reserved dough on top, introduce in your air fryer and cook at 350 °F, for 35 minutes. Leave tart to cool down, slice and serve.

---

160.   Apple Caramel Relish

Servings: 4   Cooking Time: 40 Minutes

Ingredients:

2 apples, peeled, sliced	1 tsp cinnamon
3 oz butter, melted	½ cup flour
½ cup brown sugar	1 cup caramel sauce

Directions:
Line a cake tin with baking paper. In a bowl, mix butter, sugar, cinnamon and flour until you obtain a crumbly texture. Prepare the cake mix according to the instructions (no baking). Pour the batter into the tin and arrange the apple slices on top. Spoon the caramel over the apples and add the crumble over the sauce. Cook in the air fryer for 35 minutes at 360 F; make sure to check it halfway through, so it's not overcooked.

---

161. Chocolate Biscuit Sandwich Cookies

Servings: 10   Cooking Time: 20 Minutes

Ingredients:

2 ½ cups self-rising flour	1 teaspoon vanilla essence
4 ounces brown sugar	4 ounces double cream
1 ounce honey	3 ounces dark chocolate
5 ounces butter, softened	1 teaspoon cardamom seeds, finely crushed
1 egg, beaten	

Directions:
Start by preheating your Air Fryer to 350 degrees F. In a mixing bowl, thoroughly combine the flour, brown sugar, honey, and butter. Mix until your mixture resembles breadcrumbs. Gradually, add the egg and vanilla essence. Shape your dough into small balls and place in the parchment-lined Air Fryer basket. Bake in the preheated Air Fryer for 10 minutes. Rotate the pan and bake for another 5 minutes. Transfer the freshly baked cookies to a cooling rack. As the biscuits are cooling, melt the double cream and dark chocolate in an air-fryer safe

bowl at 350 degrees F. Add the cardamom seeds and stir well. Spread the filling over the cooled biscuits and sandwich together. Bon appétit!

162. Merengues

Servings: 6   Cooking Time: 65 Minutes

Ingredients:

2 egg whites	1 teaspoon lime juice
1 teaspoon lime zest, grated	4 tablespoons Erythritol

Directions:
Whisk the egg whites until soft peaks. Then add Erythritol and lime juice and whisk the egg whites until you get strong peaks. After this, add lime zest and carefully stir the egg white mixture. Preheat the air fryer to 275F. Line the air fryer basket with baking paper. With the help of the spoon make the small merengues and put them in the air fryer in one layer. Cook the dessert for 65 minutes.

163. Orange Muffins

Servings: 5   Cooking Time: 10 Minutes

Ingredients:

1 tablespoon poppy seeds	5 eggs, beaten
1 teaspoon vanilla extract	1 teaspoon orange zest, grated
¼ teaspoon ground nutmeg	5 tablespoons coconut flour
½ teaspoon baking powder	1 tablespoon Monk fruit
1 teaspoon orange juice	2 tablespoons coconut flakes
	Cooking spray

Directions:
In the mixing bowl mix up eggs, poppy seeds, vanilla extract, ground nutmeg, baking powder, orange juice, orange zest, coconut flour, and Monk fruit. Add coconut flakes and mix up the mixture until it is homogenous and without any clumps. Preheat the air fryer to 360F. Spray the muffin molds with cooking spray from inside. Pour the muffin batter in the molds and transfer them in the air fryer. Cook the muffins for 10 minutes.

164. Mom's Orange Rolls

Servings: 6   Cooking Time: 1 Hour 20 Minutes

Ingredients:

1/2 cup milk	Filling:
1/4 cup granulated sugar	2 tablespoons butter
1 tablespoon yeast	4 tablespoons white sugar
1/2 stick butter, at room temperature	1 teaspoon ground star anise
1 egg, at room temperature	1/4 teaspoon ground cinnamon
1/4 teaspoon salt	1 teaspoon vanilla paste
2 cups all-purpose flour	1/2 cup confectioners' sugar
2 tablespoons fresh orange juice	

Directions:
Heat the milk in a microwave safe bowl and transfer the warm milk to the bowl of a stand electric mixer. Add the granulated sugar and yeast, and mix to combine well. Cover and let it sit until the yeast is foamy. Then, beat the butter on low speed. Fold in the egg and mix again. Add salt and flour. Add the orange juice and mix on medium speed until a soft dough forms. Knead the dough on a lightly floured surface. Cover it loosely and let it sit in a warm place about 1 hour or until doubled in size. Then, spritz the bottom and sides of a baking pan with cooking oil (butter flavored. Roll your dough out into a rectangle. Spread 2 tablespoons of butter all over the dough. In a mixing dish, combine the white sugar, ground star anise, cinnamon, and vanilla; sprinkle evenly over the dough. Then, roll up your dough to form a log. Cut into 6 equal rolls and place them in the parchment-lined Air Fryer basket. Bake at 350 degrees for 12 minutes, turning them halfway through the cooking time. Dust with confectioners' sugar and enjoy!

165. Raspberry-coconut Cupcake

Servings: 6   Cooking Time: 30 Minutes

Ingredients:

½ cup butter	1 tablespoon baking powder
½ teaspoon salt	
¾ cup erythritol	3 teaspoons vanilla extract
1 cup almond milk, unsweetened	7 large eggs, beaten
1 cup coconut flour	

Directions:
Preheat the air fryer for 5 minutes. Mix all ingredients using a hand mixer. Pour into hard cupcake molds. Place in the air fryer basket. Bake for 30 minutes at 350F or until a toothpick inserted in the middle comes out clean. Bake by batches if possible. Allow to chill before serving.

166. Crusty

Servings: 3   Cooking Time: 60 Minutes

Ingredients:

2 cups flour	2 large eggs
4 tsp melted butter	½ tsp salt

Directions:
Mix together the flour and butter. Add in the eggs and salt and combine well to form a dough ball. Place the dough between two pieces of parchment paper. Roll out to 10" by 16" and ¼ inch thick. Serve!

167. Lemon Mini Pies With Coconut

Servings: 8   Cooking Time: 15 Minutes + Chilling Time

Ingredients:

1 box (4-serving size lemon instant pudding filling mix	1/3 cup shredded coconut
	1 teaspoon apple pie

1 teaspoon grated lemon peel
18 wonton wrappers
1 ¼ cups cream cheese, room temperature

spice blend
1 teaspoon pure vanilla extract
1/8 teaspoon salt
1/2 teaspoon ground anise star

Directions:
Prepare a muffin pan by adding a cooking spray. Press the wonton wrappers evenly into the cups. Transfer them to your air fryer and bake at 350 degrees F just for 5 minutes. When the edges become golden, they are ready.   Meanwhile, blend all remaining ingredients using your electric mixer; place the prepared cream in the refrigerator until ready to serve.   Lastly, divide prepared cream among wrappers. Keep them refrigerated until serving time. Bon appétit!

168.   Chocolate Almond Cookies

Servings: 10   Cooking Time: 20 Minutes
Ingredients:

2 cups almond flour
1/2 cup coconut flour
5 ounces swerve
5 ounces butter, softened
1 teaspoon vanilla essence

1 egg, beaten
4 ounces double cream
3 ounces bakers' chocolate, unsweetened
1 teaspoon cardamom seeds, finely crushed

Directions:
Start by preheating your Air Fryer to 350 degrees F. In a mixing bowl, thoroughly combine the flour, swerve, and butter. Mix until your mixture resembles breadcrumbs.   Gradually, add the egg and vanilla essence. Shape your dough into small balls and place in the parchment-lined Air Fryer basket.   Bake in the preheated Air Fryer for 10 minutes. Rotate the pan and bake for another 5 minutes. Transfer the freshly baked cookies to a cooling rack.   As the biscuits are cooling, melt the double cream and bakers' chocolate in the Air Fryer safe bowl at 350 degrees F. Add the cardamom seeds and stir well.   Spread the filling over the cooled biscuits and sandwich together. Bon appétit!

169.   Hazelnut Brownie Cups

Servings: 12   Cooking Time: 30 Minutes
Ingredients:

6 oz. semisweet chocolate chips
1 stick butter, at room temperature
1 cup sugar
2 large eggs
¼ tsp. hazelnut extract

¼ cup red wine
1 tsp. pure vanilla extract
¾ cup flour
2 tbsp. cocoa powder
½ cup ground hazelnuts
Pinch of kosher salt

Directions:

Melt the butter and chocolate chips in the microwave.   In a large bowl, combine the sugar, eggs, red wine, hazelnut and vanilla extract with a whisk. Pour in the chocolate mix.   Add in the flour, cocoa powder, ground hazelnuts, and a pinch of kosher salt, continuing to stir until a creamy, smooth consistency is achieved.   Take a muffin tin and place a cupcake liner in each cup. Spoon an equal amount of the batter into each one.   Air bake at 360°F for 28 - 30 minutes, cooking in batches if necessary.   Serve with a topping of ganache if desired.

170.   Pumpkin Cookies

Servings: 27   Cooking Time: 20 Minutes
Ingredients:

1 egg
2 cups almond flour
1/2 tsp baking powder
1 tsp vanilla
1/2 cup butter

15 drops liquid stevia
1/2 tsp pumpkin pie spice
1/2 cup pumpkin puree

Directions:
Preheat the air fryer to 280 F.   In a large bowl, add all ingredients and mix until well combined. Make cookies from mixture and place into the air fryer and cook for 20 minutes.   Serve and enjoy.

171. Ricotta Cheese Cake

Servings: 8   Cooking Time: 30 Minutes
Ingredients:

3 eggs, lightly beaten
1 tsp baking powder
½ cup ghee, melted

1 cup almond flour
1/3 cup erythritol
1 cup ricotta cheese, soft

Directions:
Add all ingredients into the bowl and mix until well combined.   Pour batter into the greased air fryer baking dish and place into the air fryer.   Cook at 350 F for 30 minutes.   Slice and serve.

172. Coconut And Berries Cream

Servings: 6   Cooking Time: 30 Minutes
Ingredients:

12 ounces blackberries
6 ounces raspberries
12 ounces blueberries

¾ cup swerve
2 ounces coconut cream

Directions:
In a bowl, mix all the ingredients and whisk well. Divide this into 6 ramekins, put them in your air fryer and cook at 320 degrees F for 30 minutes. Cool down and serve it.

173. Ninja Pop-tarts

Servings: 6   Cooking Time: 1 Hour
Ingredients:

Pop-tarts:
1 cup coconut flour

2 tablespoons swerve
Lemon Glaze:

1 cup almond flour
½ cup of ice-cold water
Pop-tarts:
¼ teaspoon salt
2/3 cup very cold coconut oil
½ teaspoon vanilla extract

1¼ cups powdered swerve
2 tablespoons lemon juice
zest of 1 lemon
1 teaspoon coconut oil, melted
¼ teaspoon vanilla extract

Directions:
Pop-tarts: Preheat the Air fryer to 375F and grease an Air fryer basket.   Mix all the flours, swerve, and salt in a bowl and stir in the coconut oil. Mix well with a fork until an almond meal mixture is formed.   Stir in vanilla and 1 tablespoon of cold water and mix until a firm dough is formed.   Cut the dough into two equal pieces and spread in a thin sheet.   Cut each sheet into 12 equal sized rectangles and transfer 4 rectangles in the Air fryer basket.   Cook for about 10 minutes and repeat with the remaining rectangles.   Lemon Glaze: Meanwhile, mix all the ingredients for the lemon glaze and pour over the cooked tarts.   Top with sprinkles and serve.

174. Moon Pie

Servings: 4   Cooking Time: 10 Minutes
Ingredients:
8 squares each of dark, milk and white chocolate

8 large marshmallows

Directions:
Arrange the cracker halves on a cutting board. Put 2 marshmallows onto half of the graham cracker halves. Place 2 squares of chocolate onto the cracker with the marshmallows. Put the remaining crackers on top to create 4 sandwiches. Wrap each one in the baking paper so it resembles a parcel. Cook in the fryer for 5 minutes at 340 F.

175. Espresso Cinnamon Cookies

Servings: 12   Cooking Time: 15 Minutes
Ingredients:
8 tablespoons ghee, melted
1 cup almond flour
¼ cup brewed espresso
¼ cup swerve

½ tablespoon cinnamon powder
2 teaspoons baking powder
2 eggs, whisked

Directions:
In a bowl, mix all the ingredients and whisk well. Spread medium balls on a cookie sheet lined parchment paper, flatten them, put the cookie sheet in your air fryer and cook at 350 degrees F for 15 minutes. Serve the cookies cold.

176. Baked Plum Cream

Servings: 4   Cooking Time: 20 Minutes
Ingredients:

1 pound plums, pitted and chopped
1 tablespoon lemon juice

¼ cup swerve
1 and ½ cups heavy cream

Directions:
In a bowl, mix all the ingredients and whisk really well. Divide this into 4 ramekins, put them in the air fryer and cook at 340 degrees F for 20 minutes. Serve cold.

177. Bread Pudding

Servings: 2   Cooking Time: 12 Minutes
Ingredients:
1 cup milk
2 tablespoons raisins, soaked in hot water for about 15 minutes
2 bread slices, cut into small cubes
1 tablespoon chocolate chips

1 egg
1 tablespoon brown sugar
½ teaspoon ground cinnamon
¼ teaspoon vanilla extract
1 tablespoon sugar

Directions:
Preheat the Air fryer to 375F and grease a baking dish lightly.   Mix milk, egg, brown sugar, cinnamon and vanilla extract until well combined. Stir in the raisins and mix well.   Arrange the bread cubes evenly in the baking dish and top with the milk mixture.   Refrigerate for about 20 minutes and sprinkle with chocolate chips and sugar.   Transfer the baking pan into the Air fryer and cook for about 12 minutes.   Dish out and serve immediately.

178.   Double Chocolate Muffins

Servings: 12   Cooking Time: 30 Minutes
Ingredients:
1 1/3 cups self-rising flour
2½ tablespoons cocoa powder
2½ ounces milk chocolate, finely chopped

3½ ounces butter
5 tablespoons milk
2/3 cup plus 3 tablespoons caster sugar
½ teaspoon vanilla extract

Directions:
Preheat the Air fryer to 355F and grease 12 muffin molds lightly.   Mix flour, sugar, and cocoa powder in a bowl.   Stir in the butter, milk, vanilla extract and the chopped chocolate and mix until well combined.   Transfer the mixture evenly into the muffin molds and arrange in the Air fryer basket in 2 batches.   Cook for about 9 minutes and set the Air fryer to 320F.   Cook for about 6 minutes and remove from the Air fryer to serve.

179. Air Fried Doughnuts

Servings: 4   Cooking Time: 25 Minutes
Ingredients:

1 tsp baking powder
½ cup milk
2 ½ tbsp butter
1 egg
2 oz brown sugar

Directions:
Preheat the air fryer to 350 F, and beat the butter with the sugar, until smooth. Beat in eggs, and milk. In a bowl, combine the flour with the baking powder. Gently fold the flour into the butter mixture. Form donut shapes and cut off the center with cookie cutters. Arrange on a lined baking sheet and cook in the fryer for 15 minutes. Serve with whipped cream or icing.

180. Apple Pie In Air Fryer

Servings: 4   Cooking Time: 35 Minutes

Ingredients:

½ teaspoon vanilla extract
1 beaten egg
1 large apple, chopped
1 Pillsbury Refrigerator pie crust
1 tablespoon butter
1 tablespoon ground cinnamon
1 tablespoon raw sugar
2 tablespoon sugar
2 teaspoons lemon juice
Baking spray

Directions:
Lightly grease baking pan of air fryer with cooking spray. Spread pie crust on bottom of pan up to the sides.   In a bowl, mix vanilla, sugar, cinnamon, lemon juice, and apples. Pour on top of pie crust. Top apples with butter slices.   Cover apples with the other pie crust. Pierce with knife the tops of pie. Spread beaten egg on top of crust and sprinkle sugar. Cover with foil.   For 25 minutes, cook on 390F. Remove foil cook for 10 minutes at 330F until tops are browned.   Serve and enjoy.

181. Coffee Flavored Cookie Dough

Servings: 12   Cooking Time: 20 Minutes

Ingredients:

¼ cup butter
¼ teaspoon xanthan gum
½ teaspoon coffee espresso powder
½ teaspoon stevia powder
¾ cup almond flour
1 egg
1 teaspoon vanilla
1/3 cup sesame seeds
2 tablespoons cocoa powder
2 tablespoons cream cheese, softened

Directions:
Preheat the air fryer for 5 minutes.   Combine all ingredients in a mixing bowl.   Press into a baking dish that will fit in the air fryer.   Place in the air fryer basket and cook for 20 minutes at 400F or if a toothpick inserted in the middle comes out clean.

182. Pumpkin Bars

Servings: 6   Cooking Time: 25 Minutes

Ingredients:

¼ cup almond butter
1 tablespoon unsweetened almond
½ cup coconut flour
¼ cup swerve

milk
¾ teaspoon baking soda
½ cup dark sugar free chocolate chips, divided
1 cup canned sugar free pumpkin puree
1 teaspoon cinnamon
1 teaspoon vanilla extract
¼ teaspoon nutmeg
½ teaspoon ginger
1/8 teaspoon salt
1/8 teaspoon ground cloves

Directions:
Preheat the Air fryer to 360F and layer a baking pan with wax paper.   Mix pumpkin puree, swerve, vanilla extract, milk, and butter in a bowl. Combine coconut flour, spices, salt, and baking soda in another bowl.   Combine the two mixtures and mix well until smooth.   Add about 1/3 cup of the sugar free chocolate chips and transfer this mixture into the baking pan.   Transfer into the Air fryer basket and cook for about 25 minutes.   Microwave sugar free chocolate bits on low heat and dish out the baked cake from the pan.   Top with melted chocolate and slice to serve.

183. Berry Cookies

Servings: 4   Cooking Time: 9 Minutes

Ingredients:

2 teaspoons butter, softened
1 tablespoon Splenda
1 egg yolk
½ cup almond flour
1 oz strawberry, chopped, mashed

Directions:
In the mixing bowl mix up butter, Splenda, egg yolk, and almond flour. Knead the non-sticky dough. Then make the small balls from the dough. Use your finger to make small holes in every ball. Then fill the balls with mashed strawberries. Preheat the air fryer to 360F. Line the air fryer basket with baking paper and put the cookies inside. Cook them for 9 minutes.

184. Choco Mug Cake

Servings: 1   Cooking Time: 20 Minutes

Ingredients:

1 egg, lightly beaten
1 tbsp heavy cream
¼ tsp baking powder
2 tbsp unsweetened cocoa powder
2 tbsp Erythritol
½ tsp vanilla
1 tbsp peanut butter
1 tsp salt

Directions:
Preheat the air fryer to 400 F.   In a bowl, mix together all ingredients until well combined. Spray mug with cooking spray.   Pour batter in mug and place in the air fryer and cook for 20 minutes.   Serve and enjoy.

185. Father's Day Cranberry And Whiskey Brownies

Servings: 10   Cooking Time: 50 Minutes

Ingredients:

1/3 cup cranberries
3 tablespoons
1/2 cup coconut oil
2 eggs plus an egg

whiskey
8 ounces white chocolate
3/4 cup self-rising flour
3 tablespoons coconut flakes

yolk, whisked
3/4 cup white sugar
1/4 teaspoon ground cardamom
1 teaspoon pure rum extract

Directions:
Microwave white chocolate and coconut oil until everything's melted; allow the mixture to cool at room temperature. After that, thoroughly whisk the eggs, sugar, rum extract, and cardamom. Next step, add the rum/egg mixture to the chocolate mixture. Stir in the flour and coconut flakes; mix to combine. Mix cranberries with whiskey and let them soak for 15 minutes. Fold them into the batter. Press the batter into a lightly buttered cake pan. Air-fry for 35 minutes at 340 degrees F. Allow them to cool slightly on a wire rack before slicing and serving.

186. Almond Coconut Lemon Cake

Servings: 10   Cooking Time: 48 Minutes
Ingredients:
4 eggs
2 tbsp lemon zest
1/2 cup butter softened
2 tsp baking powder
1/4 cup coconut flour

2 cups almond flour
1/2 cup fresh lemon juice
1/4 cup swerve
1 tbsp vanilla

Directions:
Preheat the air fryer to 280 F. Spray air fryer baking dish with cooking spray and set aside. In a large bowl, beat all ingredients using a hand mixer until a smooth. Pour batter into the prepared dish and place into the air fryer and cook for 48 minutes. Slice and serve.

187. Egg Custard

Servings: 6   Cooking Time: 32 Minutes
Ingredients:
2 egg yolks
3 eggs
2 cups heavy whipping cream

1/2 cup erythritol
1/2 tsp vanilla
1 tsp nutmeg

Directions:
Preheat the air fryer to 325 F. Add all ingredients into the large bowl and beat until well combined. Pour custard mixture into the greased baking dish and place into the air fryer. Cook for 32 minutes. Let it cool completely then place in the refrigerator for 1-2 hours. Serve and enjoy.

188. Orange Carrot Cake

Servings: 8   Cooking Time: 30 Minutes
Ingredients:
2 large carrots, peeled and grated
1 ¾ cup flour
¾ cup sugar

2 cups sugar
1 tsp. mixed spice
2 tbsp. milk
4 tbsp. melted butter

2 eggs
10 tbsp. olive oil

1 small orange, rind and juice

Directions:
Set the Air Fryer to 360°F and allow to heat up for 10 minutes. Place a baking sheet inside the tin. Combine the flour, sugar, grated carrots, and mixed spice. Pour the milk, beaten eggs, and olive oil into the middle of the batter and mix well. Pour the mixture in the tin, transfer to the fryer and cook for 5 minutes. Lower the heat to 320°F and allow to cook for an additional 5 minutes. In the meantime, prepare the frosting by combining the melted butter, orange juice, rind, and sugar until a smooth consistency is achieved. Remove the cake from the fryer, allow it to cool for several minutes and add the frosting on top.

189. Homemade Coconut Banana Treat

Servings: 6   Cooking Time: 20 Minutes
Ingredients:
2 tbsp. coconut oil
¾ cup friendly bread crumbs
2 tbsp. sugar
½ tsp. cinnamon powder

¼ tsp. ground cloves
6 ripe bananas, peeled and halved
⅓ cup flour
1 large egg, beaten

Directions:
Heat a skillet over a medium heat. Add in the coconut oil and the bread crumbs, and mix together for approximately 4 minutes. Take the skillet off of the heat. Add in the sugar, cinnamon, and cloves. Cover all sides of the banana halves with the rice flour. Dip each one in the beaten egg before coating them in the bread crumb mix. Place the banana halves in the Air Fryer basket, taking care not to overlap them. Cook at 290°F for 10 minutes. You may need to complete this step in multiple batches. Serve hot or at room temperature, topped with a sprinkling of flaked coconut if desired.

190. Pumpkin Cinnamon Pudding

Servings: 4   Cooking Time: 25 Minutes
Ingredients:
3 cups pumpkin puree
3 tbsp. honey
1 tbsp. ginger
1 tbsp. cinnamon
1 tsp. clove

1 tsp. nutmeg
1 cup full-fat cream
2 eggs
1 cup sugar

Directions:
Pre-heat your Air Fryer to 390°F. In a bowl, stir all of the ingredients together to combine. Grease the inside of a small baking dish. Pour the mixture into the dish and transfer to the fryer. Cook for 15 minutes. Serve with whipped cream if desired.

191. Easy Fruitcake With Cranberries

Servings: 8   Cooking Time: 30 Minutes

Ingredients:

1 cup almond flour	2 eggs plus 1 egg yolk, beaten
1/3 teaspoon baking soda	1/2 cup cranberries, fresh or thawed
1/3 teaspoon baking powder	1 tablespoon browned butter
3/4 cup erythritol	For Ricotta Frosting:
1/2 teaspoon ground cloves	1/2 stick butter
1/3 teaspoon ground cinnamon	1/2 cup firm Ricotta cheese
1/2 teaspoon cardamom	1 cup powdered erythritol
1 stick butter	1/4 teaspoon salt
1/2 teaspoon vanilla paste	Zest of 1/2 lemon

Directions:

Start by preheating your Air Fryer to 355 degrees F. In a mixing bowl, combine the flour with baking soda, baking powder, erythritol, ground cloves, cinnamon, and cardamom.   In a separate bowl, whisk 1 stick butter with vanilla paste; mix in the eggs until light and fluffy. Add the flour/sugar mixture to the butter/egg mixture. Fold in the cranberries and browned butter.   Scrape the mixture into the greased cake pan. Then, bake in the preheated Air Fryer for about 20 minutes. Meanwhile, in a food processor, whip 1/2 stick of the butter and Ricotta cheese until there are no lumps. Slowly add the powdered erythritol and salt until your mixture has reached a thick consistency. Stir in the lemon zest; mix to combine and chill completely before using.   Frost the cake and enjoy!

---

192.   Chocolate Paradise Cake

Servings: 6   Cooking Time: 35 Minutes + Chilling Time

Ingredients:

2 eggs, beaten	1/4 cup cocoa powder
2/3 cup sour cream	1 teaspoon vanilla extract
1 cup almond flour	
2/3 cup swerve	1/2 teaspoon pure rum extract
1/3 cup coconut oil, softened	Chocolate Frosting:
2 tablespoons chocolate chips, unsweetened	1/2 cup butter, softened
	1/4 cup cocoa powder
1 ½ teaspoons baking powder	1 cup powdered swerve
	2 tablespoons milk

Directions:

Mix all ingredients for the chocolate cake with a hand mixer on low speed. Scrape the batter into a cake pan.   Bake at 330 degrees F for 25 to 30 minutes. Transfer the cake to a wire rack Meanwhile, whip the butter and cocoa until smooth. Stir in the powdered swerve. Slowly and gradually, pour in the milk until your frosting reaches desired consistency.   Whip until smooth and fluffy; then, frost the cooled cake. Place in your refrigerator for a couple of hours. Serve well chilled.

---

193.   Churros

Servings: 1   Cooking Time: 15 Minutes

Ingredients:

½ cup water	3 eggs
¼ cup butter	2 ½ tsp. sugar
½ cup flour	

Directions:

In a saucepan, bring the water and butter to a boil. Once it is bubbling, add the flour and mix to create a doughy consistency.   Remove from the heat, allow to cool, and crack the eggs into the saucepan. Blend with a hand mixer until the dough turns fluffy. Transfer the dough into a piping bag.   Pre-heat the fryer at 380°F.   Pipe the dough into the fryer in several three-inch-long segments. Cook for ten minutes before removing from the fryer and coating in the sugar.   Serve with the low-carb chocolate sauce of your choice.

---

194.   Chocolate Candies

Servings: 4   Cooking Time: 2 Minutes

Ingredients:

1 oz almonds, crushed	1 oz dark chocolate
2 tablespoons peanut butter	2 tablespoons heavy cream

Directions:

Preheat the air fryer to 390F. Chop the dark chocolate and put it in the air fryer mold. Add peanut butter and heavy cream. Stir the mixture and transfer in the air fryer. Cook it for 2 minutes or until it starts to be melt. Then line the air tray with parchment. Put the crushed almonds on the tray in one layer. Then pour the cooked chocolate mixture over the almonds. Flatten gently if needed and let it cool. Crack the cooked chocolate layer into the candies.

---

195.   Lemon Mousse

Servings: 6   Cooking Time: 10 Minutes

Ingredients:

12-ounces cream cheese, softened	¼ teaspoon salt
1 teaspoon lemon liquid stevia	1/3 cup fresh lemon juice
	1½ cups heavy cream

Directions:

Preheat the Air fryer to 345 degrees F and grease a large ramekin lightly.   Mix all the ingredients in a large bowl until well combined.   Pour into the ramekin and transfer into the Air fryer.   Cook for about 10 minutes and pour into the serving glasses. Refrigerate to cool for about 3 hours and serve chilled.

---

196.   Ginger Vanilla Cookies

Servings: 12   Cooking Time: 15 Minutes

Ingredients:

2 cups almond flour
1 cup swerve
¼ cup butter, melted
1 egg
2 teaspoons ginger, grated

1 teaspoon vanilla extract
¼ teaspoon nutmeg, ground
¼ teaspoon cinnamon powder

Directions:
In a bowl, mix all the ingredients and whisk well. Spoon small balls out of this mix on a lined baking sheet that fits the air fryer lined with parchment paper and flatten them. Put the sheet in the fryer and cook at 360 degrees F for 15 minutes. Cool the cookies down and serve.

197. Fiesta Pastries

Servings: 8   Cooking Time: 20 Minutes
Ingredients:

1 teaspoon fresh orange zest, grated finely
7.05-ounce prepared frozen puff pastry, cut into 16 squares

½ of apple, peeled, cored and chopped
½ tablespoon white sugar
½ teaspoon ground cinnamon

Directions:
Preheat the Air fryer to 390F and grease an Air fryer basket.   Mix all ingredients in a bowl except puff pastry.   Arrange about 1 teaspoon of this mixture in the center of each square.   Fold each square into a triangle and slightly press the edges with a fork.   Arrange the pastries in the Air fryer basket and cook for about 10 minutes.   Dish out and serve immediately.

198.   Avocado Cream Pudding

Servings: 6   Cooking Time: 25 Minutes
Ingredients:

4 small avocados, peeled, pitted and mashed
2 eggs, whisked
1 cup coconut milk

¾ cup swerve
1 teaspoon cinnamon powder
½ teaspoon ginger powder

Directions:
In a bowl, mix all the ingredients and whisk well. Pour into a pudding mould, put it in the air fryer and cook at 350 degrees F for 25 minutes. Serve warm.

199.   Easy 'n Delicious Brownies

Servings: 8   Cooking Time: 20 Minutes
Ingredients:

1/4 cup butter
1/2 cup white sugar
1 egg
1/2 teaspoon vanilla extract
2 tablespoons and 2 teaspoons

1 tablespoon and 1-1/2 teaspoons butter, softened
1 tablespoon and 1-1/2 teaspoons unsweetened cocoa powder

unsweetened cocoa powder
1/4 cup all-purpose flour
1/8 teaspoon salt
1/8 teaspoon baking powder

1-1/2 teaspoons honey
1/2 teaspoon vanilla extract
1/2 cup confectioners' sugar

Directions:
Lightly grease baking pan of air fryer with cooking spray. Melt ¼ cup butter for 3 minutes. Stir in vanilla, eggs, and sugar. Mix well.   Stir in baking powder, salt, flour, and cocoa mix well. Evenly spread.   For 20 minutes, cook on 300F.   In a small bowl, make the frosting by mixing well all Ingredients. Frost brownies while still warm. Serve and enjoy.

200.   Mouth-watering Strawberry Cobbler

Servings: 4   Cooking Time: 25 Minutes
Ingredients:

1 tablespoon butter, diced
1 tablespoon and 2 teaspoons butter
1-1/2 teaspoons cornstarch
1-1/2 cups strawberries, hulled
1/2 cup all-purpose flour

1/2 cup water
1-1/2 teaspoons white sugar
1/4 cup white sugar
1/4 teaspoon salt
1/4 cup heavy whipping cream
3/4 teaspoon baking powder

Directions:
Lightly grease baking pan of air fryer with cooking spray. Add water, cornstarch, and sugar. Cook for 10 minutes 390F or until hot and thick. Add strawberries and mix well. Dot tops with 1 tbsp butter.   In a bowl, mix well salt, baking powder, sugar, and flour. Cut in 1 tbsp and 2 tsp butter. Mix in cream. Spoon on top of berries.   Cook for 15 minutes at 390F, until tops are lightly browned. Serve and enjoy.

201.   Fried Pineapple Rings

Servings: 6   Cooking Time: 10 Minutes
Ingredients:

2/3 cup flour
½ tsp. baking powder
½ tsp. baking soda
Pinch of kosher salt
½ cup water
½ tsp. ground cinnamon
¼ tsp. ground anise star

1 cup rice milk
½ tsp. vanilla essence
4 tbsp. sugar
¼ cup unsweetened flaked coconut
1 medium pineapple, peeled and sliced

Directions:
Mix together all of the ingredients, minus the pineapple.   Cover the pineapple slices with the batter.   Place the slices in the Air Fryer and cook at 380°F for 6 - 8 minutes.   Pour a drizzling of

maple syrup over the pineapple and serve with a side of vanilla ice cream.

202. Marshmallow Pastries

Servings: 8   Cooking Time: 5 Minutes
Ingredients:

4-ounce butter, melted	½ cup chunky peanut butter
8 phyllo pastry sheets, thawed	8 teaspoons marshmallow fluff
Pinch of salt	

Directions:
Preheat the Air fryer to 360F and grease an Air fryer basket.   Brush butter over 1 filo pastry sheet and top with a second filo sheet.   Brush butter over second filo pastry sheet and repeat with all the remaining sheets.   Cut the phyllo layers in 8 strips and put 1 tablespoon of peanut butter and 1 teaspoon of marshmallow fluff on the underside of a filo strip.   Fold the tip of the sheet over the filling to form a triangle and fold repeatedly in a zigzag manner.   Arrange the pastries into the Air fryer basket and cook for about 5 minutes.   Season with a pinch of salt and serve warm.

203. Dark Chocolate Cheesecake

Servings: 6   Cooking Time: 34 Minutes
Ingredients:

3 eggs, whites and yolks separated	2 tablespoons cocoa powder
1 cup dark chocolate, chopped	¼ cup dates jam
½ cup cream cheese, softened	2 tablespoons powdered sugar

Directions:
Preheat the Air fryer to 285F and grease a cake pan lightly.   Refrigerate egg whites in a bowl to chill before using.   Microwave chocolate and cream cheese on high for about 3 minutes.   Remove from microwave and whisk in the egg yolks.   Whisk together egg whites until firm peaks form and combine with the chocolate mixture.   Transfer the mixture into a cake pan and arrange in the Air fryer basket.   Cook for about 30 minutes and dish out. Dust with powdered sugar and spread dates jam on top to serve.

204. Classic Mini Cheesecakes

Servings: 8   Cooking Time: 30 Minutes
Ingredients:

1/3 teaspoon grated nutmeg	For the Cheesecake:
1 ½ tablespoons erythritol	2 eggs
1 ½ cups almond meal	1/2 cups unsweetened chocolate chips
8 tablespoons melted butter	1 ½ tablespoons sour cream
1 teaspoon ground	4 ounces soft cheese
	1/2 cup swerve

cinnamon
A pinch of kosher salt

1/2 teaspoon vanilla essence

Directions:
Firstly, line eight cups of mini muffin pan with paper liners.   To make the crust, mix the almond meal together with erythritol, cinnamon, nutmeg, and kosher salt.   Now, add melted butter and stir well to moisten the crumb mixture.   Divide the crust mixture among the muffin cups and press gently to make even layers.   In another bowl, whip together the soft cheese, sour cream and swerve until uniform and smooth. Fold in the eggs and the vanilla essence. Then, divide chocolate chips among the prepared muffin cups. Then, add the cheese mix to each muffin cup.   Bake for about 18 minutes at 345 degrees F. Bake in batches if needed. To finish, transfer the mini cheesecakes to a cooling rack; store in the fridge.

205. Strawberry Jam

Servings: 6   Cooking Time: 25 Minutes
Ingredients:

Juice of 2 limes	4 cups sugar
1 pound strawberries, chopped	2 cups water

Directions:
In a pan that fits your air fryer, mix the strawberries with the sugar, lime juice and the water; stir. Place the pan in the fryer and cook at 340 degrees F for 25 minutes.   Blend the mix using an immersion blender, divide into cups, refrigerate, and serve cold.

206. Avocado Walnut Bread

Servings: 6   Cooking Time: 35 Minutes
Ingredients:

¾ cup (3 oz.) almond flour, white	1 teaspoon cinnamon ground
¼ teaspoon baking soda	½ teaspoon kosher salt
2 ripe avocados, cored, peeled and mashed	2 tablespoons vegetable oil
2 large eggs, beaten	½ cup granulated swerve
2 tablespoons (3/4 oz.) Toasted walnuts, chopped roughly	1 teaspoon vanilla extract

Directions:
Preheat the Air fryer to 310F and line a 6-inch baking pan with parchment paper.   Mix almond flour, salt, baking soda, and cinnamon in a bowl. Whisk eggs with avocado mash, yogurt, swerve, oil, and vanilla in a bowl.   Stir in the almond flour mixture and mix until well combined.   Pour the batter evenly into the pan and top with the walnuts. Place the baking pan into the Air fryer basket and cook for about 35 minutes.   Dish out in a platter and cut into slices to serve.

207. Cherry Pie

Servings: 8   Cooking Time: 35 Minutes

Ingredients:

1 tbsp. milk	21 oz. cherry pie filling
2 ready-made pie crusts	1 egg yolk

Directions:

Pre-heat the Air Fryer to 310°F.   Coat the inside of a pie pan with a little oil or butter and lay one of the pie crusts inside. Use a fork to pierce a few holes in the pastry.   Spread the pie filling evenly over the crust.   Slice the other crust into strips and place them on top of the pie filling to make the pie look more homemade.   Place in the Air Fryer and cook for 15 minutes.

208. Cheesy Orange Fritters

Servings: 8   Cooking Time: 15 Minutes

Ingredients:

1 ½ tablespoons orange juice	3/4 cup whole milk
3/4 pound cream cheese, at room temperature	1 ¼ cups all-purpose flour
1 teaspoon freshly grated orange rind	1/3 cup white sugar
1 teaspoon vanilla extract	⅓ teaspoon ground cinnamon
	1/2 teaspoon ground anise star

Directions:

Thoroughly combine all ingredients in a mixing dish. Next step, drop a teaspoonful of the mixture into the air fryer cooking basket; air-fry for 4 minutes at 340 degrees F.   Dust with icing sugar, if desired. Bon appétit!

209. Orange Sponge Cake

Servings: 6   Cooking Time: 50 Minutes

Ingredients:

9 oz self-rising flour	Frosting:
9 oz butter	4 egg whites
3 eggs	Juice of 1 orange
1 tsp baking powder	1 tsp orange food coloring
1 tsp vanilla extract	zest of 1 orange
zest of 1 orange	7 oz superfine sugar

Directions:

Preheat the air fryer to 160 F and place all cake ingredients, in a bowl and beat with an electric mixer. Transfer half of the batter into a prepared cake pan; bake for 15 minutes. Repeat the process for the other half of the batter.   Meanwhile, prepare the frosting by beating all frosting ingredients together. Spread the frosting mixture on top of one cake. Top with the other cake.

210. Apple Cake

Servings: 6   Cooking Time: 45 Minutes

Ingredients:

1 cup all-purpose flour	1/3 cup brown sugar
½ teaspoon baking soda	1 teaspoon ground cinnamon
1 egg	Salt, to taste
2 cups apples, peeled, cored and chopped	5 tablespoons plus 1 teaspoon vegetable oil
1 teaspoon ground nutmeg	¾ teaspoon vanilla extract

Directions:

Preheat the Air fryer to 355F and grease a baking pan lightly.   Mix flour, sugar, spices, baking soda and salt in a bowl until well combined.   Whisk egg with oil and vanilla extract in another bowl.   Stir in the flour mixture slowly and fold in the apples. Pour this mixture into the baking pan and cover with the foil paper.   Transfer the baking pan into the Air fryer and cook for about 40 minutes.   Remove the foil and cook for 5 more minutes.   Allow to cool completely and cut into slices to serve.

211. Grandma's Butter Cookies

Servings: 4   Cooking Time: 25 Minutes

Ingredients:

8 ounces all-purpose flour	2 ½ ounces sugar
1 teaspoon baking powder	1 large egg, room temperature.
A pinch of grated nutmeg	1 stick butter, room temperature
A pinch of coarse salt	1 teaspoon vanilla extract

Directions:

Mix the flour, sugar, baking powder, grated nutmeg, and salt in a bowl. In a separate bowl, whisk the egg, butter, and vanilla extract.   Stir the egg mixture into the flour mixture; mix to combine well or until it forms a nice, soft dough.   Roll your dough out and cut out with a cookie cutter of your choice. Bake in the preheated Air Fryer at 350 degrees F for 10 minutes. Decrease the temperature to 330 degrees F and cook for 10 minutes longer. Bon appétit!

212. Fudge Cake With Pecans

Servings: 6   Cooking Time: 30 Minutes

Ingredients:

1/2 cup butter, melted	1/2 teaspoon ground cinnamon
1/2 cup swerve	1/4 teaspoon fine sea salt
1 teaspoon vanilla essence	1 ounce bakers' chocolate, unsweetened
1 egg	
1/2 cup almond flour	
1/2 teaspoon baking powder	1/4 cup pecans, finely chopped
1/4 cup cocoa powder	

Directions:

Start by preheating your Air Fryer to 350 degrees F. Now, lightly grease six silicone molds.   In a mixing dish, beat the melted butter with the swerve until fluffy. Next, stir in the vanilla and egg and beat again. After that, add the almond flour, baking powder, cocoa powder, cinnamon, and salt. Mix until everything is well combined. Fold in the chocolate and pecans; mix to combine. Bake in the preheated Air Fryer for 20 to 22 minutes. Enjoy!

213. Enchanting Coffee-apple Cake

Servings: 6   Cooking Time: 40 Minutes

Ingredients:

2 tablespoons butter, softened	1/4 teaspoon ground cinnamon
1/4 cup and 2 tablespoons brown sugar	1/4 teaspoon baking soda
1/2 large egg	1/8 teaspoon salt
2 tablespoons sour cream	1 cup diced Granny Smith apple
2 tablespoons vanilla yogurt	2 tablespoons brown sugar
1/2 teaspoon vanilla extract	2 tablespoons all-purpose flour
1/2 cup all-purpose flour	1 tablespoon butter
	1/4 teaspoon ground cinnamon

Directions:

In blender, puree all wet Ingredients. Add dry Ingredients: except for apples and blend until smooth. Stir in apples. Lightly grease baking pan of air fryer with cooking spray. Pour batter into pan. In a small bowl mix well, all topping Ingredients: and spread on top of cake batter. Cover pan with foil. For 20 minutes, cook on 330F. Remove foil and cook for 10 minutes. Let it stand in air fryer for another 10 minutes. Serve and enjoy.

214. Zucchinis Bars

Servings: 12   Cooking Time: 15 Minutes

Ingredients:

3 tablespoons coconut oil, melted	6 eggs
3 ounces zucchini, shredded	1/2 teaspoon baking powder
2 teaspoons vanilla extract	4 ounces cream cheese
	2 tablespoons erythritol

Directions:

In a bowl, combine all the ingredients and whisk well. pour this into a baking dish that fits your air fryer lined with parchment paper, introduce in the fryer and cook at 320 degrees F, bake for 15 minutes. Slice and serve cold.

215. Crisped 'n Chewy Chonut Holes

Servings: 6   Cooking Time: 10 Minutes

Ingredients:

1/4 cup almond milk	1/2 teaspoon salt
1/4 cup coconut sugar	1 teaspoon baking powder
1/4 teaspoon cinnamon	2 tablespoon aquafaba or liquid from canned chickpeas
1 cup white all-purpose flour	
1 tablespoon coconut oil, melted	

Directions:

In a mixing bowl, mix the flour, sugar, and baking powder. Add the salt and cinnamon and mix well. In another bowl, mix together the coconut oil, aquafaba, and almond milk. Gently pour the dry ingredients to the wet ingredients. Mix together until well combined or until you form a sticky dough. Place the dough in the refrigerator to rest for at least an hour. Preheat the air fryer to 370F. Create small balls of the dough and place inside the air fryer and cook for 10 minutes. Do not shake the air fryer. Once cooked, sprinkle with sugar and cinnamon. Serve with your breakfast coffee.

216. Baked Apples With Nuts

Servings: 2   Cooking Time: 13 Minutes

Ingredients:

1 oz butter	Zest of 1 orange
2 oz breadcrumbs	2 oz mixed seeds
2 tbsp chopped hazelnuts	1 tsp cinnamon
	2 tbsp brown sugar

Directions:

Preheat the air fryer to 350 F. Core the apples. Make sure to also score their skin to prevent from splitting. Combine the remaining ingredients in a bowl; stuff the apples with the mixture and cook for 10 minutes. Serve topped with chopped hazelnuts.

217. Blackberries Cake

Servings: 4   Cooking Time: 25 Minutes

Ingredients:

2 eggs, whisked	1/4 cup almond milk
4 tablespoons swerve	1/2 teaspoon baking powder
2 tablespoons ghee, melted	1 teaspoon lemon zest, grated
1 and 1/2 cups almond flour	1 teaspoon lemon juice
1 cup blackberries, chopped	

Directions:

In a bowl, mix all the ingredients and whisk well. Pour this into a cake pan that fits the air fryer lined with parchment paper, put the pan in your air fryer and cook at 340 degrees F for 25 minutes. Cool the cake down, slice and serve.

218. Chia Chocolate Cookies

Servings: 20   Cooking Time: 8 Minutes

Ingredients:

2 1/2 tbsp ground chia	1 cup sunflower seed butter
	1 cup almond flour

2 tbsp chocolate
protein powder
Directions:
Preheat the air fryer to 325 F.   In a large bowl, add all ingredients and mix until combined.   Make cookies from bowl mixture and place into the air fryer and cook for 8 minutes.   Serve and enjoy.

219.   Old-fashioned Plum Dumplings

Servings: 4   Cooking Time: 40 Minutes
Ingredients:
1 (14-ounce) box pie crusts
2 cups plums, pitted
2 tablespoons granulated sugar
2 tablespoons coconut oil
1/4 teaspoon ground cardamom
1/2 teaspoon ground cinnamon
1 egg white, slightly beaten

Directions:
Place the pie crust on a work surface. Roll into a circle and cut into quarters.   Place 1 plum on each crust piece. Add the sugar, coconut oil, cardamom, and cinnamon. Roll up the sides into a circular shape around the plums.   Repeat with the remaining ingredients. Brush the edges with the egg white. Place in the lightly greased Air Fryer basket. Bake in the preheated Air Fryer at 360 degrees F for 20 minutes, flipping them halfway through the cooking time. Work in two batches, decorate and serve at room temperature. Bon appétit!

220.   Blackberry Crisp

Servings: 1   Cooking Time: 18 Minutes
Ingredients:
2 tbsp. lemon juice
1/3 cup powdered erythritol
¼ tsp. xantham gum
2 cup blackberries
1 cup crunchy granola

Directions:
In a bowl, combine the lemon juice, erythritol, xantham gum, and blackberries. Transfer to a round baking dish about six inches in diameter and seal with aluminum foil.   Put the dish in the fryer and leave to cook for twelve minutes at 350°F.   Take care when removing the dish from the fryer. Give the blackberries another stir and top with the granola. Return the dish to the fryer and cook for an additional three minutes, this time at 320°F. Serve once the granola has turned brown and enjoy.

221.   Birthday Chocolate Raspberry Cake

Servings: 4   Cooking Time: 30 Minutes
Ingredients:
1/3 cup monk fruit
1/4 cup unsalted butter, room temperature
1 egg plus 1 egg white,
3 ounces almond flour
1 tablespoon candied ginger
1/8 teaspoon table

lightly whisked
2 tablespoons Dutch-process cocoa powder
1/2 teaspoon ground cinnamon
salt
For the Filling:
2 ounces fresh raspberries
1/3 cup monk fruit
1 teaspoon fresh lime juice

Directions:
Firstly, set your Air Fryer to cook at 315 degrees F. Then, spritz the inside of two cake pans with the butter-flavored cooking spray.   In a mixing bowl, beat the monk fruit and butter until creamy and uniform. Then, stir in the whisked eggs. Stir in the almond flour, cocoa powder, cinnamon, ginger and salt.   Press the batter into the cake pans; use a wide spatula to level the surface of the batter. Bake for 20 minutes or until a wooden stick inserted in the center of the cake comes out completely dry. While your cake is baking, stir together all of the ingredients for the filling in a medium saucepan. Cook over high heat, stirring frequently and mashing with the back of a spoon; bring to a boil and decrease the temperature.   Continue to cook, stirring until the mixture thickens, for another 7 minutes. Let the filling cool to room temperature. Spread 1/2 of raspberry filling over the first crust. Top with another crust; spread remaining filling over top. Spread frosting over top and sides of your cake.   Enjoy!

222.   Nutty Fudge Muffins

Servings: 10   Cooking Time: 10 Minutes
Ingredients:
1 package fudge brownie mix
1 egg
2 teaspoons water
¼ cup walnuts, chopped
1/3 cup vegetable oil

Directions:
Preheat the Air fryer to 300F and grease 10 muffin tins lightly.   Mix brownie mix, egg, oil and water in a bowl.   Fold in the walnuts and pour the mixture in the muffin cups.   Transfer the muffin tins in the Air fryer basket and cook for about 10 minutes.   Dish out and serve immediately.

223.   Chocolate Molten Lava Cake

Servings: 4   Cooking Time: 25 Minutes
Ingredients:
3 ½ oz. butter, melted
3 ½ oz. chocolate, melted
3 ½ tbsp. sugar
1 ½ tbsp. flour
2 eggs

Directions:
Pre-heat the Air Fryer to 375°F.   Grease four ramekins with a little butter.   Rigorously combine the eggs and butter before stirring in the melted chocolate.   Slowly fold in the flour.   Spoon an equal amount of the mixture into each ramekin. Put them in the Air Fryer and cook for 10 minutes

Place the ramekins upside-down on plates and let the cakes fall out. Serve hot.

224. Apple-toffee Upside-down Cake

Servings: 9   Cooking Time: 30 Minutes

Ingredients:

¼ cup almond butter
¼ cup sunflower oil
½ cup walnuts, chopped
¾ cup + 3 tablespoon coconut sugar
1 ½ teaspoon mixed spice

¾ cup water
1 cup plain flour
1 lemon, zest
1 teaspoon baking soda
1 teaspoon vinegar
3 baking apples, cored and sliced

Directions:

Preheat the air fryer to 390F.   In a skillet, melt the almond butter and 3 tablespoons sugar. Pour the mixture over a baking dish that will fit in the air fryer. Arrange the slices of apples on top. Set aside.   In a mixing bowl, combine flour, ¾ cup sugar, and baking soda. Add the mixed spice.   In another bowl, mix the oil, water, vinegar, and lemon zest. Stir in the chopped walnuts.   Combine the wet ingredients to the dry ingredients until well combined.   Pour over the tin with apple slices. Bake for 30 minutes or until a toothpick inserted comes out clean.

225. Chocolate Coffee Cake

Servings: 8   Cooking Time: 40 Minutes

Ingredients:

1 ½ cups almond flour
1/2 cup coconut meal
2/3 cup swerve
1 teaspoon baking powder
1/4 teaspoon salt
1 stick butter, melted
1/2 cup hot strongly brewed coffee
1/2 teaspoon vanilla

1 egg
Topping:
1/4 cup coconut flour
1/2 cup confectioner's swerve
1/2 teaspoon ground cardamom
1 teaspoon ground cinnamon
3 tablespoons coconut oil

Directions:

Mix all dry ingredients for your cake; then, mix in the wet ingredients. Mix until everything is well incorporated.   Spritz a baking pan with cooking spray. Scrape the batter into the baking pan. Then, make the topping by mixing all ingredients. Place on top of the cake. Smooth the top with a spatula.   Bake at 330 degrees F for 30 minutes or until the top of the cake springs back when gently pressed with your fingers. Serve with your favorite hot beverage. Bon appétit!

226. Butter Custard

Servings: 2   Cooking Time: 35 Minutes

Ingredients:

1 tablespoon Erythritol
1 teaspoon coconut flour

¼ cup heavy cream
3 egg yolks
1 teaspoon butter

Directions:

Whip the heavy cream and them mix it up with Erythritol and coconut flour. Whisk the egg yolks and add them in the whipped cream mixture. Then grease 2 ramekins with butter and transfer the whipped cream mixture in the ramekins. Preheat the air fryer to 300F. Put the ramekins with custard in the air fryer and cook them for 35 minutes.

227. Ricotta And Lemon Cake Recipe

Servings: 4   Cooking Time: 1 Hour And 10 Minutes

Ingredients:

8 eggs; whisked
3 lbs. ricotta cheese
Zest from 1 lemon; grated

Zest from 1 orange; grated
1/2 lb. sugar
Butter for the pan

Directions:

In a bowl; mix eggs with sugar, cheese, lemon and orange zest and stir very well   Grease a baking pan that fits your air fryer with some batter, spread ricotta mixture, introduce in the fryer at 390 °F and bake for 30 minutes   Reduce heat at 380 °F and bake for 40 more minutes. Take out of the oven, leave cake to cool down and serve!

228. Chocolate Banana Pastries

Servings: 4   Cooking Time: 12 Minutes

Ingredients:

1 puff pastry sheet
½ cup Nutella

2 bananas, peeled and sliced

Directions:

Cut the pastry sheet into 4 equal-sized squares. Spread Nutella evenly on each square of pastry. Divide the banana slices over Nutella.   Fold each square into a triangle and with wet fingers, slightly press the edges.   Then with a fork, press the edges firmly.   Set the temperature of air fryer to 375 degrees F. Lightly, grease an air fryer basket. Arrange pastries into the prepared air fryer basket in a single layer.   Air fry for about 10-12 minutes. Remove from air fryer and transfer the pastries onto a platter.   Serve warm.

229. Mini Almond Cakes

Servings: 4   Cooking Time: 20 Minutes

Ingredients:

3 ounces dark chocolate, melted
¼ cup coconut oil, melted
2 tablespoons swerve
2 eggs, whisked

¼ teaspoon vanilla extract
1 tablespoon almond flour
Cooking spray

Directions:

In bowl, combine all the ingredients except the cooking spray and whisk really well. Divide this into 4 ramekins greased with cooking spray, put them in the fryer and cook at 360 degrees F for 20 minutes. Serve warm.

230. Coconut 'n Almond Fat Bombs

Servings: 12   Cooking Time: 15 Minutes

Ingredients:
- ¼ cup almond flour
- ½ cup shredded coconut
- 1 tablespoon coconut oil
- 1 tablespoon vanilla extract
- 2 tablespoons liquid stevia
- 3 egg whites

Directions:
Preheat the air fryer for 5 minutes.   Combine all ingredients in a mixing bowl.   Form small balls using your hands.   Place in the air fryer basket and cook for 15 minutes at 400F.

231. Pineapple Sticks

Servings: 4   Cooking Time: 20 Minutes

Ingredients:
- ½ fresh pineapple, cut into sticks
- ¼ cup desiccated coconut

Directions:
Pre-heat the Air Fryer to 400°F.   Coat the pineapple sticks in the desiccated coconut and put each one in the Air Fryer basket.   Air fry for 10 minutes.

232. White Chocolate Berry Cheesecake

Servings: 4   Cooking Time: 5-10 Minutes

Ingredients:
- 8 oz cream cheese, softened
- 2 oz heavy cream
- ½ tsp Splenda
- 1 tsp raspberries
- 1 tbsp Da Vinci Sugar-Free syrup, white chocolate flavor

Directions:
Whip together the ingredients to a thick consistency. Divide in cups.   Refrigerate.   Serve!

233. Strawberry Cheese Cake

Servings: 6   Cooking Time: 35 Minutes

Ingredients:
- 1 cup almond flour
- 3 tbsp coconut oil, melted
- ½ tsp vanilla
- 1 egg, lightly beaten
- 1 tbsp fresh lime juice
- ¼ cup erythritol
- 1 cup cream cheese, softened
- 1 lb strawberries, chopped
- 2 tsp baking powder

Directions:
Add all ingredients into the large bowl and mix until well combined.   Spray air fryer cake pan with cooking spray.   Pour batter into the prepared pan

and place into the air fryer and cook at 350 F for 35 minutes.   Allow to cool completely.   Slice and serve.

234. Pear Fritters With Cinnamon And Ginger

Servings: 4   Cooking Time: 20 Minutes

Ingredients:
- 2 pears, peeled, cored and sliced
- 1 tablespoon coconut oil, melted
- 1 ½ cups all-purpose flour
- 1 teaspoon baking powder
- A pinch of fine sea salt
- A pinch of freshly grated nutmeg
- 1/2 teaspoon ginger
- 1 teaspoon cinnamon
- 2 eggs
- 4 tablespoons milk

Directions:
Mix all ingredients, except for the pears, in a shallow bowl. Dip each slice of the pears in the batter until well coated.   Cook in the preheated Air Fryer at 360 degrees for 4 minutes, flipping them halfway through the cooking time. Repeat with the remaining ingredients.   Dust with powdered sugar if desired. Bon appétit!

235. Vanilla Soufflé

Servings: 6   Cooking Time: 40 Minutes

Ingredients:
- ¼ cup butter, softened
- ¼ cup all-purpose flour
- 1 cup milk
- 4 egg yolks
- 5 egg whites
- ½ cup sugar
- 3 teaspoons vanilla extract, divided
- 1 teaspoon cream of tartar
- 1-ounce sugar

Directions:
Preheat the Air fryer to 330F and grease 6 ramekins lightly.   Mix butter and flour in a bowl until a smooth paste is formed.   Put milk and ½ cup of sugar in a bowl on medium-low heat and cook for about 3 minutes.   Bring to a boil and stir in the flour mixture.   Let it simmer for about 4 minutes and remove from heat.   Whisk egg yolks and vanilla extract in a bowl until well combined. Combine the egg yolk mixture with milk mixture until mixed.   Mix egg whites, cream of tartar, remaining sugar and vanilla extract in another bowl. Combine the egg white mixture into milk mixture and divide this mixture into the ramekins. Transfer 3 ramekins into the Air fryer basket and cook for about 16 minutes.   Repeat with the remaining ramekins and dish out to serve.

236. Easy Blueberry Muffins

Servings: 10   Cooking Time: 20 Minutes

Ingredients:
- 1 ½ cups all-purpose flour
- 1/2 teaspoon baking soda
- 1/2 cup granulated sugar
- 1/2 cup milk
- 1/4 cup coconut oil,

1 teaspoon baking powder
1/4 teaspoon kosher salt
2 eggs, whisked

melted
1/2 teaspoon vanilla paste
1 cup fresh blueberries

Directions:
In a mixing bowl, combine the flour, baking soda, baking powder, sugar, and salt. Whisk to combine well.   In another mixing bowl, mix the eggs, milk, coconut oil, and vanilla.   Now, add the wet egg mixture to dry the flour mixture. Then, carefully fold in the fresh blueberries; gently stir to combine. Scrape the batter mixture into the muffin cups. Bake your muffins at 350 degrees F for 12 minutes or until the tops are golden brown.   Sprinkle some extra icing sugar over the top of each muffin if desired. Serve and enjoy!

237.	**Flavor-packed Clafoutis**

Servings: 4   Cooking Time: 25 Minutes

Ingredients:

1½ cups fresh cherries, pitted
¼ cup flour
1 egg
1 tablespoon butter

3 tablespoons vodka
2 tablespoons sugar
Pinch of salt
½ cup sour cream
¼ cup powdered sugar

Directions:
Preheat the Air fryer to 355F and grease a baking pan lightly.   Mix cherries and vodka in a bowl. Sift together flour, sugar and salt in another bowl. Stir in the sour cream and egg until a smooth dough is formed.   Transfer the dough evenly into the baking pan and top with the cherry mixture and butter.   Place the baking pan in the Air fryer basket and cook for about 25 minutes.   Dust with powdered sugar and serve warm.

238.	**Leche Flan Filipino Style**

Servings: 4   Cooking Time: 30 Minutes

Ingredients:

1 teaspoon vanilla extract
1/2 (14 ounce) can sweetened condensed milk

1 cup heavy cream
1/2 cup milk
2-1/2 eggs
1/3 cup white sugar

Directions:
In blender, blend well vanilla, eggs, milk, cream, and condensed milk.   Lightly grease baking pan of air fryer with cooking spray. Add sugar and heat for 10 minutes at 370F until melted and caramelized. Lower heat to 300F and continue melting and swirling.   Pour milk mixture into caramelized sugar. Cover pan with foil.   Cook for 20 minutes at 330F.   Let it cool completely in the fridge. Place a plate on top of pan and invert pan to easily remove flan.   Serve and enjoy.

239.	**Strawberry Shortcake Quickie**

Servings: 4   Cooking Time: 25 Minutes

Ingredients:

¼ teaspoon liquid stevia
¼ teaspoon salt
½ teaspoon baking powder
1 cup strawberries, halved

½ cup butter
1 teaspoon vanilla extract
1/3 cup erythritol
2/3 cup almond flour
3 large eggs, beaten

Directions:
Preheat the air fryer for 5 minutes.   In a mixing bowl, combine all ingredients except for the strawberries.   Use a hand mixer to mix everything. Pour into greased mugs.   Top with sliced strawberries   Place the mugs in the fryer basket. Bake for 25 minutes at 350F.   Place in the fridge to chill before serving.

240.	**Vanilla Bean Dream**

Servings: 1   Cooking Time: 35 Minutes

Ingredients:

½ cup extra virgin coconut oil, softened
½ cup coconut butter, softened

Juice of 1 lemon
Seeds from ½ a vanilla bean

Directions:
Whisk the ingredients in an easy-to-pour cup. Pour into a lined cupcake or loaf pan.   Refrigerate for 20 minutes. Top with lemon zest.   Serve!

241.	**Mock Cherry Pie**

Servings: 8   Cooking Time: 30 Minutes

Ingredients:

21 oz cherry pie filling

1 egg yolk
1 tbsp milk

Directions:
Preheat air fryer to 310 F.   Place one pie crust in a pie pan; poke holes into the crust. Cook for 5 minutes.   Spread the pie filling over. Cut the other pie crust into strips and arrange the pie-style over the baked crust. Whisk milk and egg yolk, and brush the mixture over the pie. Return the pie to the fryer and cook for 15 minutes.

242.	**Semolina Cake**

Servings: 8   Cooking Time: 15 Minutes

Ingredients:

2½ cups semolina
1 cup milk
1 cup Greek yogurt
2 teaspoons baking powder

½ cup walnuts, chopped
½ cup vegetable oil
1 cup sugar
Pinch of salt

Directions:
Preheat the Air fryer to 360F and grease a baking pan lightly.   Mix semolina, oil, milk, yogurt and sugar in a bowl until well combined.   Cover the bowl and keep aside for about 15 minutes.   Stir in

the baking soda, baking powder and salt and fold in the walnuts. Transfer the mixture into the baking pan and place in the Air fryer. Cook for about 15 minutes and dish out to serve.

243. Sunday Tart With Walnuts

Servings: 6   Cooking Time: 20 Minutes

Ingredients:

1 cup coconut milk	2 eggs
1/2 stick butter, at room temperature	1/4 teaspoon ground cloves
1 teaspoon vanilla essence	1/2 cup walnuts, ground
1/4 teaspoon ground cardamom	1/2 cup swerve
	1/2 cup almond flour

Directions:

Begin by preheating your Air Fryer to 360 degrees F. Spritz the sides and bottom of a baking pan with nonstick cooking spray. Mix all ingredients until well combined. Scrape the batter into the prepared baking pan. Bake approximately 13 minutes; use a toothpick to test for doneness. Bon appétit!

244. Chocolate Coconut Cake

Servings: 9   Cooking Time: 20 Minutes

Ingredients:

6 eggs	3.5 oz coconut flour
2 tsp baking powder	1 tsp vanilla
3 oz unsweetened cocoa powder	3 oz butter, melted
5 oz erythritol	11 oz heavy cream

Directions:

Preheat the air fryer to 325 F. In a bowl, mix together coconut flour, butter, 5 oz heavy cream, eggs, baking powder half cocoa powder, and 3 oz sweetener until well combined. Pour batter into the greased cake pan and place into the air fryer and cook for 20 minutes. Allow to cool completely. In a large bowl, beat remaining heavy cream, cocoa powder, and sweetener until smooth. Spread the cream on top of cake and place in the refrigerator for 30 minutes. Slice and serve.

245. Creamy Rice Pudding

Servings: 6   Cooking Time: 20 Minutes

Ingredients:

1 tablespoon butter, melted	1 tablespoon heavy cream
7 ounces white rice	1 teaspoon vanilla extract
16 ounces milk	
1/3 cup sugar	

Directions:

Place all ingredients in a pan that fits your air fryer and stir well. Put the pan in the fryer and cook at 360 degrees F for 20 minutes. Stir the pudding, divide it into bowls, refrigerate, and serve cold.

246. Spanish-style Doughnut Tejeringos

Servings: 4   Cooking Time: 20 Minutes

Ingredients:

3/4 cup water	1/4 teaspoon sea salt
1 tablespoon sugar	6 tablespoons butter
1/4 teaspoon grated nutmeg	3/4 cup all-purpose flour
1/4 teaspoon ground cloves	2 eggs

Directions:

To make the dough, boil the water in a pan over medium-high heat; now, add the sugar, salt, nutmeg, and cloves; cook until dissolved. Add the butter and turn the heat to low. Gradually stir in the flour, whisking continuously, until the mixture forms a ball. Remove from the heat; fold in the eggs one at a time, stirring to combine well. Pour the mixture into a piping bag with a large star tip. Squeeze 4-inch strips of dough into the greased Air Fryer pan. Cook at 410 degrees F for 6 minutes, working in batches. Bon appétit!

247. Hazelnut Vinegar Cookies

Servings: 6   Cooking Time: 11 Minutes

Ingredients:

1 tablespoon flaxseeds	1 teaspoon apple cider vinegar
¼ cup flax meal	3 tablespoons coconut cream
½ cup coconut flour	
½ teaspoon baking powder	1 tablespoon butter, softened
1 oz hazelnuts, chopped	3 teaspoons Splenda
	Cooking spray

Directions:

Put the flax meal in the bowl. Add flax seeds, coconut flour, baking powder, apple cider vinegar, and Splenda. Stir the mixture gently with the help of the fork and add butter, coconut cream, hazelnuts, and knead the non-sticky dough. If the dough is not sticky enough, add more coconut cream. Make the big ball from the dough and put it in the freezer for 10-15 minutes. After this, preheat the air fryer to 365F. Make the small balls (cookies) from the flax meal dough and press them gently. Spray the air fryer basket with cooking spray from inside. Arrange the cookies in the air fryer basket in one layer (cook 3-4 cookies per one time) and cook them for 11 minutes. Then transfer the cooked cookies on the plate and cool them completely. Repeat the same steps with remaining uncooked cookies. Store the cookies in the glass jar with the closed lid.

248. Raspberry Pudding Surprise

Servings: 1   Cooking Time: 40 Minutes

Ingredients:

½ cup unsweetened milk	3 tbsp chia seeds
1 scoop chocolate protein powder	¼ cup raspberries,

fresh or frozen
1 tsp honey

Directions:
Combine the milk, protein powder and chia seeds together.   Let rest for 5 minutes before stirring. Refrigerate for 30 minutes.   Top with raspberries. Serve!

249.	**Sweet Squares Recipe**

Servings: 6   Cooking Time: 40 Minutes
Ingredients:

1 cup flour	1 cup sugar
1/2 cup butter; soft	2 tsp. lemon peel;
2 tbsp. lemon juice	grated
2 eggs; whisked	1/2 tsp. baking
1/4 cup powdered	powder
sugar	

Directions:
In a bowl; mix flour with powdered sugar and butter; stir well, press on the bottom of a pan that fits your air fryer, introduce in the fryer and bake at 350 °F, for 14 minutes   In another bowl, mix sugar with

lemon juice, lemon peel, eggs and baking powder; stir using your mixer and spread over baked crust. Bake for 15 minutes more, leave aside to cool down, cut into medium squares and serve cold

---

250.	**No Flour Lime Muffins**

Servings: 6   Cooking Time: 30 Minutes
Ingredients:

Juice and zest of 2 limes	¼ cup superfine sugar
1 cup yogurt	8 oz cream cheese
	1 tsp vanilla extract

Directions:
Preheat the air fryer to 330 F, and with a spatula, gently combine the yogurt and cheese. In another bowl, beat together the rest of the ingredients. Gently fold the lime with the cheese mixture. Divide the batter between 6 lined muffin tins. Cook in the air fryer for 10 minutes.

Poultry Recipes

251. Crispy Herbed Turkey Breast

Servings: 2   Cooking Time: 30 Minutes

Ingredients:

- ½ tablespoon fresh rosemary, chopped
- ½ tablespoon fresh parsley, chopped
- 2 turkey breasts
- 1 garlic clove, minced
- 1 tablespoon ginger, minced
- 1 teaspoon five spice powder
- Salt and black pepper, to taste

Directions:

Preheat the Air fryer to 340F and grease an Air fryer basket.   Mix garlic, herbs, five spice powder, salt and black pepper in a bowl.   Brush the turkey breasts generously with garlic mixture and transfer into the Air fryer.   Cook for about 25 minutes and set the Air fryer to 390F.   Cook for about 5 more minutes and dish out to serve warm.

252. Potato Cakes & Cajun Chicken Wings

Servings: 4   Cooking Time: 40 Minutes

Ingredients:

- 4 large-sized chicken wings
- 1 tsp. Cajun seasoning
- 1 tsp. maple syrup
- ¾ tsp. sea salt flakes
- ¼ tsp. red pepper flakes, crushed
- 1 tsp. onion powder
- 1 tsp. porcini powder
- ½ tsp. celery seeds
- 1 small-seized head of cabbage, shredded
- 1 cup mashed potatoes
- 1 small-sized brown onion, coarsely grated
- 1 tsp. garlic puree
- 1 medium whole egg, well whisked
- ½ tsp. table salt
- ½ tsp. ground black pepper
- 1 ½ tbsp. flour
- ¾ tsp. baking powder
- 1 heaped tbsp. cilantro
- 1 tbsp. sesame oil

Directions:

Pre-heat your Air Fryer to 390°F.   Pat the chicken wings dry. Place them in the fryer and cook for 25 - 30 minutes, ensuring they are cooked through. Make the rub by combining the Cajun seasoning, maple syrup, sea salt flakes, red pepper, onion powder, porcini powder, and celery seeds.   Mix together the shredded cabbage, potato, onion, garlic puree, egg, table salt, black pepper, flour, baking powder and cilantro.   Separate the cabbage mixture into 4 portions and use your hands to mold each one into a cabbage-potato cake.   Douse each cake with the sesame oil.   Bake the cabbage-potato cakes in the fryer for 10 minutes, turning them once through the cooking time. You will need to do this in multiple batches.   Serve the cakes and the chicken wings together.

253. Turkey Wings With Butter Roasted Potatoes

Servings: 4   Cooking Time: 55 Minutes

Ingredients:

- 4 large-sized potatoes, peeled and cut into 1-inch chunks
- 1 tablespoon butter, melted
- 1 teaspoon rosemary
- 1 teaspoon garlic salt
- 1/2 teaspoon ground black pepper
- 1 ½ pounds turkey wings
- 2 tablespoons olive oil
- 2 garlic cloves, minced
- 1 tablespoon Dijon mustard
- 1/2 teaspoon cayenne pepper

Directions:

Add the potatoes, butter, rosemary, salt, and pepper to the cooking basket.   Cook at 400 degrees F for 12 minutes. Reserve the potatoes, keeping them warm.   Now, place the turkey wings in the cooking basket that is previously cleaned and greased with olive oil. Add the garlic, mustard, and cayenne pepper.   Cook in the preheated Air Fryer at 350 degrees f for 25 minutes. Turn them over and cook an additional 15 minutes.   Test for doneness with a meat thermometer. Serve with warm potatoes.

254. Classic Chicken Nuggets

Servings: 4   Cooking Time: 20 Minutes

Ingredients:

- 1 ½ pounds chicken tenderloins, cut into small pieces
- 1/2 teaspoon garlic salt
- 1/2 teaspoon cayenne pepper
- 4 tablespoons olive oil
- 1/4 teaspoon black pepper, freshly cracked
- 2 scoops low-carb unflavored protein powder
- 4 tablespoons Parmesan cheese, freshly grated

Directions:

Start by preheating your Air Fryer to 390 degrees F. Season each piece of the chicken with garlic salt, cayenne pepper, and black pepper.   In a mixing bowl, thoroughly combine the olive oil with protein powder and parmesan cheese. Dip each piece of chicken in the parmesan mixture.   Cook for 8 minutes, working in batches.   Later, if you want to warm the chicken nuggets, add them to the basket and cook for 1 minute more. Enjoy!

255. Malaysian Chicken Satay With Peanut Sauce

Servings: 4   Cooking Time: 25 Minutes

Ingredients:

- 1 tablespoon fish sauce
- 1/2 teaspoon granulated garlic

1 tablespoon lime juice	1/4 cup creamy peanut butter
1 tablespoon white sugar	1-pound skinless, boneless chicken breasts, cut into strips
1 tablespoon yellow curry powder	
1 teaspoon fish sauce	2 tablespoons olive oil
1 teaspoon white sugar	2 teaspoons yellow curry powder
1/2 cup chicken broth	
1/2 cup unsweetened coconut milk	3/4 cup unsweetened coconut milk

Directions:
In resealable bag, mix well garlic, 1 tsp fish sauce, 1 tsp sugar, 2 tsps. curry powder, and ½ cup coconut milk. Add chicken and toss well to coat. Remove excess air and seal bag. Marinate for 2 hours. Thread chicken into skewer and place on skewer rack. For 10 minutes, cook on 390F. Halfway through cooking time, turnover skewers. Meanwhile, make the peanut sauce by bringing remaining coconut milk to a simmer in a medium saucepan. Stir in curry powder and cook for 4 minutes. Add 1 tbsp fish sauce, lime juice, 1 tbsp sugar, peanut butter, and chicken broth. Mix well and cook until heated through. Transfer to a small bowl. Serve and enjoy with the peanut sauce.

---

256. Glazed Chicken Wings

Servings: 4   Cooking Time: 19 Minutes
Ingredients:

8 chicken wings	1 tablespoon soy sauce
2 tablespoons all-purpose flour	
1 teaspoon garlic, chopped finely	½ teaspoon dried oregano, crushed
1 tablespoon fresh lemon juice	Salt and freshly ground black pepper, to taste

Directions:
Preheat the Air fryer to 355F and grease an Air fryer basket. Mix all the ingredients except wings in a large bowl. Coat wings generously with the marinade and refrigerate for about 2 hours. Remove the chicken wings from marinade and sprinkle with flour evenly. Transfer the wings in the Air fryer tray and cook for about 6 minutes, flipping once in between. Dish out the chicken wings in a platter and serve hot.

---

257. Juicy & Spicy Chicken Wings

Servings: 4   Cooking Time: 25 Minutes
Ingredients:

2 lbs chicken wings	12 oz hot sauce
1 tsp Worcestershire sauce	1 tsp Tabasco
	6 tbsp butter, melted

Directions:
Spray air fryer basket with cooking spray. Add chicken wings into the air fryer basket and cook at 380 F for 25 minutes. Shake basket after every 5 minutes. Meanwhile, in a bowl, mix together hot sauce, Worcestershire sauce, and butter. Set aside. Add chicken wings into the sauce and toss well. Serve and enjoy.

---

258. Rosemary Lemon Chicken

Servings: 2   Cooking Time: 60 Minutes
Ingredients:

1 tbsp minced ginger	1 tbsp soy sauce
2 rosemary sprigs	½ tbsp olive oil
½ lemon, cut into wedges	1 tbsp oyster sauce
	3 tbsp brown sugar

Directions:
Add the ginger, soy sauce, and olive oil, in a bowl; add the chicken and coat well. Cover the bowl and refrigerate for 30 minutes. Preheat the air fryer to 370 F. Transfer the marinated chicken to a baking dish; cook for 6 minutes. Mix oyster sauce, rosemary, and brown sugar in a bowl. Pour the sauce over the chicken. Arrange the lemon wedges in the dish. Return to the air fryer and cook for 13 minutes.

---

259. Tasty Southwest Chicken

Servings: 2   Cooking Time: 25 Minutes
Ingredients:

1/2 lb chicken breasts, skinless and boneless	1 tbsp lime juice
	1/8 tsp garlic powder
	1/8 tsp onion powder
1/2 tsp chili powder	1/4 tsp cumin
1 tbsp olive oil	1/8 tsp salt

Directions:
Add all ingredients into the zip-lock bag and shake well to coat and place in the refrigerator for 1 hour. Add a marinated chicken wing to the air fryer basket and cook at 400 F for 25 minutes. Shake halfway through. Serve and enjoy.

---

260. Chicken Breasts & Spiced Tomatoes

Servings: 1   Cooking Time: 40 Minutes
Ingredients:

1 lb. boneless chicken breast	1 cup tomatoes, diced
Salt and pepper	1 ½ tsp. paprika
1 cup butter	1 tsp. pumpkin pie spices

Directions:
Preheat your fryer at 375°F. Cut the chicken into relatively thick slices and put them in the fryer. Sprinkle with salt and pepper to taste. Cook for fifteen minutes. In the meantime, melt the butter in a saucepan over medium heat, before adding the tomatoes, paprika, and pumpkin pie spices. Leave simmering while the chicken finishes cooking. When the chicken is cooked through, place it on a dish and pour the tomato mixture over. Serve hot.

---

261. Awesome Sweet Turkey Bake

Servings: 3   Cooking Time: 50 Minutes
Ingredients:

Salt and pepper to season
1/4 cup chicken soup cream
1/4 cup mayonnaise
2 tbsp lemon juice
1/4 cup slivered almonds, chopped
1/4 cup breadcrumbs

2 tbsp chopped green onion
2 tbsp chopped pimentos
2 Boiled eggs, chopped
1/2 cup diced celery
Cooking spray

Directions:
Preheat air fryer to 390 F. Place the turkey breasts on a clean flat surface and season with salt and pepper. Grease with cooking spray and place in the fryer's basket; cook for 13 minutes. Remove turkey back onto the chopping board, let cool, and cut into dices. In a bowl, add celery, eggs, pimentos, green onions, almonds, lemon juice, mayonnaise, diced turkey, and chicken soup cream and mix well. Grease a casserole dish with cooking spray, scoop the turkey mixture into the bowl, sprinkle the breadcrumbs on it, and spray with cooking spray. Put the dish in the fryer basket, and bake the ingredients at 390 F for 20 minutes. Remove and serve with a side of steamed asparagus.

262. Creamy Chicken Breasts With Crumbled Bacon

Servings: 4   Cooking Time: 25 Minutes
Ingredients:
1/4 cup olive oil
1 block cream cheese
8 slices of bacon, fried and crumbled

4 chicken breasts
Salt and pepper to taste

Directions:
Preheat the air fryer for 5 minutes.   Place the chicken breasts in a baking dish that will fit in the air fryer.   Add the olive oil and cream cheese. Season with salt and pepper to taste.   Place the baking dish with the chicken and cook for 25 minutes at 350F.   Sprinkle crumbled bacon after.

263. Chicken & Veggie Kabobs

Servings: 3   Cooking Time: 30 Minutes
Ingredients:
1 lb. skinless, boneless chicken thighs, cut into cubes
1/2 cup plain Greek yogurt
1 tablespoon olive oil
2 teaspoons curry powder

1/2 teaspoon smoked paprika
1/4 teaspoon cayenne pepper
Salt, to taste
2 small bell peppers, seeded and cut into large chunks
1 large red onion, cut into large chunks

Directions:
In a bowl, add the chicken, oil, yogurt, and spices and mix until well combined   Refrigerate to marinate for about 2 hours.   Thread the chicken cubes, bell pepper and onion onto pre-soaked wooden skewers.   Set the temperature of Air Fryer to 360 degrees F. Grease an Air Fryer basket. Arrange chicken skewers into the prepared Air Fryer basket in 2 batches.   Air Fry for about 15 minutes. Remove from Air Fryer and transfer the chicken skewers onto a serving platter.   Serve hot.

264. Indian Chicken Tenders

Servings: 4   Cooking Time: 15 Minutes
Ingredients:
1 lb chicken tenders, cut in half
1/4 cup parsley, chopped
1/2 tbsp garlic, minced
1/2 tbsp ginger, minced

1/4 cup yogurt
3/4 tsp paprika
1 tsp garam masala
1 tsp turmeric
1/2 tsp cayenne pepper
1 tsp salt

Directions:
Preheat the air fryer to 350 F.   Add all ingredients into the large bowl and mix well. Place in refrigerator for 30 minutes.   Spray air fryer basket with cooking spray.   Add marinated chicken into the air fryer basket and cook for 10 minutes.   Turn chicken to another side and cook for 5 minutes more. Serve and enjoy.

265. Tequila Glazed Chicken

Servings: 6   Cooking Time: 40 Minutes
Ingredients:
2 tablespoons whole coriander seeds
Salt and pepper to taste
3 pounds chicken breasts
1/3 cup orange juice

1/4 cup tequila
2 tablespoons brown sugar
2 tablespoons honey
3 cloves of garlic, minced
1 shallot, minced

Directions:
Place all ingredients in a Ziploc bag and allow to marinate for at least 2 hours in the fridge.   Preheat the air fryer at 375F.   Place the grill pan accessory in the air fryer.   Grill the chicken for at least 40 minutes.   Flip the chicken every 10 minutes for even cooking.   Meanwhile, pour the marinade in a saucepan and simmer until the sauce thickens.   Brush the chicken with the glaze before serving.

266. Spinach 'n Bacon Egg Cups

Servings: 4   Cooking Time: 10 Minutes
Ingredients:
1/4 cup spinach, chopped finely
1 bacon strip, fried and crumbled

3 tablespoons butter
4 eggs, beaten
Salt and pepper to taste

Directions:
Preheat the air fryer for 5 minutes.   In a mixing bowl, combine the eggs, butter, and spinach. Season with salt and pepper to taste.   Grease a ramekin

with cooking spray and pour the egg mixture inside. Sprinkle with bacon bits.   Place the ramekin in the air fryer.   Cook for 10 minutes at 350F.

267.   Teriyaki Chicken

Servings: 2   Cooking Time: 30 Minutes

Ingredients:

2 boneless chicken drumsticks
1 tsp. ginger, grated
1 tbsp. cooking wine
3 tbsp. teriyaki sauce

Directions:

Combine all of the ingredients in a bowl. Refrigerate for half an hour.   Place the chicken in the Air Fryer baking pan and fry at 350°F for 8 minutes. Turn the chicken over and raise the temperature to 380°F. Allow to cook for another 6 minutes. Serve hot.

268.   Lemon-butter Battered Thighs

Servings: 8   Cooking Time: 35 Minutes

Ingredients:

½ cup chicken stock
1 cup almond flour
1 egg, beaten
1 onion, diced
2 pounds chicken thighs
2 tablespoons capers
3 tablespoons olive oil
4 tablespoons butter
Juice from 2 lemons, freshly squeezed
Salt and pepper to taste

Directions:

Preheat the air fryer for 5 minutes.   Combine all ingredients in a baking dish. Make sure that all lumps are removed.   Place the baking dish in the air fryer chamber.   Cook for 35 minutes at 325F.

269.   Marinara Chicken

Servings: 6   Cooking Time: 25 Minutes

Ingredients:

1 tablespoon olive oil
2 pounds chicken breasts, skinless, boneless and cubed
Salt and black pepper to taste
¾ cup yellow onion, diced
1 cup green bell pepper, chopped
¾ cup marinara sauce
½ cup cheddar cheese, grated

Directions:

Heat up a pan that fits your air fryer with the oil over medium heat.   Add the chicken, toss, and brown for 3 minutes.   Add the salt, pepper, onions, bell peppers, and the marinara sauce; stir, and cook for 3 minutes more.   Place the pan in the air fryer and cook at 370 degrees F for 15 minutes.   Sprinkle the cheese on top, divide the mix between plates, and serve.

270.   Paprika Chicken Legs With Brussels Sprouts

Servings: 2   Cooking Time: 30 Minutes

Ingredients:

2 chicken legs
1/2 teaspoon kosher salt
1/2 teaspoon black pepper
1/2 teaspoon paprika
1 pound Brussels sprouts
1 teaspoon dill, fresh or dried

Directions:

Start by preheating your Air Fryer to 370 degrees F. Now, season your chicken with paprika, salt, and pepper. Transfer the chicken legs to the cooking basket. Cook for 10 minutes.   Flip the chicken legs and cook an additional 10 minutes. Reserve.   Add the Brussels sprouts to the cooking basket; sprinkle with dill. Cook at 380 degrees F for 15 minutes, shaking the basket halfway through.   Serve with the reserved chicken legs. Bon appétit!

271. Peanut Chicken And Pepper Wraps

Servings: 4   Cooking Time: 25 Minutes

Ingredients:

1 ½ pounds chicken breast, boneless and skinless
1 tablespoon sesame oil
1 tablespoon soy sauce
2 teaspoons rice vinegar
1 teaspoon fresh ginger, peeled and grated
1/4 cup peanut butter
1 teaspoon fresh garlic, minced
1 teaspoon brown sugar
2 tablespoons lemon juice, freshly squeezed
4 tortillas
1 bell pepper, julienned

Directions:

Start by preheating your Air Fryer to 380 degrees F. Cook the chicken breasts in the preheated Air Fryer approximately 6 minutes. Turn them over and cook an additional 6 minutes.   Meanwhile, make the sauce by mixing the peanut butter, sesame oil, soy sauce, vinegar, ginger, garlic, sugar, and lemon juice. Slice the chicken crosswise across the grain into 1/4-inch strips. Toss the chicken into the sauce. Decrease temperature to 390 degrees F. Spoon the chicken and sauce onto each tortilla; add bell peppers and wrap them tightly.   Drizzle with a nonstick cooking spray and bake about 7 minutes. Serve warm.

272.   Grilled Chicken Recipe From Korea

Servings: 4   Cooking Time: 30 Minutes

Ingredients:

½ teaspoon fresh ground black pepper
1 scallion, sliced thinly
½ cup gochujang
1 teaspoon salt
2 pounds chicken wings

Directions:
Place in a Ziploc bag the chicken wings, salt, pepper, and gochujang sauce. Allow to marinate in the fridge for at least 2 hours. Preheat the air fryer to 390F. Place the grill pan accessory in the air fryer. Grill the chicken wings for 30 minutes making sure to flip the chicken every 10 minutes. Top with scallions and serve with more gochujang.

273. Grilled Sambal Chicken

Servings: 3   Cooking Time: 25 Minutes

Ingredients:

½ cup light brown sugar	¼ cup sriracha
½ cup rice vinegar	2 teaspoons grated and peeled ginger
1/3 cup hot chili paste	1 ½ pounds chicken breasts, pounded
¼ cup fish sauce	

Directions:
Place all ingredients in a Ziploc bag and allow to marinate for at least 2 hours in the fridge. Preheat the air fryer at 375F. Place the grill pan accessory in the air fryer. Grill the chicken for 25 minutes. Flip the chicken every 10 minutes for even grilling. Meanwhile, pour the marinade in a saucepan and heat over medium heat until the sauce thickens. Before serving the chicken, brush with the sriracha glaze.

274. Easy Turkey Kabobs

Servings: 8   Cooking Time: 15 Minutes

Ingredients:

1 cup parmesan cheese, grated	1 cup chopped fresh parsley
1 ½ cups of water	2 tablespoons almond meal
14 ounces ground turkey	3/4 teaspoon salt
2 small eggs, beaten	1 heaping teaspoon fresh rosemary, finely chopped
1 teaspoon ground ginger	
2 ½ tablespoons vegetable oil	1/2 teaspoon ground allspice

Directions:
Mix all of the above ingredients in a bowl. Knead the mixture with your hands. Then, take small portions and gently roll them into balls. Now, preheat your Air Fryer to 380 degrees F. Air fry for 8 to 10 minutes in the Air Fryer basket. Serve on a serving platter with skewers and eat with your favorite dipping sauce.

275. Cheesy Potato, Broccoli 'n Ham Bake

Servings: 3   Cooking Time: 35 Minutes

Ingredients:

1 1/2 tablespoon mayonnaise	1/3 cup milk
1/3 cup canned condensed cream of mushroom soup	3/4 cup 3/cooked, cubed ham
	6-ounce frozen chopped broccoli
1/3 cup grated Parmesan cheese	6-ounce frozen French fries

Directions:
Lightly grease baking pan of air fryer with cooking spray. Evenly spread French fries on bottom of pan. Place broccoli on top in a single layer. Evenly spread ham. In a bowl, whisk well mayonnaise, milk, and soup. Pour over fries mixture. Sprinkle cheese and over pan with foil. For 25 minutes, cook on 390F. Remove foil and continue cooking for another 10 minutes. Serve and enjoy.

276. Duck Breasts With Candy Onion And Coriander

Servings: 4   Cooking Time: 25 Minutes

Ingredients:

1 ½ pounds duck breasts, skin removed	1/2 teaspoon smoked paprika
1 teaspoon kosher salt	1 tablespoon Thai red curry paste
1/2 teaspoon cayenne pepper	1 cup candy onions, halved
1/3 teaspoon black pepper	1/4 small pack coriander, chopped

Directions:
Place the duck breasts between 2 sheets of foil; then, use a rolling pin to bash the duck until they are 1-inch thick. Preheat your Air Fryer to 395 degrees F. Rub the duck breasts with salt, cayenne pepper, black pepper, paprika, and red curry paste. Place the duck breast in the cooking basket. Cook for 11 to 12 minutes. Top with candy onions and cook for another 10 to 11 minutes. Serve garnished with coriander and enjoy!

277. Pretzel Crusted Chicken With Spicy Mustard Sauce

Servings: 6   Cooking Time: 20 Minutes

Ingredients:

2 eggs	1 teaspoon paprika
1 ½ pound chicken breasts, boneless, skinless, cut into bite-sized chunks	3 tablespoons Worcestershire sauce
	3 tablespoons tomato paste
1/2 cup crushed pretzels	1 tablespoon apple cider vinegar
1 teaspoon shallot powder	2 tablespoons olive oil
Sea salt and ground black pepper, to taste	2 garlic cloves, chopped
1/2 cup vegetable broth	1 jalapeno pepper, minced
1 tablespoon cornstarch	1 teaspoon yellow mustard

Directions:
Start by preheating your Air Fryer to 390 degrees F. In a mixing dish, whisk the eggs until frothy; toss the chicken chunks into the whisked eggs and coat well. In another dish, combine the crushed pretzels with shallot powder, paprika, salt and pepper. Then, lay

the chicken chunks in the pretzel mixture; turn it over until well coated. Place the chicken pieces in the air fryer basket. Cook the chicken for 12 minutes, shaking the basket halfway through. Meanwhile, whisk the vegetable broth with cornstarch, Worcestershire sauce, tomato paste, and apple cider vinegar. Preheat a cast-iron skillet over medium flame. Heat the olive oil and sauté the garlic with jalapeno pepper for 30 to 40 seconds, stirring frequently. Add the cornstarch mixture and let it simmer until the sauce has thickened a little. Now, add the air-fried chicken and mustard; let it simmer for 2 minutes more or until heated through. Serve immediately and enjoy!

278. Turkey Meatloaf

Servings: 4   Cooking Time: 20 Minutes
Ingredients:

1 pound ground turkey	1 cup onion, chopped
1 cup kale leaves, trimmed and finely chopped	¼ cup salsa verde
	1 teaspoon red chili powder
½ cup fresh breadcrumbs	½ teaspoon ground cumin
1 cup Monterey Jack cheese, grated	½ teaspoon dried oregano, crushed
2 garlic cloves, minced	Salt and ground black pepper, as required

Directions:
Preheat the Air fryer to 400F and grease an Air fryer basket. Mix all the ingredients in a bowl and divide the turkey mixture into 4 equal-sized portions. Shape each into a mini loaf and arrange the loaves into the Air fryer basket. Cook for about 20 minutes and dish out to serve warm.

279. Turkey Strips With Cranberry Glaze

Servings: 4   Cooking Time: 20 Minutes
Ingredients:

1 tbsp Chicken seasoning	Salt and black pepper to taste
½ cup cranberry sauce	

Directions:
Preheat your Air Fryer to 390 F. Spray the air fryer basket with cooking spray. Cut the turkey into strips and season with chicken seasoning, salt, and black pepper. Spray with cooking spray and transfer to the cooking basket. Cook for 10 minutes, flipping once halfway through. Meanwhile, put a saucepan over low heat, and add the cranberry sauce and ¼ cup of water. Simmer for 5 minutes, stirring continuously. Serve the turkey topped with the sauce.

280. Lemon & Garlic Chicken

Servings: 1   Cooking Time: 25 Minutes

Ingredients:

1 chicken breast	Handful black peppercorns
1 tsp. garlic, minced	Pepper and salt to taste
1 tbsp. chicken seasoning	
1 lemon juice	

Directions:
Pre-heat the Air Fryer to 350°F. Sprinkle the chicken with pepper and salt. Massage the chicken seasoning into the chicken breast, coating it well, and lay the seasoned chicken on a sheet of aluminum foil. Top the chicken with the garlic, lemon juice, and black peppercorns. Wrap the foil to seal the chicken tightly. Cook the chicken in the fryer basket for 15 minutes.

281. Basil Mascarpone Chicken Fillets

Servings: 4   Cooking Time: 12 Minutes
Ingredients:

1 tablespoon fresh basil, chopped	1 tablespoon nut oil
4 oz Mozzarella, sliced	1 teaspoon chili flakes
12 oz chicken fillet	1 teaspoon mascarpone

Directions:
Brush the air fryer pan with nut oil. Then cut the chicken fillet on 4 servings and beat them gently with a kitchen hammer. After this, sprinkle the chicken fillets with chili flakes and put in the air fryer pan in one layer. Top the fillets with fresh basil and sprinkle with mascarpone. After this, top the chicken fillets with sliced Mozzarella. Preheat the air fryer to 375F. Put the pan with Caprese chicken fillets in the air fryer and cook them for 12 minutes.

282. Creamy Turkey Bake

Servings: 5   Cooking Time: 30 Minutes
Ingredients:

1 can (4 ounces) mushroom stems and pieces, drained	1 can (10-3/4 ounces) condensed cream of chicken soup, undiluted
1 cup chopped cooked turkey or chicken	1/2 cup frozen peas
1 tube (12 ounces) refrigerated buttermilk biscuits, cut into 4 equal slices	1/4 cup 2% milk
	Dash each ground cumin, dried basil and thyme

Directions:
Lightly grease baking pan of air fryer with cooking spray. Add all ingredients and toss well to mix except for biscuits. Top with biscuits. Cover pan with foil. For 15 minutes, cook on 390F. Remove foil and cook for 15 minutes at 330F or until biscuits are lightly browned. Serve and enjoy.

283. Eggs 'n Turkey Bake

Servings: 4   Cooking Time: 15 Minutes
Ingredients:

½ teaspoon garlic powder
½ teaspoon onion powder
1-pound leftover turkey, shredded

1 cup coconut milk
2 cups kale, chopped
4 eggs, beaten
Salt and pepper to taste

Directions:
Preheat the air fryer for 5 minutes. In a mixing bowl, combine the eggs, coconut milk, garlic powder, and onion powder. Season with salt and pepper to taste. Place the turkey meat and kale in a baking dish. Pour over the egg mixture. Place in the air fryer. Cook for 15 minutes at 350F.

284. Garlic Chicken

Servings: 4   Cooking Time: 32 Minutes
Ingredients:

2 lbs chicken drumsticks
1 fresh lemon juice
9 garlic cloves, sliced
4 tbsp butter, melted

2 tbsp parsley, chopped
2 tbsp olive oil
Pepper
Salt

Directions:
Preheat the air fryer to 400 F. Add all ingredients into the large mixing bowl and toss well. Transfer chicken wings into the air fryer basket and cook for 32 minutes. Toss halfway through. Serve and enjoy.

285. Pineapple Juice-soy Sauce Marinated Chicken

Servings: 5   Cooking Time: 20 Minutes
Ingredients:

3 tablespoons light soy sauce
1-pound chicken breast tenderloins or strips

1/2 cup pineapple juice
1/4 cup packed brown sugar

Directions:
In a small saucepan bring to a boil pineapple juice, brown sugar, and soy sauce. Transfer to a large bowl. Stir in chicken and pineapple. Let it marinate in the fridge for an hour. Thread pineapple and chicken in skewers. Place on skewer rack. For 10 minutes, cook on 360F. Halfway through cooking time, turnover chicken and baste with marinade. Serve and enjoy.

286. Dill Chicken Fritters

Servings: 8   Cooking Time: 16 Minutes
Ingredients:

1-pound chicken breast, skinless, boneless
3 oz coconut flakes
1 tablespoon ricotta cheese

1 teaspoon mascarpone
1 teaspoon dried dill
½ teaspoon salt
1 egg yolk
1 teaspoon avocado oil

Directions:

Cut the chicken breast into the tiny pieces and put them in the bowl. Add coconut flakes, ricotta cheese, mascarpone, dried dill, salt, and egg yolk. Then make the chicken fritters with the help of the fingertips. Preheat the air fryer to 360F. Line the air fryer basket with baking paper and put the chicken cakes in the air fryer. Sprinkle the chicken fritters with avocado oil and cook for 8 minutes. Then flip the chicken fritters on another side and cook them for 8 minutes more.

287. Sticky Greek-style Chicken Wings

Servings: 3   Cooking Time: 25 Minutes
Ingredients:

1 tbsp cilantro
Salt and pepper to taste
1 tbsp cashews cream
1 garlic clove, minced

1 tbsp yogurt
2 tbsp honey
½ tbsp vinegar
½ tbsp ginger, minced
½ tbsp garlic chili sauce

Directions:
Preheat air fryer to 360 F. Season the wings with salt and pepper, and place in the air fryer. Cook for 15 minutes. In a bowl, mix the remaining ingredients. Top the chicken with sauce and cook for 5 minutes.

288. Sausage Stuffed Chicken

Servings: 4   Cooking Time: 15 Minutes
Ingredients:

4 sausages, casing removed
2 tablespoons mustard sauce

4 (4-ounce) skinless, boneless chicken breasts

Directions:
Preheat the Air fryer to 375F and grease an Air fryer basket. Roll each chicken breast with a rolling pin for about 1 minute. Arrange 1 sausage over each chicken breast and roll up. Secure with toothpicks and transfer into the Air fryer basket. Cook for about 15 minutes and dish out to serve warm.

289. Tomato, Eggplant 'n Chicken Skewers

Servings: 4   Cooking Time: 25 Minutes
Ingredients:

¼ teaspoon cayenne pepper
¼ teaspoon ground cardamom
1 ½ teaspoon ground turmeric
1 can coconut milk
1 cup cherry tomatoes
1 medium eggplant, cut into cubes

2 pounds boneless chicken breasts, cut into cubes
2 tablespoons fresh lime juice
2 tablespoons tomato paste
3 teaspoons lime zest
4 cloves of garlic, minced

1 onion, cut into wedges
1-inch ginger, grated

Salt and pepper to taste

Directions:
Place in a bowl the garlic, ginger, coconut milk, lime zest, lime juice, tomato paste, salt, pepper, turmeric, cayenne pepper, cardamom, and chicken breasts. Allow to marinate in the fridge for at least for 2 hours. Preheat the air fryer to 390F. Place the grill pan accessory in the air fryer. Skewer the chicken cubes with eggplant, onion, and cherry tomatoes on bamboo skewers. Place on the grill pan and cook for 25 minutes making sure to flip the chicken every 5 minutes for even cooking.

290.   Spice Lime Chicken Tenders

Servings: 6   Cooking Time: 20 Minutes
Ingredients:

1 lime
2 pounds chicken tenderloins cut up
1 cup cornflakes, crushed
1/2 cup Parmesan cheese, grated
Sea salt and ground black pepper, to taste

1 tablespoon olive oil
1 teaspoon cayenne pepper
1/3 teaspoon ground cumin
1 teaspoon chili powder
1 egg

Directions:
Squeeze the lime juice all over the chicken. Spritz the cooking basket with a nonstick cooking spray. In a mixing bowl, thoroughly combine the cornflakes, Parmesan, olive oil, salt, black pepper, cayenne pepper, cumin, and chili powder. In another shallow bowl, whisk the egg until well beaten. Dip the chicken tenders in the egg, then in cornflakes mixture. Transfer the breaded chicken to the prepared cooking basket. Cook in the preheated Air Fryer at 380 degrees F for 12 minutes. Turn them over halfway through the cooking time. Work in batches. Serve immediately.

291.   Old-fashioned Chicken Drumettes

Servings: 3   Cooking Time: 30 Minutes
Ingredients:

1/3 cup all-purpose flour
1/2 teaspoon ground white pepper
1 teaspoon seasoning salt
1 teaspoon rosemary

1 teaspoon garlic paste
1 whole egg + 1 egg white
6 chicken drumettes
1 heaping tablespoon fresh chives, chopped

Directions:
Start by preheating your Air Fryer to 390 degrees. Mix the flour with white pepper, salt, garlic paste, and rosemary in a small-sized bowl. In another bowl, beat the eggs until frothy. Dip the chicken into the flour mixture, then into the beaten eggs; coat with the flour mixture one more time. Cook

the chicken drumettes for 22 minutes. Serve warm, garnished with chives.

292.   Fennel Duck Legs

Servings: 4   Cooking Time: 30 Minutes
Ingredients:

4 duck legs
A pinch of salt and black pepper
3 teaspoons fennel seeds, crushed

4 teaspoons thyme, dried
2 tablespoons olive oil

Directions:
In a bowl, mix the duck legs with all the other ingredients and toss well. Put the duck legs in your air fryer's basket and cook at 380 degrees F for 15 minutes on each side. Divide between plates and serve

293.   Country-fried Chicken Drumsticks

Servings: 4   Cooking Time: 20 Minutes
Ingredients:

1 tsp garlic powder
1 tsp cayenne pepper
1/2 cup flour
1/4 cup milk

1/4 tbsp lemon juice
Salt and black pepper to taste

Directions:
Preheat your Air Fryer to 390 F. Spray the air fryer basket with cooking spray. In a small bowl, mix garlic powder, cayenne pepper, salt, and black pepper. Rub the chicken drumsticks with the mixture. In a separate bowl, combine milk with lemon juice. Pour the flour on a plate. Dunk the chicken in the milk mixture, then roll in the flour to coat Place the chicken in the cooking basket and spray it with cooking spray. Cook for 6 minutes, Slide out the fryer basket and flip; cook for 6 more minutes. Serve cooled.

294.   Chicken & Pepperoni Pizza

Servings: 6   Cooking Time: 20 Minutes
Ingredients:

2 cups cooked chicken, cubed
20 slices pepperoni
1 cup sugar-free pizza sauce

1 cup mozzarella cheese, shredded
1/4 cup parmesan cheese, grated

Directions:
Place the chicken into the base of a four-cup baking dish and add the pepperoni and pizza sauce on top. Mix well so as to completely coat the meat with the sauce. Add the parmesan and mozzarella on top of the chicken, then place the baking dish into your fryer. Cook for 15 minutes at 375°F. When everything is bubbling and melted, remove from the fryer. Serve hot.

295.   Chives And Lemon Chicken

Servings: 4   Cooking Time: 20 Minutes

Ingredients:

1 pound chicken tenders, boneless, skinless	Juice of 1 lemon
	1 tablespoon chives, chopped
A pinch of salt and black pepper	A drizzle of olive oil

Directions:

In a bowl, mix the chicken tenders with all ingredients except the chives, toss, put the meat in your air fryer's basket and cook at 370 degrees F for 10 minutes on each side. Divide between plates and serve with chives sprinkled on top.

296. Chicken Wonton Rolls

Servings: 4   Cooking Time: 10 Minutes

Ingredients:

4 wonton wraps	1 garlic clove, diced
8 oz chicken fillet	¼ teaspoon chili flakes
1 teaspoon keto tomato sauce	
1 teaspoon butter, melted	½ teaspoon ground turmeric

Directions:

Slice the chicken on the small strips and sprinkle with chili flakes, ground turmeric, and butter. Preheat the air fryer to 365F. Put the sliced chicken in the air fryer and cook it for 10 minutes. Then transfer the chicken in the bowl. Add tomato sauce and diced garlic. Mix up the chicken and place it on the wonton wraps. Roll them.

297. Garlic Rosemary Roasted Chicken

Servings: 6   Cooking Time: 50 Minutes

Ingredients:

2 pounds whole chicken	1 tsp rosemary
4 cloves of garlic, minced	Salt and pepper to taste

Directions:

Season the whole chicken with garlic, salt, and pepper.   Place in the air fryer basket.   Cook for 30 minutes at 330F.   Flip the chicken in the other side and cook for another 20 minutes.

298. The Best Pizza Chicken Ever

Servings: 4   Cooking Time: 20 Minutes

Ingredients:

4 small-sized chicken breasts, boneless and skinless	Salt and pepper, to savor
1/4 cup pizza sauce	1 ½ tablespoons olive oil
1/2 cup Colby cheese, shredded	
16 slices pepperoni	1 ½ tablespoons dried oregano

Directions:

Carefully flatten out the chicken breast using a rolling pin.   Divide the ingredients among four chicken fillets. Roll the chicken fillets with the stuffing and seal them using a small skewer or two

toothpicks.   Roast in the preheated Air Fryer grill pan for 13 to 15 minutes at 370 degrees F. Bon appétit!

299. Dijon Turkey Drumstick

Servings: 2   Cooking Time: 28 Minutes

Ingredients:

4 turkey drumsticks	1/3 cup coconut milk
1/3 tsp paprika	2 tbsp Dijon mustard
1/3 cup sherry wine	Pepper
1/2 tbsp ginger, minced	Salt

Directions:

Add all ingredients into the large bowl and stir to coat. Place in refrigerator for 2 hours.   Spray air fryer basket with cooking spray.   Place marinated turkey drumsticks into the air fryer basket and cook at 380 F for 28 minutes. Turn halfway through. Serve and enjoy.

300. Honey-balsamic Orange Chicken

Servings: 3   Cooking Time: 40 Minutes

Ingredients:

½ cup balsamic vinegar	½ cup honey
1 ½ pounds boneless chicken breasts, pounded	1 teaspoon fresh oregano, chopped
	2 tablespoons extra virgin olive oil
1 tablespoon orange zest	Salt and pepper to taste

Directions:

Put the chicken in a Ziploc bag and pour over the rest of the Ingredients. Shake to combine everything. Allow to marinate in the fridge for at least 2 hours. Preheat the air fryer to 390F.   Place the grill pan accessory in the air fryer.   Grill the chicken for 40 minutes.

301. Crispy Chicken Wings

Servings: 2   Cooking Time: 25 Minutes

Ingredients:

2 lemongrass stalk (white portion), minced	1½ tablespoons honey
1 onion, finely chopped	Salt and ground white pepper, as required
1 tablespoon soy sauce	1 pound chicken wings, rinsed and trimmed
	½ cup cornstarch

Directions:

In a bowl, mix together the lemongrass, onion, soy sauce, honey, salt, and white pepper.   Add the wings and generously coat with marinade.   Cover and refrigerate to marinate overnight.   Set the temperature of Air Fryer to 355 degrees F. Grease an Air Fryer basket.   Remove the chicken wings from marinade and coat with the cornstarch. Arrange chicken wings into the prepared Air Fryer basket in a single layer. Air Fry for about 25 minutes, flipping once halfway through. Remove from Air Fryer and transfer the chicken wings onto a serving platter. Serve hot.

302.	Sun-dried Tomatoes And Chicken Mix

Servings: 4   Cooking Time: 25 Minutes

Ingredients:

4 chicken thighs, skinless, boneless	1 cup chicken stock
1 tablespoon olive oil	3 garlic cloves, minced
A pinch of salt and black pepper	½ cup coconut cream
1 tablespoon thyme, chopped	1 cup sun-dried tomatoes, chopped
	4 tablespoons parmesan, grated

Directions:
Heat up a pan that fits the air fryer with the oil over medium-high heat, add the chicken, salt, pepper and the garlic, and brown for 2-3 minutes on each side. Add the rest of the ingredients except the parmesan, toss, put the pan in the air fryer and cook at 370 degrees F for 20 minutes. Sprinkle the parmesan on top, leave the mix aside for 5 minutes, divide everything between plates and serve.

303.	Spinach Stuffed Chicken Breasts

Servings: 2   Cooking Time: 29 Minutes

Ingredients:

1¾ ounces fresh spinach	2 tablespoons cheddar cheese, grated
¼ cup ricotta cheese, shredded	1 tablespoon olive oil
2 (4-ounces) skinless, boneless chicken breasts	Salt and ground black pepper, as required
	¼ teaspoon paprika

Directions:
Preheat the Air fryer to 390F and grease an Air fryer basket. Heat olive oil in a medium skillet over medium heat and cook spinach for about 4 minutes. Add the ricotta and cook for about 1 minute. Cut the slits in each chicken breast horizontally and stuff with the spinach mixture. Season each chicken breast evenly with salt and black pepper and top with cheddar cheese and paprika. Arrange chicken breasts into the Air fryer basket in a single layer and cook for about 25 minutes. Dish out and serve hot.

304.	Almond Flour Coco-milk Battered Chicken

Servings: 4   Cooking Time: 30 Minutes

Ingredients:

¼ cup coconut milk	4 small chicken thighs
½ cup almond flour	Salt and pepper to taste
1 ½ tablespoons old bay Cajun seasoning	
1 egg, beaten	

Directions:
Preheat the air fryer for 5 minutes. Mix the egg and coconut milk in a bowl. Soak the chicken thighs in the beaten egg mixture. In a mixing bowl, combine the almond flour, Cajun seasoning, salt and pepper. Dredge the chicken thighs in the almond flour mixture. Place in the air fryer basket. Cook for 30 minutes at 350F.

305.	Peppery Turkey Sandwiches

Servings: 4   Cooking Time: 25 Minutes

Ingredients:

1 cup leftover turkey, cut into bite-sized chunks	1 tsp. hot paprika
2 bell peppers, deveined and chopped	¾ tsp. kosher salt
	½ tsp. ground black pepper
1 Serrano pepper, deveined and chopped	1 heaping tbsp. fresh cilantro, chopped
1 leek, sliced	Dash of Tabasco sauce
½ cup sour cream	4 hamburger buns

Directions:
Combine all of the ingredients except for the hamburger buns, ensuring to coat the turkey well. Place in an Air Fryer baking pan and roast for 20 minutes at 385°F. Top the hamburger buns with the turkey, and serve with mustard or sour cream as desired.

306.	Summer Meatballs With Cheese

Servings: 4   Cooking Time: 15 Minutes

Ingredients:

1 pound ground turkey	1 egg, well beaten
1/2 pound ground pork	2 tablespoons yellow onions, finely chopped
1 cup seasoned breadcrumbs	1 teaspoon fresh garlic, finely chopped
1 teaspoon dried basil	Sea salt and ground black pepper, to taste
1 teaspoon dried rosemary	
1/4 cup Manchego cheese, grated	

Directions:
In a mixing bowl, combine all the ingredients until everything is well incorporated. Shape the mixture into 1-inch balls. Cook the meatballs in the preheated Air Fryer at 380 degrees for 7 minutes. Shake halfway through the cooking time. Work in batches. Serve with your favorite pasta. Bon appétit!

307. Indian Chicken Mix

Servings: 4   Cooking Time: 30 Minutes

Ingredients:

1 yellow onion, chopped

2 tablespoons butter, melted

4 garlic cloves, minced

1 tablespoon ginger, grated

1½ teaspoons paprika

1½ teaspoons coriander, ground

1 teaspoon turmeric powder

Salt and black pepper to taste

15 ounces canned tomatoes, crushed

¼ cup lemon juice

1 pound spinach, chopped

1½ pounds chicken drumsticks

½ cup cilantro, chopped

½ cup chicken stock

½ cup heavy cream

Directions:

Place the butter in a pan that fits your air fryer and heat over medium heat.   Add the onions and the garlic, stir, and cook for 3 minutes.   Add the ginger, paprika, coriander, turmeric, salt, pepper, and the chicken; toss, and cook for 4 minutes more. Add the tomatoes and the stock, and stir.   Place the pan in the fryer and cook at 370 degrees F for 15 minutes.   Add the spinach, lemon juice, cilantro, and the cream; stir, and cook for 5-6 minutes more. Divide everything into bowls and serve.

308. Chicken Strips

Servings: 2   Cooking Time: 25 Minutes

Ingredients:

1 chicken breast, cut into strips

1 egg, beaten

¼ cup flour

¾ cup friendly bread crumbs

1 tsp. mix spice

1 tbsp. plain oats

1 tbsp. desiccated coconut

Pepper and salt to taste

Directions:

In a bowl, mix together the bread crumbs, mix spice, oats, coconut, pepper, and salt.   Put the beaten egg in a separate bowl. Pour the flour into a shallow dish.   Roll the chicken strips in the flour. Dredge each one in the egg and coat with the bread crumb mixture. Put the coated chicken strips in the Air Fryer basket and air fry at 350°F for 8 minutes. Reduce the heat to 320°F and cook for another 4 minutes. Serve hot.

309. Fried Herbed Chicken Wings

Servings: 4   Cooking Time: 11 Minutes

Ingredients:

1 tablespoon Emperor herbs chicken spices

8 chicken wings

Cooking spray

Directions:

Generously sprinkle the chicken wings with Emperor herbs chicken spices and place in the preheated to 400F air fryer. Cook the chicken wings for 6 minutes from each side.

310. Garlic Turkey And Lemon Asparagus

Servings: 4   Cooking Time: 25 Minutes

Ingredients:

1 pound turkey breast tenderloins, cut into strips

A pinch of salt and black pepper

1 tablespoon lemon juice

1 teaspoon coconut aminos

1 pound asparagus, trimmed and cut into medium pieces

2 tablespoons olive oil

2 garlic cloves, minced

¼ cup chicken stock

Directions:

Heat up a pan that fits the air fryer with the oil over medium-high heat, add the meat and brown for 2 minutes on each side. Add the rest of the ingredients, toss, put the pan in the machine and cook at 380 degrees F for 20 minutes. Divide everything between plates and serve

311. Jerk Chicken, Pineapple & Veggie Kabobs

Servings: 8   Cooking Time: 18 Minutes

Ingredients:

8 (4-ounces) boneless, skinless chicken thigh fillets, trimmed and cut into cubes

1 tablespoon jerk seasoning

8 ounces white mushrooms, stems removed

2 large zucchini, sliced

Salt and ground black pepper, as required

1 (20-ounces) can pineapple chunks, drained

1 tablespoon jerk sauce

Directions:

In a bowl, mix together the chicken cubes and jerk seasoning.   Cover the bowl and refrigerate overnight.   Sprinkle the zucchini slices, and mushrooms evenly with salt and black pepper. Thread the chicken, vegetables and pineapple onto greased metal skewers.   Set the temperature of Air Fryer to 370 degrees F. Grease an Air Fryer basket. Arrange skewers into the prepared Air Fryer basket in 2 batches.   Air Fry for about 8-9 minutes, flipping and coating with jerk sauce once halfway through.   Remove from Air Fryer and transfer the chicken skewers onto a serving platter.   Serve hot.

312. Sriracha-ginger Chicken

Servings: 3   Cooking Time: 25 Minutes

Ingredients:

¼ cup fish sauce

¼ cup sriracha

½ cup light brown sugar

½ cup rice vinegar

1/3 cup hot chili paste

1 ½ pounds chicken breasts, pounded   2 teaspoons grated and peeled ginger

Directions:

Place all Ingredients in a Ziploc bag and allow to marinate for at least 2 hours in the fridge.   Preheat the air fryer to 390F.   Place the grill pan accessory in the air fryer.   Grill the chicken for 25 minutes. Flip the chicken every 10 minutes for even grilling. Meanwhile, pour the marinade in a saucepan and heat over medium flame until the sauce thickens. Before serving the chicken, brush with the sriracha glaze.

313. Crispy 'n Salted Chicken Meatballs

Servings: 6   Cooking Time: 20 Minutes

Ingredients:

½ cup almond flour	1 tablespoon coconut milk
¾ pound skinless boneless chicken breasts, ground	2 eggs, beaten
1 ½ teaspoon herbs de Provence	Salt and pepper to taste

Directions:

Mix all ingredient in a bowl.   Form small balls using the palms of your hands.   Place in the fridge to set for at least 2 hours.   Preheat the air fryer for 5 minutes.   Place the chicken balls in the fryer basket.   Cook for 20 minutes at 325F.   Halfway through the cooking time, give the fryer basket a shake to cook evenly on all sides.

314. Kfc Like Chicken Tenders

Servings: 4   Cooking Time: 25 Minutes

Ingredients:

For Breading	
2 whole eggs, beaten	½ cup all-purpose flour
½ cup seasoned breadcrumbs	1 tbsp black pepper
	2 tbsp olive oil

Directions:

Preheat your air fryer to 330 F. Add breadcrumbs, eggs and flour in three separate bowls. Mix breadcrumbs with oil and season with salt and pepper. Dredge the tenders into flour, eggs and crumbs.   Add chicken in the air fryer and cook for 10 minutes. Increase to 390 F, and cook for 5 more minutes.

315. Adobo Seasoned Chicken With Veggies

Servings: 4   Cooking Time: 1 Hour 30 Minutes

Ingredients:

2 pounds chicken wings, rinsed and patted dry	2 tablespoons tomato powder
1 teaspoon coarse sea salt	1 tablespoon dry Madeira wine
1/4 teaspoon ground black pepper	2 stalks celery, diced
	2 cloves garlic, peeled but not chopped

1/2 teaspoon red pepper flakes, crushed	1 large Spanish onion, diced
1 teaspoon ground cumin	2 bell peppers, seeded and sliced
1 teaspoon paprika	4 carrots, trimmed and halved
1 teaspoon granulated onion	2 tablespoons olive oil
1 teaspoon ground turmeric	

Directions:

Toss all ingredients in a large bowl. Cover and let it sit for 1 hour in your refrigerator.   Add the chicken wings to a baking pan.   Roast the chicken wings in the preheated Air Fryer at 380 degrees F for 7 minutes.   Add the vegetables and cook an additional 15 minutes, shaking the basket once or twice. Serve warm.

316. Crispy Chicken Thighs

Servings: 1   Cooking Time: 35 Minutes

Ingredients:

1 lb. chicken thighs	1 cup water
Salt and pepper	1 cup flour
2 cups roasted pecans	

Directions:

Pre-heat your fryer to 400°F.   Season the chicken with salt and pepper, then set aside.   Pulse the roasted pecans in a food processor until a flour-like consistency is achieved.   Fill a dish with the water, another with the flour, and a third with the pecans. Coat the thighs with the flour. Mix the remaining flour with the processed pecans.   Dredge the thighs in the water and then press into the -pecan mix, ensuring the chicken is completely covered. Cook the chicken in the fryer for twenty-two minutes, with an extra five minutes added if you would like the chicken a darker-brown color. Check the temperature has reached 165°F before serving.

317. Ham & Cheese Chicken

Servings: 4   Cooking Time: 25 Minutes

Ingredients:

4 slices ham	1 tbsp chicken bouillon granules
4 slices Swiss cheese	
3 tbsp all-purpose flour	½ cup dry white wine
4 tbsp butter	1 cup heavy whipping cream
1 tbsp paprika	1 tbsp cornstarch

Directions:

Preheat the air fryer to 380 F. Pound the chicken breasts and put a slice of ham and cheese on each one. Fold the edges over the filling and seal the edges with toothpicks. In a medium bowl, combine the paprika and flour, and coat the chicken pieces. Transfer to the air fryer basket and cook for 15 minutes.   In a large skillet, melt the butter and add the bouillon and wine; reduce the heat to low.

Remove the chicken to the skillet. Let simmer for around 5 minutes.

318.   Chicken With Asparagus And Zucchini

Servings: 4   Cooking Time: 25 Minutes
Ingredients:

1 pound chicken thighs, boneless and skinless
2 tablespoons olive oil
3 garlic cloves, minced
1 teaspoon oregano, dried
Juice of 1 lemon
½ pound asparagus, trimmed and halved
A pinch of salt and black pepper
1 zucchinis, halved lengthwise and sliced into half-moons

Directions:
In a bowl, mix the chicken with all the ingredients except the asparagus and the zucchini, toss and leave aside for 15 minutes. Add the zucchinis and the asparagus, toss, put everything into a pan that fits the air fryer, and cook at 380 degrees F for 25 minutes. Divide everything between plates and serve.

319.   Chicken Wings And Vinegar Sauce

Servings: 4   Cooking Time: 12 Minutes
Ingredients:

4 chicken wings
1 teaspoon Erythritol
1 teaspoon water
1 teaspoon apple cider vinegar
1 teaspoon salt
¼ teaspoon ground paprika
½ teaspoon dried oregano
Cooking spray

Directions:
Sprinkle the chicken wings with salt and dried oregano. Then preheat the air fryer to 400F. Place the chicken wings in the air fryer basket and cook them for 8 minutes. Flip the chicken wings on another side after 4 minutes of cooking. Meanwhile, mix up Erythritol, water, apple cider vinegar, and ground paprika in the saucepan and bring the liquid to boil. Stir the liquid well and cook it until Erythritol is dissolved. After this, generously brush the chicken wings with sweet Erythritol liquid and cook them in the air fryer at 400F for 4 minutes more.

320.   Green Curry Hot Chicken Drumsticks

Servings: 4   Cooking Time: 25 Minutes
Ingredients:

2 tbsp green curry paste
3 tbsp coconut cream
½ fresh jalapeno chili, finely chopped
Salt and black pepper
A handful of fresh parsley, roughly chopped

Directions:

In a bowl, add drumsticks, paste, cream, salt, black pepper and jalapeno; coat the chicken well. Arrange the drumsticks in the air fryer and cook for 6 minutes at 400 F, flipping once halfway through. Serve with fresh cilantro.

321.   Chicken Fajita Casserole

Servings: 4   Cooking Time: 12 Minutes
Ingredients:

1 lb cooked chicken, shredded
1 onion, sliced
1 bell pepper, sliced
1/3 cup mayonnaise
7 oz cream cheese
7 oz cheese, shredded
2 tbsp tex-mex seasoning
Pepper
Salt

Directions:
Preheat the air fryer to 370 F.   Spray air fryer baking dish with cooking spray.   Mix all ingredients except 2 oz shredded cheese in a prepared dish.   Spread remaining cheese on top. Place dish in the air fryer and cook for 12 minutes. Serve and enjoy.

322.   Buffalo Chicken Wings

Servings: 3   Cooking Time: 37 Minutes
Ingredients:

2 lb. chicken wings
1 tsp. salt
¼ tsp. black pepper
1 cup buffalo sauce

Directions:
Wash the chicken wings and pat them dry with clean kitchen towels.   Place the chicken wings in a large bowl and sprinkle on salt and pepper.   Pre-heat the Air Fryer to 380°F.   Place the wings in the fryer and cook for 15 minutes, giving them an occasional stir throughout.   Place the wings in a bowl. Pour over the buffalo sauce and toss well to coat.   Put the chicken back in the Air Fryer and cook for a final 5 – 6 minutes.

323.   Italian-style Chicken With Roma Tomatoes

Servings: 8   Cooking Time: 45 Minutes
Ingredients:

2 teaspoons olive oil, melted
3 pounds chicken breasts, bone-in
1/2 teaspoon black pepper, freshly ground
1 teaspoon cayenne pepper
1/2 teaspoon salt
2 tablespoons fresh parsley, minced
1 teaspoon fresh basil, minced
1 teaspoon fresh rosemary, minced
4 medium-sized Roma tomatoes, halved

Directions:
Start by preheating your Air Fryer to 370 degrees F. Brush the cooking basket with 1 teaspoon of olive oil. Sprinkle the chicken breasts with all seasonings listed above.   Cook for 25 minutes or until chicken breasts are slightly browned. Work in batches.

Arrange the tomatoes in the cooking basket and brush them with the remaining teaspoon of olive oil. Season with sea salt.   Cook the tomatoes at 350 degrees F for 10 minutes, shaking halfway through the cooking time. Serve with chicken breasts. Bon appétit!

324.   Saucy Chicken With Leeks

Servings: 6   Cooking Time: 20 Minutes + Marinating Time
Ingredients:

2 large-sized tomatoes, chopped	2 leeks, sliced
3 cloves garlic, minced	½ teaspoon smoked cayenne pepper
½ teaspoon dried oregano	2 tablespoons olive oil
6 chicken legs, boneless and skinless	A freshly ground nutmeg

Directions:
In a mixing dish, thoroughly combine all ingredients, minus the leeks. Place in the refrigerator and let it marinate overnight.   Lay the leeks onto the bottom of an Air Fryer cooking basket. Top with the chicken legs.   Roast chicken legs at 375 degrees F for 18 minutes, turning halfway through. Serve with hoisin sauce.

325.   Paprika Turkey And Shallot Sauce

Servings: 4   Cooking Time: 30 Minutes
Ingredients:

1 big turkey breast, skinless, boneless and cubed	Salt and black pepper to the taste
1 tablespoon olive oil	1 cup chicken stock
¼ teaspoon sweet paprika	3 tablespoons butter, melted
	4 shallots, chopped

Directions:
Heat up a pan that fits the air fryer with the olive oil and the butter over medium high heat, add the turkey cubes, and brown for 3 minutes on each side. Add the shallots, stir and sauté for 5 minutes more. Add the paprika, stock, salt and pepper, toss, put the pan in the air fryer and cook at 370 degrees F for 20 minutes. Divide into bowls and serve.

326.   Duck And Walnut Rice

Servings: 4   Cooking Time: 20 Minutes
Ingredients:

2 ounces mushrooms, sliced	2 cups chicken stock
2 tablespoons olive oil	A pinch of salt and black pepper
2 cups cauliflower florets, riced	½ cup parsley, chopped
½ cup walnuts, toasted and chopped	2 pounds duck breasts, boneless and skin scored

Directions:

Heat up a pan that fits the air fryer with the oil over medium-high heat, add the duck breasts skin side down and brown for 4 minutes. Add the mushrooms, cauliflower, salt and pepper, and cook for 1 minute more. Add the stock, introduce the pan in the air fryer and cook at 380 degrees F for 15 minutes. Divide the mix between plates, sprinkle the parsley and walnuts on top and serve.

327.   Bacon Wrapped Chicken Breasts

Servings: 4   Cooking Time: 23 Minutes
Ingredients:

6-7 Fresh basil leaves	2 tablespoons fish sauce
2 tablespoons water	1 tablespoon palm sugar
2 (8-ounces) chicken breasts, cut each breast in half horizontally	Salt and ground black pepper, as required
12 bacon strips	1½ teaspoons honey

Directions:
Preheat the Air fryer to 365F and grease an Air fryer basket.   Cook the palm sugar in a small heavy-bottomed pan over medium-low heat for about 3 minutes until caramelized.   Stir in the basil, fish sauce and water and dish out in a bowl.   Season each chicken breast with salt and black pepper and coat with the palm sugar mixture.   Refrigerate to marinate for about 6 hours and wrap each chicken piece with 3 bacon strips.   Dip into the honey and arrange into the Air Fryer basket.   Cook for about 20 minutes, flipping once in between.   Dish out in a serving platter and serve hot.   Refrigerate to marinate for about 4-6 hours.

328.   Chicken Pockets

Servings: 4   Cooking Time: 4 Minutes
Ingredients:

2 low carb tortillas	1 tomato, chopped
2 oz Cheddar cheese, grated	2 teaspoons butter
1 teaspoon fresh cilantro, chopped	6 oz chicken fillet, boiled
½ teaspoon dried basil	1 teaspoon sunflower oil
	½ teaspoon salt

Directions:
Cut the tortillas into halves. Shred the chicken fillet with the help of the fork and put it in the bowl. Add chopped tomato, grated cheese, basil, cilantro, and alt. Then grease the tortilla halves with butter from one side. Put the shredded chicken mixture on half of every tortilla piece and fold them into the pockets. Preheat the air fryer to 400F. Brush every tortilla pocket with sunflower oil and put it in the air fryer. Cook the meal for 4 minutes.

329.   Pizza Stuffed Chicken

Servings: 4   Cooking Time: 20 Minutes
Ingredients:

4 small boneless, skinless chicken breasts	16 slices pepperoni
	Salt and pepper, to taste
¼ cup pizza sauce	
½ cup Colby cheese, shredded	1 ½ tbsp. olive oil
	1 ½ tbsp. dried oregano

Directions:
Pre-heat your Air Fryer at 370°F.   Flatten the chicken breasts with a rolling pin.   Top the chicken with equal amounts of each ingredients and roll the fillets around the stuffing. Secure with a small skewer or two toothpicks.   Roast in the fryer on the grill pan for 13 - 15 minutes.

330.	Oregano-thyme Rubbed Thighs

Servings: 4   Cooking Time: 11 Minutes

Ingredients:

4 bone-in chicken thighs with skin	1/8 teaspoon dried oregano
1/8 teaspoon garlic salt	1/8 teaspoon ground thyme
1/8 teaspoon onion salt	1/8 teaspoon ground black pepper
1/8 teaspoon paprika	

Directions:
Lightly grease baking pan of air fryer with cooking spray. Place chicken with skin side touching the bottom of pan.   In a small bowl whisk well pepper, paprika, thyme, oregano, onion salt, and garlic salt. Sprinkle all over chicken.   For 1 minute, cook on 390F.   Turnover chicken while rubbing on bottom and sides of pan for more seasoning.   Cook for 10 minutes at 390F.   Serve and enjoy.

331.	Chicken And Chickpeas Mix

Servings: 4   Cooking Time: 25 Minutes

Ingredients:

5 ounces bacon, cooked and crumbled	1 tablespoon parsley, chopped
2 tablespoons olive oil	Salt and black pepper to taste
1 cup yellow onion, chopped	2 pounds chicken thighs, boneless
8 ounces canned chickpeas, drained	1 cup chicken stock
2 carrots, chopped	1 teaspoon balsamic vinegar

Directions:
Heat up a pan that fits your air fryer with the oil over medium heat.   Add the onions, carrots, salt and pepper; stir, and sauté for 3-4 minutes.   Add the chicken, stock, vinegar, and chickpeas; then toss. Place the pan in the fryer and cook at 380 degrees F for 20 minutes.   Add the bacon and the parsley and toss again.   Divide everything between plates and serve.

332.	Beastly Bbq Drumsticks

Servings: 4   Cooking Time: 45 Minutes

Ingredients:

4 chicken drumsticks	2 tsp. sugar
½ tbsp. mustard	1 tbsp. olive oil
1 clove garlic, crushed	Freshly ground black pepper
1 tsp. chili powder	

Directions:
Pre-heat the Air Fryer to 390°F.   Mix together the garlic, sugar, mustard, a pinch of salt, freshly ground pepper, chili powder and oil.   Massage this mixture into the drumsticks and leave to marinate for a minimum of 20 minutes.   Put the drumsticks in the fryer basket and cook for 10 minutes.   Bring the temperature down to 300°F and continue to cook the drumsticks for a further 10 minutes. When cooked through, serve with bread and corn salad.

333.	Duck With Peppers And Pine Nuts Sauce

Servings: 4   Cooking Time: 25 Minutes

Ingredients:

4 duck breast fillets, skin-on	1/3 cup basil, chopped
1 tablespoon balsamic vinegar	1 tablespoon pine nuts
4 tablespoons olive oil	1 teaspoon tarragon
1 red bell pepper, roasted, peeled and chopped	1 garlic clove, minced
	1 tablespoon lemon juice

Directions:
Heat up a pan that fist your air fryer with half of the oil over medium heat, add the duck fillets skin side up and cook for 2-3 minutes. Add the vinegar, toss and cook for 2 minutes more. In a blender, combine the rest of the oil with the remaining ingredients and pulse well. Pour this over the duck, put the pan in the fryer and cook at 370 degrees F for 16 minutes. Divide everything between plates and serve.

334.	Chicken With Veggies & Rice

Servings: 3   Cooking Time: 20 Minutes

Ingredients:

3 cups cold boiled white rice	1 cup cooked chicken, diced
6 tablespoons soy sauce	½ cup frozen carrots
1 tablespoon vegetable oil	½ cup frozen peas
	½ cup onion, chopped

Directions:
In a large bowl, add the rice, soy sauce, and oil and mix thoroughly.   Add the remaining ingredients and mix until well combined.   Transfer the rice mixture into a 7" nonstick pan.   Arrange the pan into an Air Fryer basket.   Set the temperature of Air Fryer to 360 degrees F.   Air Fry for about 20 minutes.   Remove the pan from Air Fryer and transfer the rice mixture onto serving plates. Serve immediately.

335. Sweet Curried Chicken Cutlets

Servings: 3   Cooking Time: 35 Minutes
Ingredients:

1 tbsp mayonnaise	1 tbsp curry powder
2 eggs	1 tbsp sugar
1 tbsp chili pepper	1 tbsp soy sauce

Directions:
Put the chicken cutlets on a clean flat surface and use a knife to slice in diagonal pieces. Gently pound them to become thinner using a rolling pin. Place them in a bowl and add soy sauce, sugar, curry powder, and chili pepper.   Mix well and refrigerate for 1 hour; preheat the air fryer to 350 F. Remove the chicken and crack the eggs on. Add the mayonnaise and mix. Remove each chicken piece and shake well to remove as much liquid as possible. Place them in the fryer basket and cook for 8 minutes. Flip and cook further for 6 minutes. Remove onto a serving platter and continue to cook with the remaining chicken. Serve.

336. Pepper-salt Egg 'n Spinach Casserole

Servings: 6   Cooking Time: 20 Minutes
Ingredients:

½ cup red onion, chopped	3 cups frozen spinach, chopped
1 cup mushrooms, sliced	3 egg whites, beaten
	4 eggs, beaten
1 red bell pepper, seeded and julienned	Salt and pepper to taste

Directions:
Preheat the air fryer for 5 minutes.   In a mixing bowl, combine the eggs and egg whites. Whisk until fluffy.   Place the rest of the ingredients in a baking dish and pour the egg mixture.   Place in the air fryer chamber.   Cook for 20 minutes at 310F.

337. Breaded Chicken Cutlets

Servings: 4   Cooking Time: 20 Minutes
Ingredients:

4 chicken cutlets	¼ tsp pepper
⅛ tbsp paprika	1 tbsp parsley
2 tbsp panko breadcrumbs	½ tbsp garlic powder
	2 large eggs, beaten

Directions:
Preheat your air fryer to 400 F. In a bowl, mix Parmesan cheese, breadcrumbs, garlic powder, pepper, paprika and mash the mixture. Add eggs in a bowl. Dip the chicken cutlets in eggs, dredge them in cheese and panko mixture. Place the prepared cutlets in the cooking basket and cook for 15 minutes.

338. Oregano Duck Spread

Servings: 6   Cooking Time: 10 Minutes
Ingredients:

½ cup butter, softened	1 teaspoon salt
12 oz duck liver	1 tablespoon dried oregano
1 tablespoon sesame oil	½ onion, peeled

Directions:
Preheat the air fryer to 395F. Chop the onion. Put the duck liver in the air fryer, add onion, and cook the ingredients for 10 minutes. Then transfer the duck pate in the food processor and process it for 2-3 minutes or until the liver is smooth (it depends on the food processor power). Then add onion and blend the mixture for 2 minutes more. Transfer the liver mixture into the bowl. After this, add oregano, salt, sesame oil, and butter. Stir the duck liver with the help of the spoon and transfer it in the bowl. Refrigerate the pate for 10-20 minutes before serving.

339. Garlic Paprika Rubbed Chicken Breasts

Servings: 4   Cooking Time: 30 Minutes
Ingredients:

1 tablespoon stevia powder	2 tablespoons lemon juice, freshly squeezed
2 tablespoons Spanish paprika	4 boneless chicken breasts
2 teaspoon minced garlic	Salt and pepper to taste
3 tablespoons olive oil	

Directions:
Preheat the air fryer for 5 minutes.   Place all ingredients in a baking dish that will fit in the air fryer. Stir to combine.   Place the chicken pieces in the air fryer.   Cook for 30 minutes at 325F.

340. Air Fried Southern Drumsticks

Servings: 4   Cooking Time: 50 Minutes
Ingredients:

2 tbsp oregano	¼ cup milk
2 tbsp thyme	1 egg
2 oz oats	1 tbsp ground cayenne
¼ steamed cauliflower florets	Salt and pepper, to taste

Directions:
Preheat the air fryer to 350 F and season the drumsticks with salt and pepper; rub them with the milk. Place all the other ingredients, except the egg, in a food processor. Process until smooth.   Dip each drumstick in the egg first, and then in the oat mixture. Arrange half of them on a baking mat inside the air fryer. Cook for 20 minutes. Repeat with the other batch.

341. Air Fried Chicken With Honey & Lemon

Servings: 6   Cooking Time: 40 Minutes

Ingredients:

1 whole chicken, 3 lb	1 apple
2 red and peeled onions	Fresh chopped thyme
2 tbsp olive oil	Salt and pepper
2 apricots	Marinade:
1 zucchini	5 oz honey
2 cloves finely chopped garlic	juice from 1 lemon
	2 tbsp olive oil
	Salt and pepper

Directions:

For the stuffing, chop all ingredients into tiny pieces. Transfer to a large bowl and add the olive oil. Season with salt and pepper. Fill the cavity of the chicken with the stuffing, without packing it tightly.   Place the chicken in the air fryer and cook for 10 minutes at 340 F. Warm the honey and the lemon juice in a large pan; season with salt and pepper. Reduce the temperature of the air fryer to 320 F.   Brush the chicken with some of the honey-lemon marinade and return it to the fryer. Cook for another 15 minutes; brush the chicken every 5 minutes with the marinade. Serve.

342. Easy Chicken Fried Rice

Servings: 3   Cooking Time: 20 Minutes

Ingredients:

1 cup frozen peas & carrots	1/2 cup onion, diced
1 packed cup cooked chicken, diced	3 cups cold cooked white rice
1 tbsp vegetable oil	6 tbsp soy sauce

Directions:

Lightly grease baking pan of air fryer with vegetable oil. Add frozen carrots and peas.   For 5 minutes, cook on 360F.   Stir in chicken and cook for another 5 minutes.   Add remaining ingredients and toss well to mix.   Cook for another 10 minutes, while mixing halfway through.   Serve and enjoy.

343. Simple Chicken Wings

Servings: 2   Cooking Time: 25 Minutes

Ingredients:

Salt and black pepper, to taste	1 pound chicken wings

Directions:

Preheat the Air fryer to 380F and grease an Air fryer basket.   Season the chicken wings evenly with salt and black pepper.   Arrange the drumsticks into the Air Fryer basket and cook for about 25 minutes. Dish out the chicken drumsticks onto a serving platter and serve hot.

344. Lemon Grilled Chicken Breasts

Servings: 6   Cooking Time: 40 Minutes

Ingredients:

3 tablespoons fresh lemon juice	6 boneless chicken breasts, halved
2 tablespoons olive oil	Salt and pepper to taste
2 cloves of garlic, minced	

Directions:

Place all ingredients in a Ziploc bag   Allow to marinate   for   at   least   2   hours   in   the fridge.   Preheat the air fryer at 375F.   Place the grill pan accessory in the air fryer.   Grill for 40 minutes and make sure to flip the chicken every 10 minutes for even cooking.

345. Parmesan Chicken Cutlets

Servings: 4   Cooking Time: 30 Minutes

Ingredients:

¾ cup all-purpose flour	2 large eggs
1½ cups panko breadcrumbs	¼ cup Parmesan cheese, grated
4 (6-ounces) (¼-inch thick) skinless, boneless chicken cutlets	1 tablespoon mustard powder
	Salt and black pepper, to taste

Directions:

Preheat the Air fryer to 355F and grease an Air fryer basket.   Place the flour in a shallow bowl and whisk the eggs in a second bowl.   Mix the breadcrumbs, cheese, mustard powder, salt, and black pepper in a third bowl.   Season the chicken with salt and black pepper and coat the chicken with flour.   Dip the chicken into whisked eggs and finally dredge into the breadcrumb mixture. Arrange the chicken cutlets into the Air fryer basket and cook for about 30 minutes.   Dish out in a platter and immediately serve.

346. Creamy Chicken-veggie Pasta

Servings: 3   Cooking Time: 30 Minutes

Ingredients:

3 chicken tenderloins, cut into chunks	1/2 (10.75 ounce) can condensed cream of chicken soup
salt and pepper to taste	1/2 (10.75 ounce) can condensed cream of mushroom soup
garlic powder to taste	
1 cup frozen mixed vegetables	1 tablespoon and 1-1/2 teaspoons olive oil
1 tablespoon grated Parmesan cheese	1-1/2 teaspoons dried minced onion
1 tablespoon butter, melted	1-1/2 teaspoons dried basil
1/2 cup dry fusilli pasta, cooked according to manufacturer's	1-1/2 teaspoons dried parsley
	1/2 cup dry bread crumbs

Directions:

Lightly grease baking pan of air fryer with oil. Add chicken and season with parsley, basil, garlic powder, pepper, salt, and minced onion. For 10 minutes, cook on 360F. Stirring halfway through cooking time. Then stir in mixed vegetables, mushroom soup, chicken soup, and cooked pasta. Mix well. Mix well butter, Parmesan cheese, and bread crumbs in a small bowl and spread on top of casserole. Cook for 20 minutes or until tops are lightly browned. Serve and enjoy.

347. Delicious Chicken Burgers

Servings: 4   Cooking Time: 30 Minutes
Ingredients:

4 boneless, skinless chicken breasts	½ teaspoon paprika
1¾ ounces plain flour	¼ teaspoon dried tarragon
2 eggs	¼ teaspoon dried oregano
4 hamburger buns, split and toasted	1 teaspoon dried garlic
4 mozzarella cheese slices	1 teaspoon chicken seasoning
1 teaspoon mustard powder	½ teaspoon cayenne pepper
1 teaspoon Worcestershire sauce	Salt and black pepper, as required
¼ teaspoon dried parsley	

Directions:
Preheat the Air fryer to 355F and grease an Air fryer basket. Put the chicken breasts, mustard, paprika, Worcestershire sauce, salt, and black pepper in a food processor and pulse until minced. Make 4 equal-sized patties from the mixture. Place the flour in a shallow bowl and whisk the egg in a second bowl. Combine dried herbs and spices in a third bowl. Coat each chicken patty with flour, dip into whisked egg and then coat with breadcrumb mixture. Arrange the chicken patties into the Air fryer basket in a single layer and cook for about 30 minutes, flipping once in between. Place half bun in a plate, layer with lettuce leaf, patty and cheese slice. Cover with bun top and dish out to serve warm.

348. Bacon Chicken Mix

Servings: 2   Cooking Time: 25 Minutes
Ingredients:

2 chicken legs	½ teaspoon ground black pepper
4 oz bacon, sliced	
½ teaspoon salt	1 teaspoon sesame oil

Directions:
Sprinkle the chicken legs with salt and ground black pepper and wrap in the sliced bacon. After this, preheat the air fryer to 385F. Put the chicken legs in the air fryer and sprinkle with sesame oil. Cook the bacon chicken legs for 25 minutes.

349. Peppery Lemon-chicken Breast

Servings: 1   Cooking Time:
Ingredients:

1 teaspoon minced garlic	1 chicken breast
2 lemons, rinds and juice reserved	Salt and pepper to taste

Directions:
Preheat the air fryer. Place all ingredients in a baking dish that will fit in the air fryer. Place in the air fryer basket. Close and cook for 20 minutes at 400F.

350. Ginger And Coconut Chicken

Servings: 4   Cooking Time: 20 Minutes
Ingredients:

4 chicken breasts, skinless, boneless and halved	2 tablespoons stevia
	Salt and black pepper to the taste
4 tablespoons coconut aminos	¼ cup chicken stock
1 teaspoon olive oil	1 tablespoon ginger, grated

Directions:
In a pan that fits the air fryer, combine the chicken with the ginger and all the ingredients and toss.. Put the pan in your air fryer and cook at 4380 degrees F for 20, shaking the fryer halfway. Divide between plates and serve with a side salad.

351. Italian Seasoned Chicken Tenders

Servings: 2   Cooking Time: 10 Minutes
Ingredients:

2 eggs, lightly beaten	1 tsp Italian seasoning
1 1/2 lbs chicken tenders	2 tbsp ground flax seed
1/2 tsp onion powder	1 cup almond flour
1/2 tsp garlic powder	1/2 tsp pepper
1 tsp paprika	1 tsp sea salt

Directions:
Preheat the air fryer to 400 F. Season chicken with pepper and salt. In a medium bowl, whisk eggs to combine. In a shallow dish, mix together almond flour, all seasonings, and flaxseed. Dip chicken into the egg then coats with almond flour mixture and place on a plate. Spray air fryer basket with cooking spray. Place half chicken tenders in air fryer basket and cook for 10 minutes. Turn halfway through. Cook remaining chicken tenders using same steps. Serve and enjoy.

352. Basil-garlic Breaded Chicken Bake

Servings: 2   Cooking Time: 28 Minutes
Ingredients:

2 boneless skinless chicken breast halves (4 ounces each)
1 tablespoon butter, melted
1 large tomato, seeded and chopped
2 garlic cloves, minced
1 1/2 tablespoons minced fresh basil
1/2 teaspoon salt
1/2 tablespoon olive oil
1/4 cup all-purpose flour
1/4 cup egg substitute
1/4 cup grated Parmesan cheese
1/4 cup dry bread crumbs
1/4 teaspoon pepper

Directions:
In shallow bowl, whisk well egg substitute and place flour in a separate bowl. Dip chicken in flour, then egg, and then flour. In small bowl whisk well butter, bread crumbs and cheese. Sprinkle over chicken. Lightly grease baking pan of air fryer with cooking spray. Place breaded chicken on bottom of pan. Cover with foil. For 20 minutes, cook on 390F. Meanwhile, in a bowl whisk well remaining ingredient. Remove foil from pan and then pour over chicken the remaining Ingredients. Cook for 8 minutes. Serve and enjoy.

353.	Chicken With Golden Roasted Cauliflower

Servings: 4   Cooking Time: 30 Minutes
Ingredients:
2 pounds chicken legs
2 tablespoons olive oil
1 teaspoon sea salt
1/2 teaspoon ground black pepper
1 teaspoon smoked paprika
1 (1-pound head cauliflower, broken into small florets
1 teaspoon dried marjoram
2 garlic cloves, minced
1/3 cup Pecorino Romano cheese, freshly grated
1/2 teaspoon dried thyme
Salt, to taste

Directions:
Toss the chicken legs with the olive oil, salt, black pepper, paprika, and marjoram. Cook in the preheated Air Fryer at 380 degrees F for 11 minutes. Flip the chicken legs and cook for a further 5 minutes. Toss the cauliflower florets with garlic, cheese, thyme, and salt. Increase the temperature to 400 degrees F; add the cauliflower florets and cook for 12 more minutes. Serve warm.

354.	Cauliflower Stuffed Chicken

Servings: 5   Cooking Time: 25 Minutes
Ingredients:
1 ½-pound chicken breast, skinless, boneless
½ cup cauliflower, shredded
1 jalapeno pepper, chopped
¼ cup Cheddar cheese, shredded
½ teaspoon cayenne pepper
1 tablespoon cream cheese

1 teaspoon ground nutmeg
1 teaspoon salt
1 tablespoon sesame oil
½ teaspoon dried thyme

Directions:
Make the horizontal cut in the chicken breast. In the mixing bowl mix up shredded cauliflower, chopped jalapeno pepper, ground nutmeg, salt, and cayenne pepper. Fill the chicken cut with the shredded cauliflower and secure the cut with toothpicks. Then rub the chicken breast with cream cheese, dried thyme, and sesame oil. Preheat the air fryer to 380F. Put the chicken breast in the air fryer and cook it for 20 minutes. Then sprinkle it with Cheddar cheese and cook for 5 minutes more.

355.	Chicken With Veggies

Servings: 2   Cooking Time: 45 Minutes
Ingredients:
4 small artichoke hearts, quartered
4 fresh large button mushrooms, quartered
½ small onion, cut in large chunks
2 skinless, boneless chicken breasts
2 tablespoons fresh parsley, chopped
2 garlic cloves, minced
2 tablespoons chicken broth
2 tablespoons red wine vinegar
2 tablespoons olive oil
1 tablespoon Dijon mustard
1/8 teaspoon dried thyme
1/8 teaspoon dried basil
Salt and black pepper, as required

Directions:
Preheat the Air fryer to 350F and grease a baking dish lightly. Mix the garlic, broth, vinegar, olive oil, mustard, thyme, and basil in a bowl. Place the artichokes, mushrooms, onions, salt, and black pepper in the baking dish. Layer with the chicken breasts and spread half of the mustard mixture evenly on it. Transfer the baking dish into the Air fryer basket and cook for about 23 minutes. Coat the chicken breasts with the remaining mustard mixture and flip the side. Cook for about 22 minutes and serve garnished with parsley.

356.	Grilled Hawaiian Chicken

Servings: 2   Cooking Time: 25 Minutes
Ingredients:
2 garlic clove, minced
½ cup ketchup
½ tbsp ginger, minced
½ cup soy sauce
2 tbsp sherry
½ cup pineapple juice
2 tbsp apple cider vinegar
½ cup brown sugar

Directions:
Preheat your air fryer to 360 F. In a bowl, mix in ketchup, pineapple juice, sugar, cider vinegar,

ginger. Heat the sauce in a frying pan over low heat. Cover chicken with the soy sauce and sherry; pour the hot sauce on top. Set aside for 15 minutes to marinate. Place the chicken in the air fryer cooking basket and cook for 15 minutes.

357. Mixed Vegetable Breakfast Frittata

Servings: 6   Cooking Time: 45 Minutes
Ingredients:

½-pound breakfast sausage	1/2 teaspoon black pepper
1 cup cheddar cheese shredded	6 eggs
1 teaspoon kosher salt	8-ounces frozen mixed vegetables (bell peppers, broccoli, etc.), thawed
1/2 cup milk or cream	

Directions:
Lightly grease baking pan of air fryer with cooking spray. For 10 minutes, cook on 360F the breakfast sausage and crumble. Halfway through cooking time, crumble sausage some more until it looks like ground meat. Once done cooking, discard excess fat. Stir in thawed mixed vegetables and cook for 7 minutes or until heated through, stirring halfway through cooking time.   Meanwhile, in a bowl, whisk well eggs, cream, salt, and pepper.   Remove basket, evenly spread vegetable mixture, and pour in egg mixture. Cover pan with foil.   Cook for another 15 minutes, remove foil and continue cooking for another 5-10 minutes or until eggs are set to desired doneness.   Serve and enjoy.

358. Chicken, Rice & Vegetables

Servings: 4   Cooking Time: 30 Minutes
Ingredients:

1 lb. skinless, boneless chicken breasts	1 package [10 oz.] Alfredo sauce
½ lb. button mushrooms, sliced	2 cups cooked rice
1 medium onion, chopped	½ tsp. dried thyme
	1 tbsp. olive oil
	Salt and black pepper to taste

Directions:
Slice up the chicken breasts into 1-inch cubes.   In a large bowl, combine all of the ingredients. Sprinkle on salt and dried thyme and mix again.   Pre-heat the Air Fryer to 370°F and drizzle the basket with the olive oil.   Place the chicken and vegetables in the fryer and cook for 10 – 12 minutes. Stir the contents now and again.   Pour in the Alfredo sauce and allow to cook for an additional 3 – 4 minutes. Serve with rice if desired.

359. Shaking Tarragon Chicken Tenders

Servings: 2   Cooking Time: 15 Minutes
Ingredients:

Salt and pepper to taste	½ cup dried tarragon
	1 tbsp butter

Directions:
Preheat air fryer to 390 F. Lay a 12 X 12 inch cut of foil on a flat surface. Place the chicken on the foil, sprinkle the tarragon on both, and share the butter onto both breasts. Sprinkle with salt and pepper. Loosely wrap the foil around the breasts to enable airflow. Place the wrapped chicken in the basket and cook for 12 minutes. Remove the chicken and carefully unwrap the foil. Serve with the sauce extract and steamed veggies.

360. Chicken Wrapped In Bacon

Servings: 6   Cooking Time: 25 Minutes
Ingredients:

6 rashers unsmoked back bacon	1 tbsp. garlic soft cheese
1 small chicken breast	

Directions:
Cut the chicken breast into six bite-sized pieces. Spread the soft cheese across one side of each slice of bacon.   Put the chicken on top of the cheese and wrap the bacon around it, holding it in place with a toothpick.   Transfer the wrapped chicken pieces to the Air Fryer and cook for 15 minutes at 350°F.

361. Chicken Stuffed With Sage And Garlic

Servings: 2   Cooking Time: 50 Minutes
Ingredients:

1 ½ tbsp olive oil	2 cloves garlic, crushed
Salt and pepper to season	1 brown onion, chopped
1 cup breadcrumbs	3 tbsp butter
⅓ cup chopped sage	2 eggs, beaten
⅓ cup chopped thyme	

Directions:
Rinse the chicken gently, pat dry with paper towel and remove any excess fat with a knife; set aside. On a stovetop, place a pan. Add the butter, garlic and onion and sauté to brown. Add the eggs, sage, thyme, pepper, and salt.   Mix well. Cook for 20 seconds and turn the heat off. Stuff the chicken with the mixture into the cavity. Then, tie the legs of the spatchcock with a butcher's twine and brush with olive oil. Rub the top and sides of the chicken generously with salt and pepper. Preheat the air fryer to 390 F.   Place the spatchcock into the fryer basket and roast for 25 minutes. Turn the chicken over and continue cooking for 10-15 minutes more; check throughout the cooking time to ensure it doesn't dry or overcooks. Remove onto a chopping board and wrap it with aluminum foil; let rest for 10 minutes. Serve with a side of steamed broccoli.

362. Parmesan Chicken Nuggets

Servings: 4   Cooking Time: 10 Minutes
Ingredients:

1 pound chicken breast, ground
1 teaspoon hot paprika
2 teaspoon sage, ground
1/3 teaspoon powdered ginger
1/2 teaspoon dried thyme
1/3 teaspoon ground black pepper, to taste
1 teaspoon kosher salt
2 tablespoons melted butter
3 eggs, beaten
1/2 cup parmesan cheese, grated

Directions:
In a mixing bowl, thoroughly combine ground chicken together with spices and an egg. After that, stir in the melted butter; mix to combine well. Whisk the remaining eggs in a shallow bowl. Form the mixture into chicken nugget shapes; now, coat them with the beaten eggs; then, dredge them in the grated parmesan cheese.   Cook in the preheated Air Fryer at 405 degrees F for 8 minutes. Bon appétit!

363.   Tasty Caribbean Chicken

Servings: 8   Cooking Time: 10 Minutes
Ingredients:

3 lbs chicken thigh, skinless and boneless
1 tbsp coriander powder
3 tbsp coconut oil, melted
½ tsp ground nutmeg
½ tsp ground ginger
1 tbsp cayenne
1 tbsp cinnamon
Pepper
Salt

Directions:
In a small bowl, mix together all spices and rub all over the chicken.   Spray air fryer basket with cooking spray.   Place chicken into the air fryer basket and cook at 390 F for 10 minutes.   Serve and enjoy.

364.   Chinese-style Sticky Turkey Thighs

Servings: 6   Cooking Time: 35 Minutes
Ingredients:

1 tablespoon sesame oil
2 pounds turkey thighs
1 teaspoon Chinese Five-spice powder
1 teaspoon pink Himalayan salt
6 tablespoons honey
1/4 teaspoon Sichuan pepper
1 tablespoon Chinese rice vinegar
2 tablespoons soy sauce
1 tablespoon sweet chili sauce
1 tablespoon mustard

Directions:
Preheat your Air Fryer to 360 degrees F.   Brush the sesame oil all over the turkey thighs. Season them with spices.   Cook for 23 minutes, turning over once or twice. Make sure to work in batches to ensure even cooking   In the meantime, combine the remaining ingredients in a wok (or similar type pan that is preheated over medium-high heat. Cook

and stir until the sauce reduces by about a third. Add the fried turkey thighs to the wok; gently stir to coat with the sauce.   Let the turkey rest for 10 minutes before slicing and serving. Enjoy!

365.   Graceful Mango Chicken

Servings: 2   Cooking Time: 20 Minutes
Ingredients:

1 large mango, cubed
1 medium avocado, sliced
1 red pepper, chopped
5 tbsp balsamic vinegar
4 garlic cloves, minced
15 tbsp olive oil
1 tbsp oregano
1 tbsp parsley, chopped
A pinch of mustard powder
Salt and pepper to taste

Directions:
In a bowl, mix whole mango, garlic, oil, and balsamic vinegar. Add the mixture to a blender and blend well. Pour the liquid over chicken cubes and soak for 3 hours. Take a pastry brush and rub the mixture over breasts as well.   Preheat your air fryer to 360 F. Place the chicken cubes in the cooking basket, and cook for 12 minutes. Add avocado, pork chops mango and pepper and toss well. Drizzle balsamic vinegar and garnish with chopped parsley.

366.   Chicken Bbq Recipe From Peru

Servings: 4   Cooking Time: 40 Minutes
Ingredients:

½ teaspoon dried oregano
1 teaspoon paprika
1/3 cup soy sauce
2 ½ pounds chicken, quartered
2 tablespoons fresh lime juice
2 teaspoons ground cumin
5 cloves of garlic, minced

Directions:
Place all Ingredients in a Ziploc bag and shake to mix everything.   Allow to marinate for at least 2 hours in the fridge.   Preheat the air fryer to 390F. Place the grill pan accessory in the air fryer.   Grill the chicken for 40 minutes making sure to flip the chicken every 10 minutes for even grilling.

367.   Quick 'n Easy Brekky Eggs 'n Cream

Servings: 2   Cooking Time: 15 Minutes
Ingredients:

2 tablespoons coconut cream
A dash of Spanish paprika
2 eggs
Salt and pepper to taste

Directions:
Preheat the air fryer for 5 minutes.   Place the eggs and coconut cream in a bowl. Season with salt and pepper to taste then whisk until fluffy   Pour into greased ramekins and sprinkle with Spanish paprika. Place in the air fryer.   Bake for 15 minutes at 350F.

368. Sweet & Sour Chicken Thighs

Servings: 2   Cooking Time: 20 Minutes

Ingredients:

1 scallion, finely chopped	1 teaspoon sugar
1 garlic clove, minced	Salt and ground black pepper, as required
½ tablespoon soy sauce	2 (4-ounces) skinless, boneless chicken thighs
½ tablespoon rice vinegar	½ cup corn flour

Directions:

Mix together all the ingredients except chicken, and corn flour in a bowl.   Add the chicken thighs and generously coat with marinade.   Add the corn flour in another bowl.   Remove the chicken thighs from marinade and coat with corn flour.   Set the temperature of Air Fryer to 390 degrees F. Grease an Air Fryer basket.   Arrange chicken thighs into the prepared Air Fryer basket, skin side down.   Air Fry for about 10 minutes and then another 10 minutes at 355 degrees F.   Remove from Air Fryer and transfer the chicken thighs onto a serving platter.   Serve hot.

369. Sweet And Sour Grilled Chicken

Servings: 6   Cooking Time: 40 Minutes

Ingredients:

6 chicken drumsticks	¾ cup sugar
1 cup water	¾ cup minced onion
¼ cup tomato paste	¼ cup minced garlic
1 cup soy sauce	Salt and pepper to taste
1 cup white vinegar	

Directions:

Place all ingredients in a Ziploc bag   Allow to marinate for at least 2 hours in the fridge.   Preheat the air fryer at 375F.   Place the grill pan accessory in the air fryer.   Grill the chicken for 40 minutes.   Flip the chicken every 10 minutes for even grilling.   Meanwhile, pour the marinade in a saucepan and heat over medium flame until the sauce thickens.   Before serving the chicken, brush with the glaze.

370. Chicken And Ghee Mix

Servings: 4   Cooking Time: 30 Minutes

Ingredients:

12 oz chicken legs	1 teaspoon ground turmeric
1 teaspoon nutritional yeast	½ teaspoon ground paprika
1 teaspoon chili flakes	1 teaspoon Splenda
½ teaspoon ground cumin	¼ cup coconut flour
½ teaspoon garlic powder	1 tablespoon ghee, melted

Directions:

In the mixing bowl mix up nutritional yeast, chili flakes, ground cumin, garlic powder, ground turmeric, ground paprika, Splenda, and coconut flour. Then brush every chicken leg with ghee and coat well in the coconut flour mixture. Preheat the air fryer to 380F. Place the chicken legs in the air fryer in one layer. Cook them for 15 minutes. Then flip the chicken legs on another side and cook them for 15 minutes more.

371. Simple Turkey Breasts

Servings: 5   Cooking Time: 35 Minutes

Ingredients:

6 – 7 lb. skinless, boneless turkey breast	1 tsp. black pepper
2 tsp. salt	½ tsp. dried cumin
	2 tbsp. olive oil

Directions:

Massage all of the other ingredients into the turkey breast.   Pre-heat the Air Fryer to 340°F,   Cook the turkey breast for 15 minutes. Turn it over and cook for an additional 10 – 15 minutes, until cooked through and crispy.   Slice and serve the turkey with rice or fresh vegetables.

372. Air Fried Cheese Chicken

Servings: 6   Cooking Time: 15 Minutes

Ingredients:

6 tbsp seasoned breadcrumbs	½ cup mozzarella cheese, shredded
2 tbsp Parmesan cheese, grated	1 tbsp marinara sauce
1 tbsp melted butter	Cooking spray as needed

Directions:

Preheat your air fryer to 390 F. Grease the cooking basket with cooking spray. In a small bowl, mix breadcrumbs and Parmesan cheese. Brush the chicken pieces with butter and dredge into the breadcrumbs. Add chicken to the cooking basket and cook for 6 minutes. Turn over and top with marinara sauce and shredded mozzarella; cook for 3 more minutes.

373. Duck Breast With Fig Sauce Recipe

Servings: 4   Cooking Time: 30 Minutes

Ingredients:

2 duck breasts; skin on, halved	1/4 tsp. sweet paprika
1 tbsp. white flour	1 cup beef stock
1 tbsp. olive oil	3 tbsp. butter; melted
1/2 tsp. thyme; chopped	1 shallot; chopped
1/2 cup port wine	4 tbsp. fig preserves
1/2 tsp. garlic powder	Salt and black pepper to the taste

Directions:

Season duck breasts with salt and pepper, drizzle half of the melted butter, rub well, put in your air fryer's basket and cook at 350 °F, for 5 minutes on each side.   Meanwhile; heat up a pan with the olive oil and the rest of the butter over medium high heat, add shallot; stir and cook for 2 minutes.   Add thyme, garlic powder, paprika, stock, salt, pepper, wine and figs; stir and cook for 7-8 minutes.   Add flour; stir well, cook until sauce thickens a bit and take off heat.   Divide duck breasts on plates, drizzle figs sauce all over and serve.

---

374.   Chinese Chili Chicken

Servings: 6   Cooking Time: 20 Minutes

Ingredients:

6 chicken wings	1 teaspoon salt
1 tablespoon coconut aminos	2 tablespoons apple cider vinegar
1 teaspoon ground ginger	1 tablespoon olive oil
1 teaspoon minced garlic	1 chili pepper, chopped

Directions:
Put the chicken wings in the bowl and sprinkle with coconut aminos and ground ginger. Add salt, minced garlic, apple cider vinegar, olive oil, and chopped chili. Mix up the chicken wings and leave them for 15 minutes to marinate. Meanwhile, preheat the air fryer to 380F. Place the marinated chicken wings in the air fryer and cook them for 20 minutes. Flip the chicken wings from time to time to avoid the burning.

---

375.   Chili And Paprika Chicken Wings

Servings: 5   Cooking Time: 12 Minutes

Ingredients:

1 teaspoon ground paprika	1-pound chicken wings
1 teaspoon chili powder	½ teaspoon salt
	1 tablespoon sunflower oil

Directions:
Pour the sunflower oil in the shallow bowl. Add chili powder and ground paprika. Gently stir the mixture. Sprinkle the chicken wings with red chili mixture and salt. Preheat the air fryer to 400F. Place the chicken wings in the preheated air fryer in one layer and cook for 6 minutes. Then flip the wings on another side and cook for 6 minutes more.

---

376.   Crusted Chicken

Servings: 2   Cooking Time: 30 Minutes

Ingredients:

¼ cup slivered s	2 tbsp. full-fat mayonnaise
2x 6-oz. boneless skinless chicken breasts	1 tbsp. Dijon mustard

Directions:
Pulse the s in a food processor until they are finely chopped. Spread the s on a plate and set aside. Cut each chicken breast in half lengthwise.   Mix the mayonnaise and mustard together and then spread evenly on top of the chicken slices.   Place the chicken into the plate of chopped s to coat completely, laying each coated slice into the basket of your fryer.   Cook for 25 minutes at 350°F until golden. Test the temperature, making sure the chicken has reached 165°F. Serve hot.

---

377.   Greek Chicken Meatballs

Servings: 1   Cooking Time: 15 Minutes

Ingredients:

½ oz. finely ground pork rinds	1/3 cup feta, crumbled
1 lb. ground chicken	1/3 cup frozen spinach, drained and thawed
1 tsp. Greek seasoning	

Directions:
Place all the ingredients in a large bowl and combine using your hands. Take equal-sized portions of this mixture and roll each into a 2-inch ball. Place the balls in your fryer.   Cook the meatballs at 350°F for twelve minutes, in several batches if necessary. Once they are golden, ensure they have reached an ideal temperature of 165°F and remove from the fryer. Keep each batch warm while you move on to the next one. Serve with Tzatziki if desired.

---

378.   Buffalo Chicken

Servings: 4   Cooking Time: 25 Minutes

Ingredients:

½ cup yogurt	1 tbsp hot sauce
1 lb chicken breasts cut into strips	2 beaten eggs
1 tbsp ground cayenne	1 tbsp sweet paprika
	1 tbsp garlic powder

Directions:
Preheat air fryer to 390 F. Whisk eggs along with the hot sauce and yogurt. In a shallow bowl, combine the breadcrumbs, paprika, pepper, and garlic powder. Line a baking dish with parchment paper.   Dip the chicken in the egg/yogurt mixture first, and then coat with breadcrumbs. Arrange on the sheet and bake in the air fryer for 8 minutes. Flip the chicken over and bake for 8 more minutes. Serve.

---

379.   Bacon-wrapped Turkey With Cheese

Servings: 12   Cooking Time: 20 Minutes

Ingredients:

1 ½ small-sized turkey breast, chop into 12 pieces	Paprika, to taste
12 thin slices Asiago cheese	Fine sea salt and ground black pepper, to savor
	12 rashers bacon

Directions:
Lay out the bacon rashers; place 1 slice of Asiago cheese on each bacon piece.   Top with turkey, season with paprika, salt, and pepper, and roll them up; secure with a cocktail stick.   Air-fry at 365 degrees F for 13 minutes. Bon appétit!

380. Creamy Scrambled Eggs With Broccoli

Servings: 2   Cooking Time: 20 Minutes

Ingredients:

3 Eggs	Black Pepper to taste
2 tbsp Cream	1/2 cup Broccoli
2 tbsp Parmesan	small florets
Cheese grated or	1/2 cup Bell Pepper
cheddar cheese	cut into small pieces
Salt to taste	

Directions:

Lightly grease baking pan of air fryer with cooking spray. Spread broccoli florets and bell pepper on bottom and for 7 minutes, cook on 360F. Meanwhile, in a bowl whisk eggs. Stir in cream. Season with pepper and salt.   Remove basket and toss the mixture a bit. Pour egg mixture over. Cook for another 10 minutes.   Sprinkle cheese and let it rest for 3 minutes.   Serve and enjoy.

381. Sweet Chili Chicken Wings

Servings: 4   Cooking Time: 20 Minutes

Ingredients:

1 tsp garlic powder	¼ cup sweet chili
1 tbsp tamarind	sauce
powder	

Directions:

Preheat your Air Fryer to 390 F. Spray the air fryer basket with cooking spray.   Rub the chicken wings with tamarind and garlic powders. Spray with cooking spray and place in the cooking basket. Cook for 6 minutes, Slide out the fryer basket and cover with sweet chili sauce; cook for 8 more minutes. Serve cooled.

382. Chicken Pizza Crusts

Servings: 1   Cooking Time: 35 Minutes

Ingredients:

½ cup mozzarella,	¼ cup parmesan
shredded	cheese, grated
1 lb. ground chicken	

Directions:

In a large bowl, combine all the ingredients and then spread the mixture out, dividing it into four parts of equal size.   Cut a sheet of parchment paper into four circles, roughly six inches in diameter, and put some of the chicken mixture onto the center of each piece, flattening the mixture to fill out the circle. Depending on the size of your fryer, cook either one or two circles at a time at 375°F for 25 minutes. Halfway through, turn the crust over to cook on the other side. Keep each batch warm while you move onto the next one.   Once all the crusts are cooked, top with cheese and the toppings of your choice. If desired, cook the topped crusts for an additional five minutes.   Serve hot, or freeze and save for later!

383. Nacho-fried Chicken Burgers

Servings: 4   Cooking Time: 25 Minutes

Ingredients:

1 palmful dried basil	Toppings, to serve
1/3 cup parmesan	1 teaspoon sea salt
cheese, grated	flakes
2 teaspoons dried	1 pound chicken
marjoram	meat, ground
1/3 teaspoon ancho	2 teaspoons cumin
chili powder	powder
2 teaspoons dried	1/3 teaspoon red
parsley flakes	pepper flakes,
1/2 teaspoon onion	crushed
powder	1 teaspoon freshly
1/3 teaspoon porcini	cracked black pepper
powder	

Directions:

Generously grease an Air Fryer cooking basket with a thin layer of vegetable oil.   In a mixing dish, combine chicken meat with all seasonings. Shape into 4 patties and coat them with grated parmesan cheese.   Cook chicken burgers in the preheated Air Fryer for 15 minutes at 345 degrees F, working in batches, flipping them once.   Serve with toppings of choice. Bon appétit!

384. Holiday Colby Turkey Meatloaf

Servings: 6   Cooking Time: 50 Minutes

Ingredients:

1 pound turkey mince	1 tablespoon tamari
1/2 cup scallions,	sauce
finely chopped	Salt and black
2 garlic cloves, finely	pepper, to your liking
minced	1/4 cup roasted red
1 teaspoon dried	pepper tomato sauce
thyme	1 teaspoon brown
1/2 teaspoon dried	sugar
basil	3/4 tablespoons olive
3/4 cup Colby cheese,	oil
shredded	1 medium-sized egg,
3/4 cup crushed	well beaten
saltines	

Directions:

In a nonstick skillet, that is preheated over a moderate heat, sauté the turkey mince, scallions, garlic, thyme, and basil until just tender and fragrant.   Then set your Air Fryer to cook at 360 degrees. Combine sautéed mixture with the cheese, saltines and tamari sauce; then form the mixture into a loaf shape.   Mix the remaining items and pour them over the meatloaf. Cook in the Air Fryer baking pan for 45 to 47 minutes. Eat warm.

385. Bacon 'n Egg-substitute Bake

Servings: 4   Cooking Time: 35 Minutes

Ingredients:

1 (6 ounce) package	1/4 teaspoon salt
Canadian bacon,	3/4 cup and 2
quartered	tablespoons egg
1/2 cup 2% milk	substitute (such as
1/4 teaspoon ground	Egg Beaters®

mustard
2 cups shredded
Cheddar-Monterey
Jack cheese blend

Southwestern Style)
4 frozen hash brown
patties

Directions:
Lightly grease baking pan of air fryer with cooking spray. Evenly spread hash brown patties on bottom of pan. Top evenly with bacon and then followed by cheese. In a bowl, whisk well mustard, salt, milk, and egg substitute. Pour over bacon mixture. Cover air fryer baking pan with foil. Preheat air fryer to 330F. Cook for another 20 minutes, remove foil and continue cooking for another 15 minutes or until eggs are set. Serve and enjoy.

---

386. Flavorful Cornish Hen

Servings: 3   Cooking Time: 25 Minutes

Ingredients:
1 Cornish hen, wash
and pat dry
1 tbsp olive oil
1 tsp smoked paprika

1/2 tsp garlic powder
Pepper
Salt

Directions:
Coat Cornish hen with olive oil and rub with paprika, garlic powder, pepper, and salt. Place Cornish hen in the air fryer basket. Cook at 390 F for 25 minutes. Turn halfway through. Slice and serve.

---

387. Chicken Bbq On Kale Salad

Servings: 4   Cooking Time: 30 Minutes

Ingredients:
¼ cup Greek yogurt
¼ cup parmesan
cheese, grated
½ cup cherry
tomatoes, halved
½ teaspoon
Worcestershire sauce
1 large bunch Tuscan
kale, cleaned and
torn

1 clove of garlic,
minced
3 tablespoons extra
virgin olive oil
4 large chicken
breasts, pounded
Juice from 2 lemons,
divided
Salt and pepper to
taste

Directions:
Place all Ingredients in a bowl except for the kale and tomatoes. Allow to marinate in the fridge for at least 2 hours. Preheat the air fryer to 390F. Place the grill pan accessory in the air fryer. Grill the chicken for 30 minutes. Once cooked, slice the chicken and toss together with the kale and tomatoes.

---

388. Tomato, Cheese 'n Broccoli Quiche

Servings: 2   Cooking Time: 24 Minutes

Ingredients:
½ cup Cheddar
Cheese grated
½ cup Whole Milk
1 Large Carrot, peeled
and diced

1 small Broccoli, cut
into florets
1 Tsp Parsley
1 Tsp Thyme
2 Large Eggs

1 Large Tomato,
chopped

2 tbsp Feta Cheese
Salt & Pepper

Directions:
Lightly grease baking pan of air fryer with cooking spray. Spread carrots, broccoli, and tomato in baking pan. For 10 minutes, cook on 330F. Meanwhile, in a medium bowl whisk well eggs and milk. Season generously with pepper and salt. Whisk in parsley and thyme. Remove basket and toss the mixture a bit. Sprinkle cheddar cheese. Pour egg mixture over vegetables and cheese. Cook for another 12 minutes or until set to desired doneness. Sprinkle feta cheese and let it sit for 2 minutes. Serve and enjoy.

---

389. Creamy Onion Chicken

Servings: 4   Cooking Time: 20 Minutes

Ingredients:
1 ½ cup onion soup
mix

1 cup mushroom soup
½ cup cream

Directions:
Preheat Fryer to 400 F. Add mushrooms, onion mix and cream in a frying pan. Heat on low heat for 1 minute. Pour the warm mixture over chicken slices and allow to sit for 25 minutes. Place the marinated chicken in the air fryer cooking basket and cook for 15 minutes. Serve with the remaining cream.

---

390. Sweet Turmeric Chicken Wings

Servings: 8   Cooking Time: 15 Minutes

Ingredients:
8 chicken wings
1 teaspoon Splenda
1 teaspoon ground
turmeric

½ teaspoon cayenne
pepper
1 tablespoon avocado
oil

Directions:
Mix up Splenda and avocado oil and stir the mixture until Splenda is dissolved. Then rub the chicken wings with ground turmeric and cayenne pepper. Brush the chicken wings with sweet avocado oil from both sides. Preheat the air fryer to 390F. Place the chicken wings in the air fryer and cook them for 15 minutes.

---

391. Mouthwatering Turkey Roll

Servings: 4   Cooking Time: 40 Minutes

Ingredients:
1 pound turkey breast
fillet, deep slit cut
lengthwise with knife
1 small red onion,
chopped finely
1 garlic clove, crushed
1½ teaspoons ground
cumin

3 tablespoons fresh
parsley, chopped
finely
1 teaspoon ground
cinnamon
½ teaspoon red chili
powder
Salt, to taste
2 tablespoons olive
oil

Directions:
Preheat the Air fryer to 355F and grease an Air fryer basket. Mix garlic, parsley, onion, spices and olive oil in a bowl. Coat the open side of fillet with onion mixture and roll the fillet tightly. Coat the outer side of roll with remaining spice mixture and transfer into the Air fryer. Cook for about 40 minutes and dish out to serve warm.

---

392. Chinese Chicken Drumsticks

Servings: 4   Cooking Time: 20 Minutes
Ingredients:

4 (6-ounces) chicken drumsticks	1 cup corn flour
1 tablespoon oyster sauce	½ teaspoon sesame oil
1 teaspoon light soy sauce	1 teaspoon Chinese five spice powder
	Salt and white pepper, as required

Directions:
Preheat the Air fryer to 390F and grease an Air fryer basket. Mix the sauces, oil, five spice powder, salt, and black pepper in a bowl. Rub the chicken drumsticks with marinade and refrigerate for about 40 minutes. Arrange the drumsticks into the Air Fryer basket in a single layer and cook for about 20 minutes. Dish out the chicken drumsticks onto a serving platter and serve hot.

---

393. Bbq Turkey Meatballs With Cranberry Sauce

Servings: 4   Cooking Time: 25 Minutes
Ingredients:

1 ½ tablespoons water	1 1/2 tablespoons barbecue sauce
2 teaspoons cider vinegar	1/3 cup cranberry sauce
1 tsp salt and more to taste	1/4-pound ground bacon
1-pound ground turkey	

Directions:
In a bowl, mix well with hands the turkey, ground bacon and a tsp of salt. Evenly form into 16 equal sized balls. In a small saucepan boil cranberry sauce, barbecue sauce, water, cider vinegar, and a dash or two of salt. Mix well and simmer for 3 minutes. Thread meatballs in skewers and baste with cranberry sauce. Place on skewer rack in air fryer. For 15 minutes, cook on 360F. Every after 5 minutes of cooking time, turnover skewers and baste with sauce. If needed, cook in batches. Serve and enjoy.

---

394. Sriracha-vinegar Marinated Chicken

Servings: 4   Cooking Time: 40 Minutes
Ingredients:

¼ cup Thai fish sauce	2 pounds chicken breasts
¼ cups sriracha sauce	Juice from 1 lime, freshly squeezed
½ cup rice vinegar	Salt and pepper to taste
1 tablespoons sugar	
2 garlic cloves, minced	

Directions:
Place all Ingredients in a Ziploc bag except for the corn. Allow to marinate in the fridge for at least 2 hours. Preheat the air fryer to 390F. Place the grill pan accessory in the air fryer. Grill the chicken for 40 minutes and make sure to flip the chicken to grill evenly. Meanwhile, place the marinade in a saucepan and heat over medium flame until it thickens. Brush the chicken with the glaze and serve with cucumbers if desired.

---

395. Chicken Gruyere

Servings: 4   Cooking Time: 20 Minutes
Ingredients:

¼ cup Gruyere cheese, grated	½ cup flour
1 pound chicken breasts, boneless, skinless	2 eggs, beaten
	Sea salt and black pepper to taste
	4 lemon slices

Directions:
Preheat your Air Fryer to 370 F. Spray the air fryer basket with cooking spray. Mix the breadcrumbs with Gruyere cheese in a bowl, pour the eggs in another bowl, and the flour in a third bowl. Toss the chicken in the flour, then in the eggs, and then in the breadcrumb mixture. Place in the fryer basket, close and cook for 12 minutes. At the 6-minute mark, turn the chicken over. Once golden brown, remove onto a serving plate and serve topped with lemon slices.

---

396. Easy How-to Hard Boil Egg In Air Fryer

Servings: 6   Cooking Time: 15 Minutes
Ingredients:
6 eggs
Directions:
Preheat the air fryer for 5 minutes. Place the eggs in the air fryer basket. Cook for 15 minutes at 360F. Remove from the air fryer basket and place in cold water.

---

397. Chicken Popcorn

Servings: 6   Cooking Time: 10 Minutes
Ingredients:

4 eggs	1 tsp onion powder
1 1/2 lbs chicken breasts, cut into small chunks	2 1/2 cups pork rind, crushed
1 tsp paprika	1/4 cup coconut flour
1/2 tsp garlic powder	Pepper
	Salt

Directions:

In a small bowl, mix together coconut flour, pepper, and salt.   In another bowl, whisk eggs until combined.   Take one more bowl and mix together pork panko, paprika, garlic powder, and onion powder.   Add chicken pieces in a large mixing bowl. Sprinkle coconut flour mixture over chicken and toss well.   Dip chicken pieces in the egg mixture and coat with pork panko mixture and place on a plate.   Spray air fryer basket with cooking spray.   Preheat the air fryer to 400 F.   Add half prepared chicken in air fryer basket and cook for 10-12 minutes. Shake basket halfway through.   Cook remaining half using the same method.   Serve and enjoy.

398.   Vermouth Bacon And Turkey Burgers

Servings: 4   Cooking Time: 30 Minutes
Ingredients:

2 tablespoons vermouth	1/2 shallot, minced
1 tablespoon honey	1 teaspoon red pepper flakes
2 strips Canadian bacon, sliced	4 soft hamburger rolls
1 pound ground turkey	4 tablespoons tomato ketchup
2 garlic cloves, minced	4 tablespoons mayonnaise
2 tablespoons fish sauce	4 (1-ounce slices Cheddar cheese
Sea salt and ground black pepper, to taste	4 lettuce leaves

Directions:
Start by preheating your Air Fryer to 400 degrees F. Whisk the vermouth and honey in a mixing bowl; brush the Canadian bacon with the vermouth mixture.   Cook for 3 minutes. Flip the bacon over and cook an additional 3 minutes.   Then, thoroughly combine the ground turkey, shallots, garlic, fish sauce, salt, black pepper, and red pepper. Form the meat mixture into 4 burger patties. Bake in the preheated Air Fryer at 370 degrees F for 10 minutes. Flip them over and cook another 10 minutes.   Spread the ketchup and mayonnaise on the inside of the hamburger rolls and place the burgers on the rolls; top with bacon, cheese and lettuce; serve immediately.

399.   Coconut Chicken Bake

Servings: 6   Cooking Time: 20 Minutes
Ingredients:

2 tbsp garlic powder	¾ cup shredded coconut
1 tbsp salt	1 pound chicken tenders
½ tbsp ground black pepper	Cooking spray
¾ cup breadcrumbs	

Directions:
Preheat your fryer to 400 F. Spray a baking sheet with cooking spray. In a wide dish, whisk in garlic powder, eggs, pepper and salt. In another bowl, mix the breadcrumbs and coconut.   Dip your chicken tenders in egg, then in the coconut mix; shake off any excess. Place the prepared chicken tenders in your air fryer's cooking basket and cook for 12-14 minutes until golden brown.

400.   Thyme And Sage Turkey Breasts

Servings: 4   Cooking Time: 25 Minutes
Ingredients:

2 turkey breasts, skinless, boneless and halved	1 tablespoons rosemary, chopped
4 tablespoons butter, melted	2 tablespoons parsley, chopped
2 tablespoons thyme, chopped	A pinch of salt and black pepper
2 tablespoons sage, chopped	2 cups chicken stock
	2 celery stalks, chopped

Directions:
Heat up a pan that fits your air fryer with the butter over medium-high heat, add the turkey and brown for 2-3 minutes on each side. Add the herbs, stock, celery, salt and pepper, toss, put the pan in your air fryer, cook at 390 degrees F for 20 minutes. Divide between plates and serve.

Beef,pork & Lamb Recipes

401. Asian-style Round Steak

Servings: 4   Cooking Time: 40 Minutes + Marinating Time

Ingredients:

2 pounds top round steak, cut into bite-sized strips	Salt and black pepper, to taste
2 garlic cloves, sliced	1 tablespoon olive oil
1 teaspoon dried marjoram	1 red onion, sliced
1/4 cup red wine	2 bell peppers, sliced
1 tablespoon tamari sauce	1 celery stalk, sliced

Directions:
Place the top round, garlic, marjoram, red wine, tamari sauce, salt and pepper in a bowl, cover and let it marinate for 1 hour.   Preheat your Air Fryer to 390 degrees F and add the oil.   Once hot, discard the marinade and cook the beef for 15 minutes. Add the onion, peppers, carrot, and garlic and continue cooking until tender about 15 minutes more.   Open the Air Fryer every 5 minutes and baste the meat with the remaining marinade. Serve immediately.

402. Rich Meatball And Mushroom Cassoulet

Servings: 4   Cooking Time: 41 Minutes

Ingredients:

1/2 cup celery, peeled and grated	1 teaspoon saffron
1 ½ cup mushrooms, sliced	2 teaspoons fennel seeds
1/2 cup heavy cream	1 medium-sized lees, finely chopped
1/2 cup Monterey Jack cheese, preferably freshly grated	1/teaspoon dried dill weed
Meatballs:	2 small-sized egg
2 tablespoons pork rinds	1/2 teaspoon cumin
12 ounces lean ground pork	½ teaspoon fine sea salt
	Freshly ground black pepper, to taste

Directions:
Begin by preheating the Air Fryer to 400 degrees F. In a bowl, mix the ingredients for the meatballs. Shape the mixture into mini meatballs.   In an Air Fryer baking dish, toss the celery and mushrooms with the cream; cook for 23 minutes in the preheated Air Fryer.   Pause the machine and place the reserved meatballs in a single layer on top of the celery/mushroom mixture.   Top with the grated Monterey Jack cheese; bake for 9 minutes longer. Serve warm.

403. Cinnamon Lamb Meatloaf

Servings: 4   Cooking Time: 35 Minutes

Ingredients:

A pinch of salt and black pepper	2 pounds lamb, ground
½ teaspoon hot paprika	¼ teaspoon cinnamon powder
A drizzle of olive oil	1 teaspoon coriander, ground
2 tablespoons parsley, chopped	1 egg
2 tablespoons cilantro, chopped	2 tablespoons keto tomato sauce
1 teaspoon cumin, ground	4 scallions, chopped
	1 teaspoon lemon juice

Directions:
In a bowl, combine the lamb with the rest of the ingredients except the oil and stir really well. Grease a loaf pan that fits the air fryer with the oil, add the lamb mix and shape the meatloaf. Put the pan in the air fryer and cook at 380 degrees F for 35 minutes. Slice and serve.

404. Spiced Lamb Steaks

Servings: 3   Cooking Time: 15 Minutes

Ingredients:

½ onion, roughly chopped	1 teaspoon ground fennel
1½ pounds boneless lamb sirloin steaks	½ teaspoon ground cumin
5 garlic cloves, peeled	½ teaspoon ground cinnamon
1 tablespoon fresh ginger, peeled	½ teaspoon cayenne pepper
1 teaspoon garam masala	Salt and black pepper, to taste

Directions:
Preheat the Air fryer to 330F and grease an Air fryer basket.   Put the onion, garlic, ginger, and spices in a blender and pulse until smooth.   Coat the lamb steaks with this mixture on both sides and refrigerate to marinate for about 24 hours. Arrange the lamb steaks in the Air fryer basket and cook for about 15 minutes, flipping once in between. Dish out the steaks in a platter and serve warm.

405. Top Chuck With Mustard And Herbs

Servings: 3   Cooking Time: 1 Hour

Ingredients:

1 ½ pounds top chuck	1 teaspoon dried marjoram
2 teaspoons olive oil	1 teaspoon dried thyme
1 tablespoon Dijon	

mustard
Sea salt and ground
black pepper, to taste

1/2 teaspoon fennel
seeds

Directions:
Start by preheating your Air Fryer to 380 degrees F
Add all ingredients in a Ziploc bag; shake to mix well.
Next, spritz the bottom of the Air Fryer basket with
cooking spray.   Place the beef in the cooking
basket and cook for 50 minutes, turning every 10 to
15 minutes.   Let it rest for 5 to 7 minutes before
slicing and serving. Enjoy!

406.   Paprika Burgers With Blue Cheese

Servings: 6   Cooking Time: 44 Minutes
Ingredients:

1 cup blue cheese,
sliced
2 teaspoons dried
basil
1 teaspoon smoked
paprika
2 pounds ground
pork
2 tablespoons tomato
puree

2 small-sized onions,
peeled and chopped
1/2 teaspoon ground
black pepper
3 garlic cloves,
minced
1 teaspoon fine sea
salt

Directions:
Start by preheating your Air Fryer to 385 degrees F.
In a mixing dish, combine the pork, onion, garlic,
tomato puree, and seasonings; mix to combine well.
Form the pork mixture into six patties; cook the
burgers for 23 minutes. Pause the machine, turn the
temperature to 365 degrees F and cook for 18 more
minutes.   Place the prepared burgers on a serving
platter; top with blue cheese and serve warm.

407.   Pork Belly Marinated In Onion-coconut Cream

Servings: 3   Cooking Time: 25 Minutes
Ingredients:

1/2 pork belly, sliced
to thin strips
1 onion, diced
1 tablespoon butter

4 tablespoons
coconut cream
Salt and pepper to
taste

Directions:
Place all ingredients in a mixing bowl and allow to
marinate in the fridge for 2 hours.   Preheat the air
fryer for 5 minutes.   Place the pork strips in the air
fryer and bake for 25 minutes at 350F.

408.   Herbed Crumbed Filet Mignon

Servings: 4   Cooking Time: 20 Minutes
Ingredients:

1/2 pound filet
mignon
1/2 teaspoon cayenne
pepper
1 teaspoon dried basil

Sea salt and ground
black pepper, to your
liking
1 tablespoon sesame
oil

1 teaspoon dried
rosemary
1 teaspoon dried
thyme

1 small-sized egg,
well-whisked
1/2 cup seasoned
breadcrumbs

Directions:
Season the filet mignon with salt, black pepper,
cayenne pepper, basil, rosemary, and thyme. Brush
with sesame oil.   Put the egg in a shallow plate.
Now, place the breadcrumbs in another plate.
Coat the filet mignon with the egg; then, lay it into
the crumbs. Set your Air Fryer to cook at 360
degrees F.   Cook for 10 to 13 minutes or until
golden. Serve with mixed salad leaves and enjoy!

409.   Beef & Kale Omelet

Servings: 4   Cooking Time: 20 Minutes
Ingredients:

Cooking spray
1/2 lb. leftover beef,
coarsely chopped
2 garlic cloves,
pressed
1 cup kale, torn into
pieces and wilted
1 tomato, chopped
1/4 tsp. sugar

4 eggs, beaten
4 tbsp. heavy cream
1/2 tsp. turmeric
powder
Salt and ground black
pepper to taste
1/8 tsp. ground
allspice

Directions:
Grease four ramekins with cooking spray.   Place
equal amounts of each of the ingredients into each
ramekin and mix well.   Air-fry at 360°F for 16
minutes, or longer if necessary. Serve immediately.

410.   Bolognese Sauce With A Twist

Servings: 4   Cooking Time: 19 Minutes
Ingredients:

1 teaspoon kosher
salt
1/3 teaspoon cayenne
pepper
1½ pounds ground
pork
3 cloves garlic,
minced
1/2 medium-sized
white onion, peeled
and chopped

1/3 cup tomato paste
1/3 tablespoon fresh
cilantro, chopped
1/2 tablespoon extra-
virgin olive oil
1/3 teaspoon freshly
cracked black pepper
1/2 teaspoon grated
fresh ginger

Directions:
Begin by preheating your Air Fryer to 395 degrees F.
Then, thoroughly combine all the ingredients until
the mixture is uniform.   Transfer the meat
mixture to the Air Fryer baking dish and cook for
about 14 minutes. Serve with zucchini noodles and
enjoy.

411. Ginger And Turmeric Lamb

Servings: 4   Cooking Time: 25 Minutes
Ingredients:

16 oz rack of lamb
1 teaspoon ginger
paste

1/2 teaspoon salt

1/4 teaspoon ground

½ teaspoon ground ginger
½ teaspoon ground paprika
turmeric
1 tablespoon butter, melted
1 teaspoon olive oil

Directions:
In the mixing bowl mix up ground ginger, ginger paste, salt, ground paprika, turmeric, butter, and olive oil. Then brush the rack of lamb with the butter mixture and put it in the air fryer. Cook the rack of lamb for 25 minutes at 380F.

412. Crispy Roast Garlic-salt Pork

Servings: 4   Cooking Time: 45 Minutes
Ingredients:
1 teaspoon Chinese five spice powder
1 teaspoon white pepper
2 pounds pork belly
2 teaspoons garlic salt

Directions:
Preheat the air fryer to 390F.   Mix all the spices in a bowl to create the dry rub.   Score the skin of the pork belly with a knife and season the entire pork with the spice rub.   Place in the air fryer basket and cook for 40 to 45 minutes until the skin is crispy. Chop before serving.

413. Beef And Broccoli

Servings: 4   Cooking Time: 25 Minutes
Ingredients:
1 broccoli head, florets separated
2 tablespoons olive oil
1 teaspoon coconut aminos
1 pound beef, cubed
1 teaspoon stevia
1/3 cup balsamic vinegar
2 garlic cloves, minced

Directions:
In a pan that fits your air fryer, mix the beef with the rest of the ingredients, toss, put the pan in the fryer and cook at 390 degrees F for 225 minutes. Divide into bowls and serve hot.

414. Meaty Pasta Bake From The Southwest

Servings: 6   Cooking Time: 45 Minutes
Ingredients:
1 can (14-1/2 ounces each) diced tomatoes, undrained
1 cup shredded Monterey Jack cheese
1 cup uncooked elbow macaroni, cooked according to manufacturer's Directions:
1 jalapeno pepper, seeded and chopped
1 large onion, chopped
1 teaspoons salt
1/2 can (16 ounces) kidney beans, rinsed and drained
1/2 can (4 ounces) chopped green chilies, drained
1/2 can (6 ounces) tomato paste
1/2 teaspoon ground cumin
1/2 teaspoon pepper
1-pound ground beef
2 garlic cloves, minced

1 teaspoon chili powder

Directions:
Lightly grease baking pan of air fryer with cooking spray. Add ground beef, onion, and garlic. For 10 minutes, cook on 360F. Halfway through cooking time, stir and crumble beef.   Mix in diced tomatoes, kidney beans, tomato paste, green chilies, salt, chili powder, cumin, and pepper. Mix well. Cook for another 10 minutes.   Stir in macaroni and mix well. Top with jalapenos and cheese. Cover pan with foil.   Cook for 15 minutes at 390F, remove foil and continue cooking for another 10 minutes until tops are lightly browned.   Serve and enjoy.

415. Spicy Pork With Herbs And Candy Onions

Servings: 4   Cooking Time: 1 Hour
Ingredients:
1 rosemary sprig, chopped
1 thyme sprig, chopped
1 teaspoon dried sage, crushed
Sea salt and ground black pepper, to taste
1 teaspoon cayenne pepper
2 teaspoons sesame oil
2 pounds pork leg roast, scored
1/2 pound candy onions, peeled
2 chili peppers, minced
4 cloves garlic, finely chopped

Directions:
Start by preheating your Air Fryer to 400 degrees F. Then, mix the seasonings with the sesame oil. Rub the seasoning mixture all over the pork leg. Cook in the preheated Air Fryer for 40 minutes. Add the candy onions, peppers and garlic and cook an additional 12 minutes. Slice the pork leg. Afterwards, spoon the pan juices over the meat and serve with the candy onions. Bon appétit!

416. Pork Chops Marinate In Honey-mustard

Servings: 4   Cooking Time: 25 Minutes
Ingredients:
2 tablespoons honey
2 tablespoons minced garlic
4 pork chops
4 tablespoons mustard
Salt and pepper to taste

Directions:
Preheat the air fryer to 330F.   Place the air fryer basket.   Season the pork chops with the rest of the Ingredients.   Place inside the basket.   Cook for 20 to 25 minutes until golden.

417. Tamales

Servings: 6   Cooking Time: 20 Minutes
Ingredients:
10 oz pork stew meat
1 teaspoon almond butter
1 egg, beaten
1 tablespoon almond flour

½ teaspoon dried parsley
1 teaspoon salsa Verde
¼ teaspoon garlic powder
1 cup cauliflower, shredded

1 tablespoon flax meal
½ teaspoon cayenne pepper
3 oz Cheddar cheese, shredded
Cooking spray

Directions:
Grind the pork stew meat and put it in the skillet. Add almond butter and dried parsley and cook the meat on medium heat for 10 minutes. Stir it from time to time. After this, add salsa Verde, and garlic powder and stir the ingredients well. Remove the skillet from the heat. Make the tamale dough: in the mixing bowl, mix up shredded cauliflower, egg, almond flour, flax meal, and cayenne pepper. When the mixture is homogenous, add Cheddar cheese. Mix up the mixture well. After this, cut the foil into medium size squares and spray it with cooking spray. Put the tamale dough in the prepared foil squares. Then top the dough with cooked meat. Roll the foil in the shape of tamales. Preheat the air fryer to 395F. Put the tamales in foil in the air fryer in one layer. Cook the meal for 8 minutes.

418. Flatiron Steak Grill On Parsley Salad

Servings: 4   Cooking Time: 45 Minutes
Ingredients:
½ cup parmesan cheese, grated
1 ½ pounds flatiron steak
1 tablespoon fresh lemon juice

2 cups parsley leaves
3 tablespoons olive oil
Salt and pepper to taste

Directions:
Preheat the air fryer to 390F.   Place the grill pan accessory in the air fryer.   Mix together the steak, oil, salt and pepper.   Grill for 15 minutes per batch and make sure to flip the meat halfway through the cooking time.   Meanwhile, prepare the salad by combining in a bowl the parsley leaves, parmesan cheese and lemon juice. Season with salt and pepper.

419. Beef Roast In Worcestershire-rosemary

Servings: 6   Cooking Time: 2 Hours
Ingredients:
1 onion, chopped
1 tablespoon butter
1 tablespoon Worcestershire sauce
1 teaspoon rosemary
1 teaspoon thyme
1-pound beef chuck roast

2 cloves of garlic, minced
2 tablespoons olive oil
3 cups water
3 stalks of celery, sliced

Directions:
Preheat the air fryer for 5 minutes.   Place all ingredients in a deep baking dish that will fit in the air fryer.   Bake for 2 hours at 350F.   Braise the meat with its sauce every 30 minutes until cooked.

420. Champagne-vinegar Marinated Skirt Steak

Servings: 2   Cooking Time: 40 Minutes
Ingredients:
¼ cup Dijon mustard
1 tablespoon rosemary leaves
1-pound skirt steak, trimmed

2 tablespoons champagne vinegar
Salt and pepper to taste

Directions:
Place all ingredients in a Ziploc bag and marinate in the fridge for 2 hours.   Preheat the air fryer to 390F.   Place the grill pan accessory in the air fryer. Grill the skirt steak for 20 minutes per batch.   Flip the beef halfway through the cooking time.

421. Hickory Smoked Beef Jerky

Servings: 2   Cooking Time: 1 Hour
Ingredients:
¼ cup Worcestershire sauce
½ cup brown sugar
½ teaspoon black pepper
½ teaspoon smoked paprika
1 tablespoon chili pepper sauce

½ cup soy sauce
1 tablespoon liquid smoke, hickory
1 teaspoon garlic powder
1 teaspoon onion powder
1-pound ground beef, sliced thinly

Directions:
Combine all Ingredients in a mixing bowl or Ziploc bag.   Marinate in the fridge overnight.   Preheat the air fryer to 330F.   Place the beef slices on the double layer rack.   Cook for one hour until the beef jerky is very dry.

422. Beef, Pearl Onions And Cauliflower

Servings: 4   Cooking Time: 20 Minutes + Marinating Time
Ingredients:
1 ½ pounds New York strip, cut into strips
1 (1-pound) head cauliflower, broken into florets
1 cup pearl onion, sliced
Marinade:

1 tablespoon olive oil
2 cloves garlic, minced
1 teaspoon of ground ginger
1/4 cup tomato paste
1/2 cup red wine

Directions:
Mix all ingredients for the marinade. Add the beef to the marinade and let it sit in your refrigerator for 1 hour.   Preheat your Air Fryer to 400 degrees F. Transfer the meat to the Air Fryer basket. Add the cauliflower and onions.   Drizzle a few tablespoons of marinade all over the meat and vegetables. Cook

for 12 minutes, shaking the basket halfway through the cooking time. Serve warm.

423. Pork Tenderloin With Bacon & Veggies

Servings: 3   Cooking Time: 28 Minutes
Ingredients:

3 potatoes
¾ pound frozen green beans
6 bacon slices
3 (6-ounces) pork tenderloins
2 tablespoons olive oil

Directions:
Set the temperature of air fryer to 390 degrees F. Grease an air fryer basket.   With a fork, pierce the potatoes.   Place potatoes into the prepared air fryer basket and air fry for about 15 minutes. Wrap one bacon slice around 4-6 green beans. Coat the pork tenderloins with oil   After 15 minutes, add the pork tenderloins into air fryer basket with potatoes and air fry for about 5-6 minutes.   Remove the pork tenderloins from basket.   Place bean rolls into the basket and top with the pork tenderloins.   Air fry for another 7 minutes.   Remove from air fryer and transfer the pork tenderloins onto a platter.   Cut each tenderloin into desired size slices.   Serve alongside the potatoes and green beans rolls.

424. Air Fryer Beef Casserole

Servings: 4   Cooking Time: 30 Minutes
Ingredients:

1 green bell pepper, seeded and chopped
1 onion, chopped
1-pound ground beef
3 cloves of garlic, minced
3 tablespoons olive oil
6 cups eggs, beaten
Salt and pepper to taste

Directions:
Preheat the air fryer for 5 minutes.   In a baking dish that will fit in the air fryer, mix the ground beef, onion, garlic, olive oil, and bell pepper. Season with salt and pepper to taste.   Pour in the beaten eggs and give a good stir.   Place the dish with the beef and egg mixture in the air fryer.   Bake for 30 minutes at 325F.

425. Saucy Beef With Cotija Cheese

Servings: 3   Cooking Time: 27 Minutes
Ingredients:

2 ounces Cotija cheese, cut into sticks
2 teaspoons dried thyme
1/2 cup shallots, peeled and chopped
3 beef tenderloins, cut in half lengthwise
2 teaspoons dried basil
2 teaspoons paprika
2 tablespoon olive oil
3 cloves garlic, minced
1 ½ cups tomato puree, no sugar added
1 teaspoon ground black pepper, or more to taste

1/3 cup homemade bone stock
1 teaspoon fine sea salt, or more to taste

Directions:
Firstly, season the beef tenderloin with the salt, ground black pepper, and paprika; place a piece of the Cotija cheese in the middle.   Now, tie each tenderloin with a kitchen string; drizzle with olive oil and reserve.   Stir the garlic, shallots, bone stock, tomato puree into an oven safe bowl; cook in the preheated Air Fryer at 375 degrees F for 7 minutes. Add the reserved beef along with basil and thyme. Set the timer for 14 minutes. Eat warm and enjoy!

426. Korean Beef Bulgogi Burgers

Servings: 4   Cooking Time: 20 Minutes
Ingredients:

1 ½ pounds ground beef
1 teaspoon garlic, minced
2 tablespoons scallions, chopped
1 teaspoon Gochugaru (Korean chili powder)
1/2 teaspoon dried marjoram
1 teaspoon dried thyme
Sea salt and cracked black pepper, to taste
1 teaspoon mustard seeds
1/2 teaspoon shallot powder
1/2 teaspoon cumin powder
1/2 teaspoon paprika
1 tablespoon liquid smoke flavoring

Directions:
In a mixing bowl, thoroughly combine all ingredients until well combined.   Shape into four patties and spritz them with cooking oil on both sides. Bake at 357 degrees F for 18 minutes, flipping over halfway through the cooking time.   Serve warm. Bon appétit!

427. Beefy Bell Pepper'n Egg Scramble

Servings: 4   Cooking Time: 30 Minutes
Ingredients:

1 green bell pepper, seeded and chopped
1 onion, chopped
1-pound ground beef
3 cloves of garlic, minced
3 tablespoons olive oil
6 cups eggs, beaten
Salt and pepper to taste

Directions:
Preheat the air fryer for 5 minutes with baking pan insert.   In a baking dish mix the ground beef, onion, garlic, olive oil, and bell pepper. Season with salt and pepper to taste.   Pour in the beaten eggs and give a good stir.   Place the dish with the beef and egg mixture in the air fryer.   Bake for 30 minutes at 330F.

428. Ground Beef On Deep Dish Pizza

Servings: 4   Cooking Time: 25 Minutes
Ingredients:

1 can (10-3/4 ounces) condensed tomato soup, undiluted
1 can (8 ounces) mushroom stems and pieces, drained
1 cup shredded part-skim mozzarella cheese
1 cup warm water (110°F to 115°F)
1 package (1/4 ounce) active dry yeast
1 small green pepper, julienned

1 teaspoon dried rosemary, crushed
1 teaspoon each dried basil, oregano and thyme
1 teaspoon salt
1 teaspoon sugar
1/4 teaspoon garlic powder
1-pound ground beef, cooked and drained
2 tablespoons canola oil
2-1/2 cups all-purpose flour

Directions:
In a large bowl, dissolve yeast in warm water. Add the sugar, salt, oil and 2 cups flour. Beat until smooth. Stir in enough remaining flour to form a soft dough. Cover and let rest for 20 minutes. Divide into two and store half in the freezer for future use. On a floured surface, roll into a square the size of your air fryer. Transfer to a greased air fryer baking pan. Sprinkle with beef. Mix well seasonings and soup in a small bowl and pour over beef. Sprinkle top with mushrooms and green pepper. Top with cheese. Cover pan with foil. For 15 minutes, cook on 390F. Remove foil, cook for another 10 minutes or until cheese is melted. Serve and enjoy.

429.	Spicy Mexican Beef With Cotija Cheese

Servings: 6   Cooking Time: 20 Minutes
Ingredients:

3 eggs, whisked
1/3 cup finely grated cotija cheese
1 cup parmesan cheese
2 tablespoons Mexican spice blend

6 minute steaks
1 ½ tablespoons olive oil
Fine sea salt and ground black pepper, to taste

Directions:
Begin by sprinkling minute steaks with Mexican spice blend, salt and pepper. Take a mixing dish and thoroughly combine the oil, cotija cheese, and parmesan cheese. In a separate mixing dish, beat the eggs. Firstly, dip minute steaks in the egg; then, dip them in the cheese mixture. Air-fry for 15 minutes at 345 degrees F; work in batches. Bon appétit!

430.	Spicy And Saucy Pork Sirloin

Servings: 3   Cooking Time: 55 Minutes
Ingredients:

2 teaspoons peanut oil
1 ½ pounds pork sirloin

Coarse sea salt and ground black pepper, to taste
1/4 cup prepared salsa sauce

1 tablespoon smoked paprika

Directions:
Start by preheating your Air Fryer to 360 degrees F. Drizzle the oil all over the pork sirloin. Sprinkle with salt, black pepper, and paprika. Cook for 50 minutes in the preheated Air Fryer. Remove the roast from the Air Fryer and shred with two forks. Mix in the salsa sauce. Enjoy!

431.	Cheesy Sausage'n Grits Bake From Down South

Servings: 4   Cooking Time: 30 Minutes
Ingredients:

1/2 cup uncooked grits
1/4-pound ground pork sausage
1-1/2 cups water
2 tablespoons butter, divided

2 tablespoons milk
3 eggs
3/4 cup shredded Cheddar cheese, divided
salt and pepper to taste

Directions:
In a large saucepan bring water to a boil. Stir in grits and simmer until liquid is absorbed, around 5 minutes. Stir in ¼ cup cheese and 1 tbsp butter. Mix well until thoroughly incorporated. Lightly grease baking pan of air fryer with cooking spray. Add pork sausage and for 5 minutes, cook on 360F. Crumble sausage and discard excess fat. Transfer grits into pan of sausage. In a bowl whisk well, milk and eggs and pour into pan. Mix well. Dot the top with butter and sprinkle cheese. Season with pepper and salt. Cook until tops are browned, around 20 minutes. Serve and enjoy.

432.	Garlic Burgers

Servings: 4   Cooking Time: 15 Minutes
Ingredients:

2 spring onions, diced
¼ teaspoon garlic powder
1 teaspoon ground black pepper

1-pound ground beef
1 teaspoon salt
1 tablespoon flax meal
1 egg yolk
1 teaspoon nut oil

Directions:
In the mixing bowl mix up ground beef, spring onion, garlic powder, ground black pepper, salt, flax meal, and egg yolk. Stir the mixture to get the homogenous texture. After this, make 4 burgers with the help of the fingertips. Put the prepared burgers in the freezer for 5 minutes. Meanwhile, preheat the air fryer to 370F. Then put the burgers in the hot air fryer and sprinkle them with nut oil. Cook the burgers for 8 minutes. Then flip them on another side and cook for 7 minutes more.

433.	Sweet & Sour Pork Chops

Servings: 6   Cooking Time: 16 Minutes
Ingredients:

6 pork loin chops
Salt and ground black pepper, as required
2 garlic cloves, minced
2 tablespoons honey
2 tablespoons soy sauce
1 tablespoon balsamic vinegar
¼ teaspoon ground ginger

Directions:
With a meat tenderizer, tenderize the chops completely and then, sprinkle each with salt and black pepper. In a large bowl, mix the remaining ingredients. Add the chops and generously coat with marinade. Cover and refrigerate for about 2-8 hours. Set the temperature of air fryer to 355 degrees F. Grease an air fryer basket. Arrange chops into the prepared air fryer basket in a single layer. Air fry for about 6-8 minutes per side. Remove from air fryer and transfer the chops onto plates. Serve hot.

434. Gourmet Meatloaf

Servings: 4   Cooking Time: 25 Minutes

Ingredients:
14-ounce lean ground beef
1 chorizo sausage, chopped finely
1 small onion, chopped
2 tablespoons fresh mushrooms, sliced thinly
3 tablespoons breadcrumbs
1 garlic clove, minced
Salt and black pepper, to taste
2 tablespoons olive oil

Directions:
Preheat the Air fryer to 390F and grease an Air fryer basket. Mix all the ingredients in a large bowl except mushrooms. Place the beef mixture in the pan and smooth the surface with the back of spatula. Top with mushroom slices and press into the meatloaf gently. Drizzle evenly with oil and arrange in the Air fryer basket. Cook for about 25 minutes and cut into desires size wedges to serve.

435. Almond Flour 'n Egg Crusted Beef

Servings: 1   Cooking Time: 15 Minutes

Ingredients:
½ cup almond flour
1 egg, beaten
1 slice of lemon, to serve
1/2-pound beef schnitzel
2 tablespoons vegetable oil

Directions:
Preheat the air fryer for 5 minutes. Mix the oil and almond flour together. Dip the schnitzel into the egg and dredge in the almond flour mixture. Press the almond flour so that it sticks on to the beef. Place in the air fryer and cook for 15 minutes at 350F. Serve with a slice of lemon.

436. Cajun Pork And Peppers Mix

Servings: 2   Cooking Time: 35 Minutes

Ingredients:
1 pound pork stew meat, cut into strips
1 tablespoon Cajun seasoning
2 red bell peppers, sliced
1 pound tomatoes, chopped
4 garlic cloves, minced
2 tablespoons coconut oil, melted
A pinch of salt and black pepper

Directions:
Heat up a pan that fits the air fryer with the oil over medium-high heat, add the pork meat, seasoning, garlic, salt and pepper, toss and brown for 5 minutes. Add the remaining ingredients, toss, put the pan in the fryer and cook at 390 degrees F for 30 minutes. Divide everything between plates and serve.

437. Bbq Skirt Steak

Servings: 5   Cooking Time: 20 Minutes + Marinating Time

Ingredients:
2 pounds skirt steak
2 tablespoons tomato paste
1 tablespoon olive oil
1 tablespoon coconut aminos
1 tablespoon fish sauce
1/4 cup rice vinegar
Sea salt, to taste
1/2 teaspoon dried dill
1/2 teaspoon dried rosemary
1/4 teaspoon black pepper, freshly cracked

Directions:
Place all ingredients in a large ceramic dish; let it marinate for 3 hours in your refrigerator. Coat the sides and bottom of the Air Fryer with cooking spray. Add your steak to the cooking basket; reserve the marinade. Cook the skirt steak in the preheated Air Fryer at 400 degrees F for 12 minutes, turning over a couple of times, basting with the reserved marinade. Bon appétit!

438. Moist Stuffed Pork Roll

Servings: 4   Cooking Time: 15 Minutes

Ingredients:
1 scallion, chopped
¼ cup sun-dried tomatoes, chopped finely
4 (6-ounce) pork cutlets, pounded slightly
2 tablespoons fresh parsley, chopped
Salt and black pepper, to taste
2 teaspoons paprika
½ tablespoon olive oil

Directions:
Preheat the Air fryer to 390F and grease an Air fryer basket. Mix scallion, tomatoes, parsley, salt and black pepper in a large bowl. Coat the cutlets with tomato mixture and roll each cutlet. Secure the cutlets with cocktail sticks and rub with paprika, salt and black pepper. Coat evenly with oil and transfer into the Air fryer basket. Cook for about 15 minutes, flipping once in between and dish out to serve hot.

439. Top Loin Beef Strips With Blue Cheese

Servings: 4   Cooking Time: 50 Minutes

Ingredients:

- 1 tablespoon pine nuts, toasted
- 2 pounds crumbled blue cheese
- 2 tablespoons butter, softened
- 2 tablespoons cream cheese
- 4 boneless beef top loin steaks
- Salt and pepper to taste

Directions:

Preheat the air fryer to 390F.   Place the grill pan accessory in the air fryer.   Season the beef with salt and pepper. Brush all sides with butter.   Grill for 25 minutes per batch making sure to flip halfway through the cooking time.   Slice the beef and serve with blue cheese, cream cheese and pine nuts.

440. Beef And Garlic Onions Sauce

Servings: 6   Cooking Time: 20 Minutes

Ingredients:

- 2-pound beef shank
- 1 teaspoon ground black pepper
- 1 teaspoon salt
- 1 oz crushed tomatoes
- 1 teaspoon sesame oil
- 3 tablespoons apple cider vinegar
- 1 garlic clove, diced
- 3 tablespoons water
- 3 spring onions, chopped

Directions:

Sprinkle the beef shank with ground black pepper and salt and put in the air fryer. Sprinkle the meat with sesame oil. Cook it for 20 minutes at 390F. Flip the meat on another side after 10 minutes of cooking. Meanwhile, make the sauce: put crushed tomatoes in the saucepan. Add apple cider vinegar, garlic clove, water, and spring onions. Bring the liquid to boil and remove it from the heat. When the meat is cooked, chop it into the servings and sprinkle with hot sauce.

441. Garlic Pork And Bok Choy

Servings: 4   Cooking Time: 35 Minutes

Ingredients:

- 4 pork chops, boneless
- 1 bok choy head, torn
- 2 cups chicken stock
- 2 tablespoons coconut aminos
- 2 garlic cloves, minced
- A pinch of salt and black pepper
- 2 tablespoons coconut oil, melted

Directions:

Heat up a pan that fits the air fryer with the oil over medium-high heat, add the pork chops and brown for 5 minutes. Add the garlic, salt and pepper and cook for another minute. Add the rest of the ingredients except the bok choy and cook at 380 degrees F for 25 minutes. Add the bok choy, cook for 5 minutes more, divide everything between plates and serve.

442. Pork Tenderloin With Bell Peppers

Servings: 3   Cooking Time: 15 Minutes

Ingredients:

- 1 large red bell pepper, seeded and cut into thin strips
- 1 red onion, thinly sliced
- 10½-ounces pork tenderloin, cut into 4 pieces
- 2 teaspoons Herbs de Provence
- Salt and ground black pepper, as required
- 1 tablespoon olive oil
- ½ tablespoon Dijon mustard

Directions:

Preheat the Air fryer to 390F and grease an Air fryer pan.   Mix the bell pepper, onion, Herbs de Provence, salt, black pepper, and ½ tablespoon of oil in a bowl.   Rub the tenderloins evenly with mustard, salt, and black pepper and drizzle with the remaining oil.   Place bell pepper mixture in the Air fryer basket and top with the pork tenderloin. Cook for about 15 minutes, flipping once in between. Dish out the steaks and cut into desired size slices to serve.

443. Herbed Beef Roast

Servings: 5   Cooking Time: 45 Minutes

Ingredients:

- 1 tablespoon olive oil
- 1 teaspoon dried rosemary, crushed
- 2 pounds beef roast
- 1 teaspoon dried thyme, crushed
- Salt, to taste

Directions:

Preheat the Air fryer to 360F and grease an Air fryer basket.   Rub the roast generously with herb mixture and coat with olive oil.   Arrange the roast in the Air fryer basket and cook for about 45 minutes. Dish out the roast and cover with foil for about 10 minutes.   Cut into desired size slices and serve.

444. Garlic Fillets

Servings: 4   Cooking Time: 15 Minutes

Ingredients:

- 1-pound beef filet mignon
- 1 teaspoon minced garlic
- ½ teaspoon salt
- 1 tablespoon peanut oil
- 1 teaspoon dried oregano

Directions:

Chop the beef into the medium size pieces and sprinkle with salt and dried oregano. Then add minced garlic and peanut oil and mix up the meat well. Place the bowl with meat in the fridge for 10 minutes to marinate. Meanwhile, preheat the air fryer to 400F. Put the marinated beef pieces in the air fryer and cook them for 10 minutes Then flip the beef on another side and cook for 5 minutes more.

445. Simple New York Strip Steak

Servings: 2   Cooking Time: 10 Minutes

Ingredients:

1 (9½-ounces) New York strip steak	1 teaspoon olive oil
Crushed red pepper flakes, to taste	Salt and black pepper, to taste

Directions:

Preheat the Air fryer to 400F and grease an Air fryer basket.   Rub the steak generously with red pepper flakes, salt and black pepper and coat with olive oil. Transfer the steak in the Air fryer basket and cook for about 10 minutes, flipping once in between. Dish out the steak and cut into desired size slices to serve.

---

446.   Spicy Buttered Steaks

Servings: 4   Cooking Time: 17 Minutes

Ingredients:

1-pound beef rib eye steak, bone-in (4 steaks)	1 tablespoon butter
1 teaspoon garlic, diced	½ teaspoon ground ginger
½ teaspoon lime zest, grated	½ teaspoon chipotle powder
½ teaspoon ground paprika	1 teaspoon salt
	½ teaspoon chili flakes

Directions:

Rub the meat steaks with garlic, lime zest, ground paprika, ground ginger, chipotle powder, salt, and chili flakes, Then melt the butter and brush the meat with it. Put the steaks in the air fryer and cook them for 17 minutes at 400F. Flip the meat on another side after 10 minutes of cooking.

---

447.   Mustard Beef And Garlic Spinach

Servings: 4   Cooking Time: 20 Minutes

Ingredients:

3 garlic cloves, minced	2 cups baby spinach
1 and ½ pound beef, cut into strips	2 tablespoons chives, chopped
2 tablespoons coconut oil, melted	4 tablespoons mustard
	Salt and black pepper to the taste

Directions:

In a pan that fits the air fryer, combine all the ingredients, put the pan in the air fryer and cook at 390 degrees F for 20 minutes. Divide between plates and serve.

---

448.   Marinated Flank Steak

Servings: 4   Cooking Time: 15 Minutes

Ingredients:

¾ lb. flank steak	1 tsp. honey
1 ½ tbsp. sake	2 cloves garlic, pressed
1 tbsp. brown miso paste	1 tbsp. olive oil

Directions:

Put all of the ingredients in a Ziploc bag. Shake to cover the steak well with the seasonings and refrigerate for at least 1 hour.   Coat all sides of the steak with cooking spray.   Put the steak in the Air Fryer baking pan.   Cook at 400°F for 12 minutes, turning the steak twice during the cooking time, then serve immediately.

---

449.   Coffee Flavored Steaks Recipe

Servings: 4   Cooking Time: 25 Minutes

Ingredients:

1 ½ tbsp. coffee; ground	1/2 tbsp. sweet paprika
4 rib eye steaks	2 tbsp. chili powder
2 tsp. onion powder	2 tsp. garlic powder
1/4 tsp. ginger; ground	A pinch of cayenne pepper
1/4 teaspoon; coriander, ground	Black pepper to the taste

Directions:

In a bowl; mix coffee with paprika, chili powder, garlic powder, onion powder, ginger, coriander, cayenne and black pepper; stir, rub steaks with this mix, put in preheated air fryer and cook at 360 °F, for 15 minutes. Divide steaks on plates and serve with a side salad.

---

450.   Saffron Spiced Rack Of Lamb

Servings: 4   Cooking Time: 1 Hour And 10 Minutes

Ingredients:

½ teaspoon crumbled saffron threads	2 racks of lamb, rib bones frenched
1 cup plain Greek yogurt	2 tablespoons olive oil
1 teaspoon lemon zest	Salt and pepper to taste
2 cloves of garlic, minced	

Directions:

Preheat the air fryer to 390F.   Place the grill pan accessory in the air fryer.   Season the lamb meat with salt and pepper to taste. Set aside.   In a bowl, combine the rest of ingredients.   Brush the mixture onto the lamb.   Place on the grill pan and cook for 1 hour and 10 minutes.

---

451.   Balsamic London Broil With Garlic

Servings: 8   Cooking Time: 30 Minutes + Marinating Time

Ingredients:

2 pounds London broil	2 tablespoons olive oil
3 large garlic cloves, minced	Sea salt and ground black pepper, to taste
3 tablespoons balsamic vinegar	1/2 teaspoon dried hot red pepper flakes
3 tablespoons whole-grain mustard	

Directions:

Score both sides of the cleaned London broil. Thoroughly combine the remaining ingredients; massage this mixture into the meat to coat it on all sides. Let it marinate for at least 3 hours.   Set the Air Fryer to cook at 400 degrees F; Then cook the London broil for 15 minutes. Flip it over and cook another 10 to 12 minutes. Bon appétit!

452.   Teriyaki Steak With Fresh Herbs

Servings: 4   Cooking Time: 40 Minutes

Ingredients:

2 heaping tablespoons fresh parsley, roughly chopped	For the Sauce: 1/4 cup rice vinegar 1 tablespoon fresh ginger, grated
1 pound beef rump steaks	1 ½ tablespoons mirin
2 heaping tablespoons fresh chives, roughly chopped	3 garlic cloves, minced
Salt and black pepper (or mixed peppercorns), to savor	2 tablespoon rice bran oil 1/3 cup soy sauce A few drops of liquid Stevia

Directions:

Firstly, steam the beef rump steaks for 8 minutes (use the method of steaming that you prefer). Season the beef with salt and black pepper; scatter the chopped parsley and chives over the top. Roast the beef rump steaks in an Air Fryer basket for 28 minutes at 345 degrees, turning halfway through. While the beef is cooking, combine the ingredients for the teriyaki sauce in a sauté pan. Then, let it simmer over low heat until it has thickened.   Toss the beef with the teriyaki sauce until it is well covered and serve. Enjoy!

453.   Italian Beef Meatballs

Servings: 6   Cooking Time: 15 Minutes

Ingredients:

2 large eggs	1 teaspoon dried oregano
2 pounds ground beef	1 small garlic clove, chopped
¼ cup fresh parsley, chopped	Salt and black pepper, to taste
1¼ cups panko breadcrumbs	1 teaspoon vegetable oil
¼ cup Parmigiano Reggiano, grated	

Directions:

Preheat the Air fryer to 350F and grease an Air fryer basket.   Mix beef with all other ingredients in a bowl until well combined.   Make equal-sized balls from the mixture and arrange the balls in the Air fryer basket.   Cook for about 13 minutes and dish out to serve warm.

454.   Easy Beef Medallions With Parsley And Peppers

Servings: 4   Cooking Time: 30 Minutes

Ingredients:

2 tablespoons olive oil	3 bell peppers, seeded and sliced
2 small bunch parsley, roughly chopped	1 sprig rosemary Umami dust seasoning, to taste
1 ½ pounds beef medallions	Salt and ground black pepper, to taste
2 sprigs thyme	

Directions:

Firstly, arrange the vegetables on the bottom of the air fry Air Fryer basket; add seasonings and drizzle with olive oil. Roast for 8 minutes and pause the machine.   Now, place beef medallions on top of the vegetables.   Roast for 18 minutes longer at 375 degrees, stirring once halfway through. To serve, sprinkle with umami dust seasoning and enjoy!

455.   Stuffed Pork Steaks Recipe

Servings: 4   Cooking Time: 30 Minutes

Ingredients:

Zest from 2 limes; grated	1 cup mint; chopped
Zest from 1 orange; grated	1 tsp. oregano; dried
Juice from 1 orange	2 tsp. cumin; ground
Juice from 2 limes	4 pork loin steaks
4 tsp. garlic; minced	2 pickles; chopped
3/4 cup olive oil	4 ham slices
1 cup cilantro; chopped.	6 Swiss cheese slices
	2 tbsp. mustard
	Salt and black pepper to the taste

Directions:

In your food processor, mix lime zest and juice with orange zest and juice, garlic, oil, cilantro, mint, oregano, cumin, salt and pepper and blend well.   Season steaks with salt and pepper, place them into a bowl, add marinade and toss to coat.   Place steaks on a working surface, divide pickles, cheese, mustard and ham on them, roll and secure with toothpicks.   Put stuffed pork steaks in your air fryer and cook at 340 °F, for 20 minutes. Divide among plates and serve with a side salad.

456.   Cumin-paprika Rubbed Beef Brisket

Servings: 12   Cooking Time: 2 Hours

Ingredients:

¼ teaspoon cayenne pepper	2 teaspoons dry mustard
1 ½ tablespoons paprika	2 teaspoons ground black pepper
1 teaspoon garlic powder	2 teaspoons salt
1 teaspoon ground cumin	5 pounds brisket roast
	5 tablespoons olive oil

1 teaspoon onion powder

Directions:
Place all ingredients in a Ziploc bag and allow to marinate in the fridge for at least 2 hours. Preheat the air fryer for 5 minutes. Place the meat in a baking dish that will fit in the air fryer. Place in the air fryer and cook for 2 hours at 350F.

457.	Saucy Lemony Beef Steaks

Servings: 2   Cooking Time: 25 Minutes

Ingredients:

1 pound beef steaks	1/3 cup beef broth
4 tablespoons white wine	2 tablespoons canola oil
2 teaspoons crushed coriander seeds	1/2 lemon, cut into wedges
½ teaspoon fennel seeds	Salt flakes and freshly ground black pepper, to taste
2 tablespoons lemon zest, grated	

Directions:
Heat the oil in a saucepan over a moderate flame. Then, cook the garlic for 1 minute, or until just fragrant. Remove the pan from the heat; add the beef broth, wine, lemon zest, coriander seeds, fennel, salt flakes, and freshly ground black. Pour the mixture into a baking dish. Add beef steaks to the baking dish; toss to coat well. Now, tuck the lemon wedges among the beef steaks. Bake for 18 minutes at 335 degrees F. Serve warm.

458.	Bacon With Shallot And Greens

Servings: 2   Cooking Time: 10 Minutes

Ingredients:

8 thick slices pork bacon	7 ounces mixed greens
2 shallots, peeled and diced	Nonstick cooking spray

Directions:
Begin by preheating the air fryer to 345 degrees F. Now, add the shallot and bacon to the Air Fryer cooking basket; set the timer for 2 minutes. Spritz with a nonstick cooking spray. After that, pause the Air Fryer; throw in the mixed greens; give it a good stir and cook an additional 5 minutes. Serve warm.

459.	Marjoram Lamb

Servings: 4   Cooking Time: 25 Minutes

Ingredients:

4 lamb chops	3 garlic cloves, minced
2 tablespoons olive oil	1 teaspoon thyme, dried
Salt and black pepper to the taste	½ cup keto tomato sauce
1 tablespoon marjoram, chopped	

Directions:

Heat up a pan that fits the air fryer with the oil over medium-high heat, add the lamb chops and brown for 5 minutes. Add the rest of the ingredients, toss, put the pan in the fryer and cook at 390 degrees F for 20 minutes more. Divide into bowls and serve right away.

460.	Steak Rolls

Servings: 4   Cooking Time: 18 Minutes

Ingredients:

12 oz pork steaks (3 oz each steak)	¼ teaspoon salt
1 green bell pepper	1 teaspoon sunflower oil
2 oz asparagus, trimmed	1 teaspoon chili flakes
1 teaspoon ground black pepper	1 teaspoon avocado oil

Directions:
Beat every pork steak with the kitchen hammer gently. Then sprinkle the meat with chili flakes and avocado oil and place it in the air fryer in one layer. Cook the meat for 8 minutes at 375F. Then remove the meat from the air fryer and cool to the room temperature. Meanwhile, cut the bell pepper on the thin wedges. Mix up together pepper wedges and asparagus. Add ground black pepper, salt, and sunflower oil. Mix up the vegetables. After this, place the vegetables on the pork steaks and roll them. Secure the meat with toothpicks if needed. Then transfer the steak bundles in the air fryer in one layer and cook them for 10 minutes at 365F.

461.	Italian Pork

Servings: 2   Cooking Time: 50 Minutes

Ingredients:

8 oz pork loin	½ teaspoon salt
1 tablespoon sesame oil	1 teaspoon Italian herbs

Directions:
In the shallow bowl mix up Italian herbs, salt, and sesame oil. Then brush the pork loin with the Italian herbs mixture and wrap in the foil. Preheat the air fryer to 350F. Put the wrapped pork loin in the air fryer and cook it for 50 minutes. When the time is over, remove the meat from the air fryer and discard the foil. Slice the pork loin into the servings.

462.	Favorite Beef Stroganoff

Servings: 4   Cooking Time: 20 Minutes + Marinating Time

Ingredients:

1 ¼ pounds beef sirloin steak, cut into small-sized strips	2 cloves garlic, crushed
1/4 cup balsamic vinegar	1 teaspoon cayenne pepper
1 tablespoon brown mustard	Sea salt flakes and crushed red pepper, to taste
1 tablespoon butter	1 cup sour cream

1 cup beef broth
1 cup leek, chopped

2 ½ tablespoons tomato paste

Directions:
Place the beef along with the balsamic vinegar and the mustard in a mixing dish; cover and marinate in your refrigerator for about 1 hour.   Butter the inside of a baking dish and put the beef into the dish. Add the broth, leeks and garlic. Cook at 380 degrees for 8 minutes. Pause the machine and add the cayenne pepper, salt, red pepper, sour cream and tomato paste; cook for additional 7 minutes.   Bon appétit!

463.   Spicy Pork

Servings: 6   Cooking Time: 20 Minutes
Ingredients:

2-pound pork shoulder, boneless
1 teaspoon salt
1 teaspoon chili powder
1 teaspoon five spices powder
1 tablespoon apple cider vinegar

1 teaspoon Erythritol
¼ teaspoon keto tomato sauce
1 teaspoon ground black pepper
2 tablespoons water
1 tablespoon avocado oil

Directions:
Pierce the pork shoulder with the help of the knife. Then make the sauce: in the mixing bowl mix up salt, chili powder, five spices powder, apple cider vinegar, Erythritol, tomato sauce, ground black pepper, and water. Whisk the mixture until it is smooth. Then put the pork shoulder in the sauce and coat well. Leave the meat in the sauce for 8 hours. When the time is finished, preheat the air fryer to 390F. Brush the marinated meat with avocado oil and put it in the preheated air fryer. Cook the meat for 15 minutes. Then flip it on another side and cook for 5 minutes more. Let the cooked pork shoulder rest for 10 minutes before serving.

464.   Scrumptious Lamb Chops

Servings: 4   Cooking Time: 8 Minutes
Ingredients:

2 tablespoons fresh mint leaves, minced
4 (6-ounce) lamb chops
2 carrots, peeled and cubed
1 parsnip, peeled and cubed
1 fennel bulb, cubed

1 garlic clove, minced
2 tablespoons dried rosemary
3 tablespoons olive oil
Salt and black pepper, to taste

Directions:
Preheat the Air fryer to 390F and grease an Air fryer basket.   Mix herbs, garlic and oil in a large bowl and coat chops generously with this mixture. Marinate in the refrigerator for about 3 hours. Soak the vegetables in a large pan of water for about 15 minutes.   Arrange the chops in the Air fryer basket and cook for about 2 minutes.   Remove the

chops and place the vegetables in the Air fryer basket.   Top with the chops and cook for about 6 minutes.   Dish out and serve warm.

465.   Easy Cheeseburger Meatballs

Servings: 3   Cooking Time: 15 Minutes
Ingredients:

1 pound ground pork
1 tablespoon coconut aminos
2 tablespoons spring onions, finely chopped

1 teaspoon garlic, minced
1/2 cup pork rinds
1/2 cup parmesan cheese, preferably freshly grated

Directions:
Combine the ground pork, coconut aminos, garlic, and spring onions in a mixing dish. Mix until everything is well incorporated.   Form the mixture into small meatballs.   In a shallow bowl, mix the pork rinds and grated parmesan cheese. Roll the meatballs over the parmesan mixture.   Cook at 380 degrees F for 3 minutes; shake the basket and cook an additional 4 minutes or until meatballs are browned on all sides. Bon appétit!

466.   Spicy Meatloaf With Peppers And Parmesan Cheese

Servings: 4   Cooking Time: 35 Minutes
Ingredients:

1/2 pound beef sausage, crumbled
1/2 pound ground beef
1/4 cup pork rinds
2 tablespoons Parmesan, preferably freshly grated
1 shallot, finely chopped

2 garlic cloves, minced
Sea salt and ground black pepper, to taste
1 red bell pepper, finely chopped
1 serrano pepper, finely chopped

Directions:
Start by preheating your Air Fryer to 390 degrees F. Mix all ingredients in a bowl. Knead until everything is well incorporated.   Shape the mixture into a meatloaf and place in the baking pan that is previously greased with cooking oil.   Cook for 24 minutes in the preheated Air Fryer.   Let it stand on a cooling rack for 6 minutes before slicing and serving. Enjoy!

467.   Cardamom Lamb Mix

Servings: 2   Cooking Time: 20 Minutes
Ingredients:

1 oz fresh ginger, sliced
2 oz spring onions, chopped
¼ teaspoon ground cinnamon
½ teaspoon ground cardamom

10 oz lamb sirloin
½ teaspoon fennel seeds
½ teaspoon chili flakes
¼ teaspoon salt

1 tablespoon avocado oil

Directions:
Put the fresh ginger in the blender. Add onion, ground cardamom, cinnamon, fennel seeds, chili flakes, salt, and avocado oil. Blend the mixture until you get the smooth mass. After this, make the small cuts in the lamb sirloin. Rub the meat with the blended spice mixture and leave it for 20 minutes to marinate. Meanwhile, preheat the air fryer to 350F. Put the marinated lamb sirloin in the air fryer and cook it for 20 minutes. Flip the meat on another side in halfway. Slice the cooked meat.

---

468. Sausage 'n Cauliflower Frittata

Servings: 3   Cooking Time: 27 Minutes

Ingredients:

1-pound hot pork sausage, diced	3 large eggs
½ cup shredded Cheddar cheese	1/2 (30 ounce) package frozen hash brown potatoes, thawed
1 teaspoons salt	
½ cup milk	1/2 teaspoon ground black pepper
1 small cauliflower, riced	

Directions:
Lightly grease baking pan of air fryer with cooking spray. And add diced sausage and cook for 10 minutes on 360F.   Add hash brown and riced cauliflower.   Cook   for   another   5   minutes. Meanwhile, whisk well eggs, salt, pepper, and milk. Remove basket and toss the mixture a bit. Evenly spread cheese and pour eggs.   Cook for another 12 minutes or until set   Serve and enjoy.

---

469. Sriracha-hoisin Glazed Grilled Beef

Servings: 5   Cooking Time: 16 Minutes

Ingredients:

1-pound flank steak, sliced at an angle 1" x ¼" thick	1-1/2 teaspoons honey
1 tablespoon lime juice	1/2 teaspoon sesame oil (optional)
1 chopped green onions	1/2 teaspoon chile-garlic sauce (such as Sriracha®)
1/2 clove garlic, minced	1-1/2 teaspoons toasted sesame seeds
1/2 teaspoon kosher salt	1/4 cup hoisin sauce
1/2 teaspoon peeled and grated fresh ginger root	1/4 teaspoon crushed red pepper flakes
	1/8 teaspoon ground black pepper

Directions:
In a shallow dish, mix well pepper, red pepper flakes, chile-garlic sauce, sesame oil, ginger, salt, honey, lime juice, and hoisin sauce. Add steak and toss well to coat. Marinate in the ref for 3 hours.   Thread steak in skewers. Place on skewer rack in air fryer.

For 8 minutes, cook on 360F. If needed, cook in batches.   Serve and enjoy with a drizzle of green onions and sesame seeds.

---

470. Tomato Stuffed Pork Roll

Servings: 4   Cooking Time: 15 Minutes

Ingredients:

¼ cup sun-dried tomatoes, chopped finely	1 scallion, chopped
2 tablespoons fresh parsley, chopped	Salt and freshly ground black pepper, to taste
4 (6-ounce) pork cutlets, pounded slightly	2 teaspoons paprika
	½ tablespoon olive oil

Directions:
Preheat the Air fryer to 390F and grease an Air fryer basket.   Mix scallion, tomatoes, parsley, salt and black pepper in a bowl.   Coat each cutlet with tomato mixture and roll up the cutlet, securing with cocktail sticks.   Coat the rolls with oil and rub with paprika, salt and black pepper.   Arrange the rolls in the Air fryer basket and cook for about 15 minutes, flipping once in between.   Dish out in a platter and serve warm.

---

471. Coriander, Mustard 'n Cumin Rubbed Flank Steak

Servings: 3   Cooking Time: 45 Minutes

Ingredients:

½ teaspoon coriander	1 teaspoon garlic powder
½ teaspoon ground cumin	1 teaspoon mustard powder
1 ½ pounds flank steak	2 tablespoons sugar
1 tablespoon chili powder	2 tablespoons black pepper
1 tablespoon paprika	2 teaspoons salt

Directions:
Preheat the air fryer to 390F.   Place the grill pan accessory in the air fryer.   In a small bowl, combine all the spices and rub all over the flank steak.   Place on the grill and cook for 15 minutes per batch.   Make sure to flip the meat every 8 minutes for even grilling.

---

472. Fat Burger Bombs

Servings: 6   Cooking Time: 20 Minutes

Ingredients:

½ pound ground beef	3 tablespoons olive oil
1 cup almond flour	Salt and pepper to taste
12 slices uncured bacon, chopped	
2 eggs, beaten	

Directions:
In a mixing bowl, combine all ingredients except for the olive oil.   Use your hands to form small balls with the mixture. Place in a baking sheet and allow to set in the fridge for at least 2 hours.   Preheat the

air fryer for 5 minutes.   Brush the meat balls with olive oil on all sides.   Place in the air fryer basket. Cook for 20 minutes at 350F.   Halfway through the cooking time, shake the fryer basket for a more even cooking.

---

473.   Cilantro Steak

Servings: 4   Cooking Time: 25 Minutes

Ingredients:

1-pound flank steak	½ green bell pepper, chopped
1 oz fresh cilantro, chopped	1 tablespoon avocado oil
1 garlic clove, diced	
1 oz fresh parsley, chopped	½ teaspoon salt
1 egg, hard-boiled, peeled	½ teaspoon ground black pepper
	1 teaspoon peanut oil

Directions:

In the mixing bowl, mix up fresh cilantro, diced garlic, parsley, and avocado oil. Then slice the flank steak in one big fillet (square) and brush it with a cilantro mixture. Then chop the egg roughly and put it on the steak. Add chopped bell pepper. After this, roll the meat and secure it with the kitchen thread. Carefully rub the meat roll with salt and ground black pepper. Then sprinkle the meat roll with peanut oil. Preheat the air fryer to 400F. Put the meat in the air fryer basket and cook it for 25 minutes.

---

474.   Orange Carne Asada

Servings: 4   Cooking Time: 14 Minutes

Ingredients:

¼ lime	1 tablespoon apple cider vinegar
2 tablespoons orange juice	½ teaspoon chili paste
1 teaspoon dried cilantro	
1 chili pepper, chopped	½ teaspoon ground cumin
1 tablespoon sesame oil	½ teaspoon salt
	1-pound beef skirt steak

Directions:

Chop the lime roughly and put it in the blender. Add orange juice, dried cilantro, chili pepper, sesame oil, apple cider vinegar, chili paste, ground cumin, and salt. Blend the mixture until smooth. Cut the skirt steak on 4 servings. Then brush every steak with blended lime mixture and leave for 10 minutes to marinate. Meanwhile, preheat the air fryer to 400F. Put the steaks in the air fryer in one layer and cook them for 7 minutes. Flip the meat on another side and cook it for 7 minutes more.

---

475.   Beef Schnitzel

Servings: 1   Cooking Time: 30 Minutes

Ingredients:

1 egg	1 parsley, roughly chopped
1 thin beef schnitzel	
3 tbsp. friendly bread crumbs	½ lemon, cut in wedges
2 tbsp. olive oil	

Directions:

Pre-heat your Air Fryer to the 360°F.   In a bowl combine the bread crumbs and olive oil to form a loose, crumbly mixture.   Beat the egg with a whisk. Coat the schnitzel first in the egg and then in the bread crumbs, ensuring to cover it fully.   Place the schnitzel in the Air Fryer and cook for 12 – 14 minutes. Garnish the schnitzel with the lemon wedges and parsley before serving.

---

476.   Classic Skirt Steak Strips With Veggies

Servings: 4   Cooking Time: 17 Minutes

Ingredients:

1 (12-ounce) skirt steak, cut into thin strips	¼ cup olive oil, divided
½ pound fresh mushrooms, quartered	2 tablespoons soy sauce
6-ounce snow peas	2 tablespoons honey
1 onion, cut into half rings	Salt and black pepper, to taste

Directions:

Preheat the Air fryer to 390F and grease an Air fryer basket.   Mix 2 tablespoons of oil, soy sauce and honey in a bowl and coat steak strips with this marinade.   Put vegetables, remaining oil, salt and black pepper in another bowl and toss well. Transfer the steak strips and vegetables in the Air fryer basket and cook for about 17 minutes.   Dish out and serve warm.

---

477.   Sloppy Joes With A Twist

Servings: 4   Cooking Time: 45 Minutes

Ingredients:

1 tablespoon olive oil	Keto Buns:
1 shallot, chopped	1/3 cup ricotta cheese, crumbled
2 garlic cloves, minced	2/3 cup part skim mozzarella cheese, shredded
1 bell pepper, chopped	
1 pound ground pork	1 egg
1 ripe medium-sized tomato, pureed	1/3 cup coconut flour
	1/2 cup almond flour
1 tablespoon poultry seasoning blend	1 teaspoon baking soda
Dash ground allspice	1 ½ tablespoons plain whey protein isolate

Directions:

Start by preheating your Air Fryer to 390 degrees F. Heat the olive oil for a few minutes.   Once hot, sauté the shallots until just tender. Add the garlic and bell pepper; cook for 4 minutes more or until they are aromatic. Add the ground pork and cook for 5 minutes more, crumbling with a fork. Next step, stir in the pureed tomatoes and spices. Decrease the temperature to 365 degrees F and cook another 10 minutes. Reserve. To make the keto buns, microwave the cheese for 1 minute 30 seconds, stirring twice. Add the cheese to the bowl of a food processor and blend well. Fold in the egg and mix again. Add in the flour, baking soda, and plain whey protein isolate; blend again. Scrape the batter onto the center of a lightly greased cling film. Form the dough into a disk and transfer to your freezer to cool; cut into 4 pieces and transfer to a parchment-lined baking pan (make sure to grease your hands). Bake in the preheated oven at 400 degrees F for about 14 minutes. Spoon the meat mixture into keto buns and transfer them to the cooking basket. Cook for 7 minutes or until thoroughly warmed.

478. Buttered Filet Mignon

Servings: 4   Cooking Time: 14 Minutes
Ingredients:

2 (6-ounces) filet mignon steaks	Salt and black pepper, to taste
1 tablespoon butter, softened	

Directions:
Preheat the Air fryer to 390F and grease an Air fryer basket. Rub the steak generously with salt and black pepper and coat with butter. Arrange the steaks in the Air fryer basket and cook for about 14 minutes. Dish out the steaks and cut into desired size slices to serve.

479. Beef And Thyme Cabbage Mix

Servings: 4   Cooking Time: 25 Minutes
Ingredients:

2 pounds beef, cubed	A pinch of salt and black pepper
½ pound bacon, chopped	2 tablespoons olive oil
2 shallots, chopped	
1 napa cabbage, shredded	1 teaspoon thyme, dried
2 garlic cloves, minced	1 cup beef stock

Directions:
Heat up a pan that fits the air fryer with the oil over medium-high heat, add the beef and brown for 3 minutes. Add the bacon, shallots and garlic and cook for 2 minutes more. Add the rest of the ingredients, toss, put the pan in the air fryer and cook at 390 degrees F for 20 minutes. Divide between plates and serve.

480. Easy Corn Dog Bites

Servings: 2   Cooking Time: 10 Minutes
Ingredients:

½ cup all-purpose flour	1 ½ cup crushed cornflakes
2 large beef hot dogs, cut in half crosswise	2 large eggs, beaten
	Salt and pepper to taste

Directions:
Preheat the air fryer to 330F. Skewer the hot dogs using the metal skewers included in the double layer rack accessory. In a mixing bowl, combine the flour and eggs to form a batter. Season with salt and pepper to taste. Add water if too dry. Dip the skewered hot dogs in the batter and dredge in cornflakes. Place on the double layer rack accessory and cook for 10 minutes.

481. Bjorn's Beef Steak

Servings: 1   Cooking Time: 15 Minutes
Ingredients:

1 steak, 1-inch thick	Black pepper to taste
1 tbsp. olive oil	Sea salt to taste

Directions:
Place the baking tray inside the Air Fryer and pre-heat for about 5 minutes at 390°F. Brush or spray both sides of the steak with the oil. Season both sides with salt and pepper. Take care when placing the steak in the baking tray and allow to cook for 3 minutes. Flip the meat over, and cook for an additional 3 minutes. Take it out of the fryer and allow to sit for roughly 3 minutes before serving.

482. Max's Meatloaf

Servings: 4   Cooking Time: 35 Minutes
Ingredients:

1 large onion, peeled and diced	1 tbsp. basil
2 kg. minced beef	1 tbsp. oregano
1 tsp. Worcester sauce	1 tbsp. mixed herbs
3 tbsp. tomato ketchup	1 tbsp. friendly bread crumbs
	Salt & pepper to taste

Directions:
In a large bowl, combine the mince with the herbs, Worcester sauce, onion and tomato ketchup, incorporating every component well. Pour in the breadcrumbs and give it another stir. Transfer the mixture to a small dish and cook for 25 minutes in the Air Fryer at 350°F.

483. Bacon Stuffing

Servings: 6   Cooking Time: 10 Minutes
Ingredients:

10 oz uncured bacon, chopped, cooked	2 oz celery stalk, chopped
3 oz hazelnuts, chopped	1/3 cup coconut flour
1 teaspoon dried sage	¼ teaspoon baking powder
½ teaspoon salt	3 tablespoons coconut oil, softened
½ teaspoon ground	

black pepper
1 egg yolk

1 egg, beaten
1 teaspoon sesame oil

Directions:
Make the cornbread: in the mixing bowl mix up coconut flour, baking powder, coconut oil, and beaten egg. Stir the mixture until it is smooth and homogenous. After this, brush the air fryer pan with sesame oil. Put the cornbread mixture in the air fryer pan and flatten it well. Preheat the air fryer to 385F. Put the pan with cornbread in the air fryer and cook it for 5 minutes or until it is light brown. Then remove the cornbread from the air fryer and let it cool well. Meanwhile, in the mixing bowl mix up chopped bacon, hazelnuts, dried sage, salt, and ground black pepper. Add celery stalk and egg yolk, Then crumble the cooked cornbread and add it in the bacon mixture. Stir it well and transfer in the pan. Flatten the mixture well. Cook it in the air fryer at 400F for 5 minutes.

---

484. Curry Pork Roast In Coconut Sauce

Servings: 6   Cooking Time: 60 Minutes
Ingredients:

½ teaspoon curry powder
½ teaspoon ground turmeric powder
1 can unsweetened coconut milk
2 tablespoons fish sauce

1 tablespoons sugar
2 tablespoons soy sauce
3 pounds pork shoulder
Salt and pepper to taste

Directions:
Place all Ingredients in bowl and allow the meat to marinate in the fridge for at least 2 hours.   Preheat the air fryer to 390F.   Place the grill pan accessory in the air fryer.   Grill the meat for 20 minutes making sure to flip the pork every 10 minutes for even grilling and cook in batches.   Meanwhile, pour the marinade in a saucepan and allow to simmer for 10 minutes until the sauce thickens. Baste the pork with the sauce before serving.

---

485. Mexican Beef Mix Recipe

Servings: 8   Cooking Time: 1 Hour And 20 Minutes
Ingredients:

2 yellow onions; chopped.
2 tbsp. cilantro; chopped.
6 garlic cloves; minced
2 lbs. beef roast; cubed
2 green bell peppers; chopped.
1 habanero pepper; chopped.

2 tbsp. olive oil
4 jalapenos; chopped.
14 oz. canned tomatoes; chopped.
1/2 cup water
1 ½ tsp. cumin; ground
1/2 cup black olives; pitted and chopped.
1 tsp. oregano; dried
Salt and black pepper to the taste

Directions:

In a pan that fits your air fryer, combine beef with oil, green bell peppers, onions, jalapenos, habanero pepper, tomatoes, garlic, water, cilantro, oregano, cumin, salt and pepper; stir, put in your air fryer and cook at 300 °F, for 1 hour and 10 minutes. Add olives; stir, divide into bowls and serve.

---

486. Cheesy Mini Meatloaves

Servings: 4   Cooking Time: 50 Minutes
Ingredients:

1 pound ground pork
1/2 pound ground beef
1 package onion soup mix
1/2 cup Romano cheese, grated
2 eggs
1 bell pepper, chopped
1 serrano pepper, minced
2 scallions, chopped

2 cloves garlic, finely chopped
Sea salt and black pepper, to your liking
Glaze:
1/2 cup tomato paste
1 tablespoon brown mustard
1 teaspoon smoked paprika

Directions:
In a large mixing bowl, thoroughly combine all ingredients for meatloaves. Mix with your hands until everything is well incorporated.   Then, shape the mixture into four mini loaves. Transfer them to the cooking basket previously generously greased with cooking oil.   Cook in the preheated Air Fryer at 385 degrees F approximately 43 minutes.   Mix all ingredients for the glaze. Spread the glaze over mini meatloaves and cook for another 6 minutes. Bon appétit!

---

487. Herbed Pork Chops

Servings: 4   Cooking Time: 12 Minutes
Ingredients:

2 garlic cloves, minced
½ tablespoon fresh cilantro, chopped
½ tablespoon fresh rosemary, chopped
½ tablespoon fresh parsley, chopped
1 teaspoon sugar

2 tablespoons olive oil
¾ tablespoon Dijon mustard
1 tablespoon ground coriander
Salt, to taste
2 (6-ounces) (1-inch thick) pork chops

Directions:
In a bowl, mix together the garlic, herbs, oil, mustard, coriander, sugar, and salt.   Add the pork chops and generously coat with marinade.   Cover and refrigerate for about 2-3 hours.   Remove chops from the refrigerator and set aside at room temperature for about 30 minutes.   Set the temperature of air fryer to 390 degrees F. Grease an air fryer basket.   Arrange chops into the prepared air fryer basket in a single layer.   Air fry for about 10-12 minutes.   Remove from air fryer and transfer the chops onto plates.   Serve hot.

488. Fried Sausage And Mushrooms Recipe

Servings: 6   Cooking Time: 50 Minutes
Ingredients:

3 red bell peppers; chopped	2 lbs. pork sausage; sliced
2 sweet onions; chopped.	Salt and black pepper to the taste
1 tbsp. brown sugar	2 lbs. Portobello mushrooms; sliced
1 tsp. olive oil	

Directions:

In a baking dish that fits your air fryer, mix sausage slices with oil, salt, pepper, bell pepper, mushrooms, onion and sugar, toss, introduce in your air fryer and cook at 300 °F, for 40 minutes. Divide among plates and serve right away.

489. Beef Sausage And Vegetable Medley

Servings: 4   Cooking Time: 25 Minutes
Ingredients:

1 pound beef sausage	2 garlic cloves, minced
2 red bell peppers, cut lengthwise	1/2 pound broccoli, cut into chunks
1 poblano pepper, minced	½ celery stalk, sliced
1 sprig rosemary, chopped	½ teaspoon caraway seeds
2 shallots, cut into wedges	1 teaspoon salt

Directions:

Place all the ingredients on the bottom of the Air Fryer basket. Toss until everything is well combined. Roast for approximately 32 minutes at 385 degrees F, stirring once halfway through. Serve warm on a serving platter.

490. Pork Butt With Herb-garlic Sauce

Servings: 4   Cooking Time: 35 Minutes + Marinating Time
Ingredients:

1 pound pork butt, cut into pieces 2-inches long	1 tablespoon olive oil
1 teaspoon golden flaxseed meal	1 tablespoon coconut aminos
1 egg white, well whisked	3 garlic cloves, peeled
Salt and ground black pepper, to taste	1/3 cup fresh parsley leaves
1 teaspoon lemon juice, preferably freshly squeezed	1/3 cup fresh coriander leaves
For the Coriander-Garlic Sauce:	1/2 tablespoon salt
	1 teaspoon lemon juice
	1/3 cup extra-virgin olive oil

Directions:

Combine the pork strips with the flaxseed meal, egg white, salt, pepper, olive oil, coconut aminos, and lemon juice. Cover and refrigerate for 30 to 45 minutes.   After that, spritz the pork strips with a nonstick cooking spray.   Set your Air Fryer to cook at 380 degrees F. Press the power button and air-fry for 15 minutes; pause the machine, shake the basket and cook for 15 more minutes.   Meanwhile, puree the garlic in a food processor until finely minced. Now, puree the parsley, coriander, salt, and lemon juice. With the machine running, carefully pour in the olive oil.   Serve the pork with well-chilled sauce with and enjoy!

491. Classic Keto Cheeseburgers

Servings: 4   Cooking Time: 15 Minutes
Ingredients:

1 ½ pounds ground chuck	1 envelope onion soup mix
Kosher salt and freshly ground black pepper, to taste	1 teaspoon paprika
	4 slices Monterey-Jack cheese

Directions:

In a mixing dish, thoroughly combine ground chuck, onion soup mix, salt, black pepper, and paprika. Then, set your Air Fryer to cook at 385 degrees F. Shape the mixture into 4 patties. Air-fry them for 10 minutes.   Next step, place the slices of cheese on the top of the warm burgers. Air-fry for one minute more.   Serve with mustard and pickled salad of choice. Bon appétit!

492. Grilled Steak On Tomato-olive Salad

Servings: 5   Cooking Time: 50 Minutes
Ingredients:

¼ cup extra virgin olive oil	1 teaspoon paprika
¼ teaspoon cayenne pepper	2 ½ pound flank
½ cup green olives, pitted and sliced	2 pounds cherry tomatoes, halved
1 cup red onion, chopped	2 tablespoons Sherry vinegar
1 tablespoon oil	Salt and pepper to taste

Directions:

Preheat the air fryer to 390F.   Place the grill pan accessory in the air fryer.   Season the steak with salt, pepper, paprika, and cayenne pepper. Brush with oil   Place on the grill pan and cook for 45 to 50 minutes.   Meanwhile, prepare the salad by mixing the remaining ingredients.   Serve the beef with salad.

493. Italian Fennel Lamb

Servings: 6   Cooking Time: 22 Minutes
Ingredients:

18 oz rack of lamb	1 teaspoon fennel seeds
1 teaspoon Italian seasonings	½ teaspoon lemon zest, grated
½ teaspoon cayenne pepper	

½ teaspoon dried thyme
½ teaspoon dried cumin

1 tablespoon coconut oil, melted
½ teaspoon onion powder

Directions:
Sprinkle the rack of lamb with Italian seasonings, cayenne pepper, dried thyme, cumin, fennel seeds, and onion powder. Then sprinkle the meat with lemon zest and coconut oil. Preheat the air fryer to 385F. Put the rack off the lamb in the air fryer basket and cook it for 22 minutes.

494. Beef Bulgogi

Servings: 1   Cooking Time: 15 Minutes
Ingredients:
½ cup sliced mushrooms
1 tbsp diced onion

2 tbsp bulgogi marinade

Directions:
Cut the beef into small pieces and place them in a bowl. Add the bulgogi and mix to coat the beef completely. Cover the bowl and place in the fridge for 3 hours. Preheat the air fryer to 350 F. Transfer the beef to a baking dish; stir in the mushroom and onion. Cook for 10 minutes, until nice and tender. Serve with some roasted potatoes and a green salad.

495. Beef Recipe Texas-rodeo Style

Servings: 6   Cooking Time: 1 Hour
Ingredients:
½ cup honey
½ teaspoon dry mustard
1 clove of garlic, minced
1 tablespoon chili powder

½ cup ketchup
2 onion, chopped
3 pounds beef steak sliced
Salt and pepper to taste

Directions:
Place all ingredients in a Ziploc bag and allow to marinate in the fridge for at least 2 hours.   Preheat the air fryer to 390F.   Place the grill pan accessory in the air fryer.   Grill the beef for 15 minutes per batch making sure that you flip it every 8 minutes for even grilling.   Meanwhile, pour the marinade on a saucepan and allow to simmer over medium heat until the sauce thickens.   Baste the beef with the sauce before serving.

496. Lamb And Vinaigrette

Servings: 4   Cooking Time: 30 Minutes
Ingredients:
A pinch of salt and black pepper
3 garlic cloves, minced
2 teaspoons thyme, chopped

4 lamb loin slices
1/3 cup parsley, chopped
1/3 cup sun-dried tomatoes, chopped
2 tablespoons

2 tablespoons olive oil

balsamic vinegar
2 tablespoons water

Directions:
In a blender, combine all the ingredients except the lamb slices and pulse well. In a bowl, mix the lamb with the tomato vinaigrette and toss well. Put the lamb in your air fryer's basket and cook at 380 degrees F for 15 minutes on each side. Divide everything between plates and serve.

497. Caraway, Sichuan 'n Cumin Lamb Kebabs

Servings: 3   Cooking Time: 1 Hour
Ingredients:
1 ½ pounds lamb shoulder, bones removed and cut into pieces
1 tablespoon Sichuan peppercorns
2 tablespoons cumin seeds, toasted

1 teaspoon sugar
2 teaspoons caraway seeds, toasted
2 teaspoons crushed red pepper flakes
Salt and pepper to taste

Directions:
Place all ingredients in bowl and allow the meat to marinate in the fridge for at least 2 hours.   Preheat the air fryer to 390F.   Place the grill pan accessory in the air fryer.   Grill the meat for 15 minutes per batch.   Flip the meat every 8 minutes for even grilling.

498. Pork With Padrón Peppers And Green Olives

Servings: 4   Cooking Time: 30 Minutes
Ingredients:
1 tablespoon olive oil
8 ounces Padrón peppers
2 pounds pork loin, sliced
1 teaspoon paprika

1 teaspoon Celtic salt
1 heaped tablespoon capers, drained
8 green olives, pitted and halved

Directions:
Drizzle olive oil all over the Padrón peppers; cook them in the preheated Air Fryer at 400 degrees F for 10 minutes, turning occasionally, until well blistered all over and tender-crisp.   Then, turn the temperature to 360 degrees F.   Season the pork loin with salt and paprika. Add the capers and cook for 16 minutes, turning them over halfway through the cooking time.   Serve with olives and the reserved Padrón peppers. Bon appétit!

499. Italian Peperonata With A Twist

Servings: 4   Cooking Time: 35 Minutes
Ingredients:
2 teaspoons canola oil
2 bell peppers, sliced
1 green bell pepper,

1 shallot, sliced
1/2 dried thyme
1 teaspoon dried rosemary

sliced
1 serrano pepper,
sliced
Sea salt and pepper,
to taste

1/2 teaspoon mustard
seeds
1 teaspoon fennel
seeds
2 pounds thin beef
parboiled sausage

Directions:
Brush the sides and bottom of the cooking basket with 1 teaspoon of canola oil. Add the peppers and shallot to the cooking basket.   Toss them with the spices and cook at 390 degrees F for 15 minutes, shaking the basket occasionally. Reserve.   Turn the temperature to 380 degrees F   Then, add the remaining 1 teaspoon of oil. Once hot, add the sausage and cook in the preheated Air Frye for 15 minutes, flipping them halfway through the cooking time.   Serve with reserved pepper mixture. Bon appétit!

500.   Lamb Racks And Fennel Mix Recipe

Servings: 4   Cooking Time: 26 Minutes
Ingredients:
12 oz. lamb racks
2 fennel bulbs; sliced
2 tbsp. olive oil
1/8 cup apple cider
vinegar

1 tbsp. brown sugar
4 figs; cut into halves
Salt and black pepper
to the taste

Directions:
In a bowl; mix fennel with figs, vinegar, sugar and oil, toss to coat well, transfer to a baking dish that fits your air fryer, introduce in your air fryer and cook at 350 °F, for 6 minutes.   Season lamb with salt and pepper, add to the baking dish with the fennel mix and air fry for 10 minutes more. Divide everything on plates and serve.

Fish & Seafood Recipes

501.   Crumbed Cod

Servings: 4   Cooking Time: 7 Minutes

Ingredients:

1 cup flour
4 (4-ounce) skinless
codfish fillets, cut
into rectangular
pieces
6 eggs
2 green chilies, finely
chopped

6 scallions, finely
chopped
4 garlic cloves,
minced
Salt and black
pepper, to taste
2 teaspoons soy sauce

Directions:

Preheat the Air fryer to 375F and grease an Air fryer basket.   Place the flour in a shallow dish and mix remaining ingredients except cod in another shallow dish.   Coat each cod fillet into the flour and then dip in the egg mixture.   Arrange the cod fillets in the Air fryer basket and cook for about 7 minutes. Dish out and serve warm.

502.   Fish Packets

Servings: 2   Cooking Time: 15 Minutes

Ingredients:

2 cod fish fillets
1/2 tsp dried tarragon
1/2 cup bell peppers,
sliced
1/4 cup celery, cut
into julienne

1/2 cup carrots, cut
into julienne
1 tbsp olive oil
1 tbsp lemon juice
2 pats butter, melted
Pepper
Salt

Directions:

In a bowl, mix together butter, lemon juice, tarragon, and salt. Add vegetables and toss well. Set aside. Take two parchments paper pieces to fold vegetables and fish.   Spray fish with cooking spray and season with pepper and salt.   Place a fish fillet on each parchment paper piece and top with vegetables. Fold parchment paper around the fish and vegetables.   Place veggie fish packets into the air fryer basket and cook at 350 F for 15 minutes. Serve and enjoy.

503.   Cod And Shallot Frittata

Servings: 3   Cooking Time: 20 Minutes

Ingredients:

2 cod fillets
6 eggs
1/2 cup milk
1 shallot, chopped
2 garlic cloves,
minced

Sea salt and ground
black pepper, to taste
1/2 teaspoon red
pepper flakes,
crushed

Directions:

Bring a pot of salted water to a boil. Boil the cod fillets for 5 minutes or until it is opaque. Flake the fish into bite-sized pieces.   In a mixing bowl, whisk the eggs and milk. Stir in the shallots, garlic,

salt, black pepper, and red pepper flakes. Stir in the reserved fish.   Pour the mixture into the lightly greased baking pan.   Cook in the preheated Air Fryer at 360 degrees F for 9 minutes, flipping over halfway through. Bon appétit!

504.   Butterflied Prawns With Garlic-sriracha

Servings: 2   Cooking Time: 15 Minutes

Ingredients:

1 tablespoon lime
juice
1 tablespoon sriracha
1-pound large
prawns, shells
removed and cut
lengthwise or
butterflied

1teaspoon fish sauce
2 tablespoons melted
butter
2 tablespoons minced
garlic
Salt and pepper to
taste

Directions:

Preheat the air fryer to 390F.   Place the grill pan accessory in the air fryer.   Season the prawns with the rest of the ingredients.   Place on the grill pan and cook for 15 minutes. Make sure to flip the prawns halfway through the cooking time.

505.   Lobster Tails With Olives And Butter

Servings: 5   Cooking Time: 20 Minutes

Ingredients:

2 pounds fresh
lobster tails, cleaned
and halved, in shells
2 tablespoons butter,
melted
1 teaspoon onion
powder

1 teaspoon cayenne
pepper
Salt and ground black
pepper, to taste
2 garlic cloves,
minced
1 cup green olives

Directions:

In a plastic closeable bag, thoroughly combine all ingredients; shake to combine well.   Transfer the coated lobster tails to the greased cooking basket. Cook in the preheated Air Fryer at 390 degrees for 6 to 7 minutes, shaking the basket halfway through. Work in batches.   Serve with green olives and enjoy!

506.   Butter Flounder Fillets

Servings: 4   Cooking Time: 20 Minutes

Ingredients:

4 flounder fillets,
boneless
A pinch of salt and
black pepper
1 cup parmesan,
grated

4 tablespoons butter,
melted
2 tablespoons olive
oil

Directions:

In a bowl, mix the parmesan with salt, pepper, butter and the oil and stir well. Arrange the fish in a pan that fits the air fryer, spread the parmesan mix all over, introduce in the fryer and cook at 400 degrees F for 20 minutes. Divide between plates and serve with a side salad.

507. Fried Anchovies

Servings: 4   Cooking Time: 6 Minutes
Ingredients:

1-pound anchovies	1 teaspoon salt
¼ cup coconut flour	1 tablespoon lemon
2 eggs, beaten	juice
1 teaspoon ground	1 tablespoon sesame
black pepper	oil

Directions:
Trim and wash anchovies if needed and put in the big bowl. Add salt and ground black pepper. Mix up the anchovies. Then add eggs and stir the fish until you get a homogenous mixture. After this coat every anchovies fish in the coconut flour. Brush the air fryer pan with sesame oil. Place the anchovies in the pan in one layer. Preheat the air fryer to 400F. Put the pan with anchovies in the air fryer and cook them for 6 minutes or until anchovies are golden brown.

508. Rich Crab Croquettes

Servings: 4   Cooking Time: 30 Minutes
Ingredients:

1 ½ lb lump crab meat	½ tsp chopped tarragon
3 egg whites, beaten	½ tsp chopped
⅓ cup sour cream	chives
⅓ cup mayonnaise	1 tsp chopped parsley
1 ½ tbsp olive oil	1 tsp cayenne pepper
1 red pepper, chopped finely	Breading:
⅓ cup chopped red onion	1 ½ cup breadcrumbs
2 ½ tbsp chopped celery	2 tsp olive oil
	1 cup flour
	4 eggs, beaten
	Salt to taste

Directions:
Place a skillet over medium heat on a stovetop, add 1 ½ tbsp olive oil, red pepper, onion, and celery. Sauté for 5 minutes or until sweaty and translucent. Turn off heat. Add the breadcrumbs, the remaining olive oil, and salt to a food processor. Blend to mix evenly; set aside. In 2 separate bowls, add the flour and 4 eggs respectively, set aside.   In a separate bowl, add crabmeat, mayo, egg whites, sour cream, tarragon, chives, parsley, cayenne pepper, and celery sauté and mix evenly. Form bite-sized balls from the mixture and place onto a plate.   Preheat the air fryer to 390 F. Dip each crab meatball (croquettes) in the egg mixture and press them in the breadcrumb mixture. Place the croquettes in the fryer basket, avoid overcrowding. Close the air fryer and cook for 10 minutes or until golden brown. Remove them and plate them. Serve the crab

croquettes with tomato dipping sauce and a side of vegetable fries.

509.   Baked Scallops With Garlic Aioli

Servings: 4   Cooking Time: 10 Minutes
Ingredients:

1 cup bread crumbs	4 tablespoons olive
1/4 cup chopped parsley	oil
16 sea scallops, rinsed and drained	5 cloves garlic, minced
2 shallots, chopped	5 tablespoons butter, melted
3 pinches ground nutmeg	salt and pepper to taste

Directions:
Lightly grease baking pan of air fryer with cooking spray.   Mix in shallots, garlic, melted butter, and scallops. Season with pepper, salt, and nutmeg. In a small bowl, whisk well olive oil and bread crumbs. Sprinkle over scallops.   For 10 minutes, cook on 390F until tops are lightly browned. Serve and enjoy with a sprinkle of parsley.

510.   Italian Sardinas Fritas

Servings: 4   Cooking Time: 1 Hour 15 Minutes
Ingredients:

1 ½ pounds sardines, cleaned and rinsed	1 tablespoon lemon juice
Salt and ground black pepper, to savor	1 tablespoon soy sauce
1 tablespoon Italian seasoning mix	2 tablespoons olive oil

Directions:
Firstly, pat the sardines dry with a kitchen towel. Add salt, black pepper, Italian seasoning mix, lemon juice, soy sauce, and olive oil; marinate them for 30 minutes.   Air-fry the sardines at 350 degrees F for approximately 5 minutes. Increase the temperature to 385 degrees F and air-fry them for further 7 to 8 minutes.   Then, place the sardines in a nice serving platter. Bon appétit!

511. Butter Mussels

Servings: 5   Cooking Time: 2 Minutes
Ingredients:

2-pounds mussels	1 shallot, chopped
1 tablespoon minced garlic	1 teaspoon salt
1 tablespoon butter, melted	1 tablespoon fresh parsley, chopped
1 teaspoon sunflower oil	½ teaspoon chili flakes

Directions:
Clean and wash mussels and put them in the big bowl. Add shallot, minced garlic, butter, sunflower oil, salt, and chili flakes. Shake the mussels well. Preheat the air fryer to 390F. Put the mussels in the air fryer basket and cook for 2 minutes. Then

transfer the cooked meal in the serving bowl and top it with chopped fresh parsley.

512. Swordfish With Roasted Peppers And Garlic Sauce

Servings: 3   Cooking Time: 30 Minutes

Ingredients:

3 bell peppers	2 garlic cloves,
3 swordfish steaks	minced
1 tablespoon butter,	1/2 teaspoon cayenne
melted	pepper
Sea salt and freshly	1/2 teaspoon ginger
ground black pepper,	powder
to taste	

Directions:
Start by preheating your Air Fryer to 400 degrees F. Brush the Air Fryer basket lightly with cooking oil. Then, roast the bell peppers for 5 minutes. Give the peppers a half turn; place them back in the cooking basket and roast for another 5 minutes.   Turn them one more time and roast until the skin is charred and soft or 5 more minutes. Peel the peppers and set aside.   Then, add the swordfish steaks to the lightly greased cooking basket and cook at 400 degrees F for 10 minutes.   Meanwhile, melt the butter in a small saucepan. Cook the garlic until fragrant and add the salt, pepper, cayenne pepper, and ginger powder. Cook until everything is thoroughly heated.   Plate the peeled peppers and the roasted swordfish; spoon the sauce over them and serve warm.

513. Crispy Tilapia Fillets

Servings: 5   Cooking Time: 20 Minutes

Ingredients:

5 tablespoons all-	2 tablespoons extra
purpose flour	virgin olive oil
Sea salt and white	1/2 cup cornmeal
pepper, to taste	5 tilapia fillets, slice
1 teaspoon garlic	into halves
paste	

Directions:
Combine the flour, salt, white pepper, garlic paste, olive oil, and cornmeal in a Ziploc bag. Add the fish fillets and shake to coat well.   Spritz the Air Fryer basket with cooking spray. Cook in the preheated Air Fryer at 400 degrees F for 10 minutes; turn them over and cook for 6 minutes more. Work in batches. Serve with lemon wedges if desired. Enjoy!

514. English-style Flounder Fillets

Servings: 2   Cooking Time: 20 Minutes

Ingredients:

2 flounder fillets	1/2 teaspoon lemon
1/4 cup all-purpose	pepper
flour	1/2 teaspoon coarse
1 egg	sea salt
1/2 teaspoon	1/4 teaspoon chili
Worcestershire sauce	powder
1/2 cup bread crumbs	

Directions:
Rinse and pat dry the flounder fillets.   Place the flour in a large pan.   Whisk the egg and Worcestershire sauce in a shallow bowl. In a separate bowl, mix the bread crumbs with the lemon pepper, salt, and chili powder.   Dredge the fillets in the flour, shaking off the excess. Then, dip them into the egg mixture. Lastly, coat the fish fillets with the breadcrumb mixture until they are coated on all sides.   Spritz with cooking spray and transfer to the Air Fryer basket. Cook at 390 degrees for 7 minutes.   Turn them over, spritz with cooking spray on the other side, and cook another 5 minutes. Bon appétit!

515. Monkfish With Sautéed Vegetables And Olives

Servings: 2   Cooking Time: 20 Minutes

Ingredients:

2 teaspoons olive oil	2 monkfish fillets
2 carrots, sliced	2 tablespoons lime
2 bell peppers, sliced	juice
1 teaspoon dried	Coarse salt and
thyme	ground black pepper,
1/2 teaspoon dried	to taste
marjoram	1 teaspoon cayenne
1/2 teaspoon dried	pepper
rosemary	1/2 cup Kalamata
1 tablespoon soy	olives, pitted and
sauce	sliced

Directions:
In a nonstick skillet, heat the olive oil for 1 minute. Once hot, sauté the carrots and peppers until tender, about 4 minutes. Sprinkle with thyme, marjoram, and rosemary and set aside.   Toss the fish fillets with the soy sauce, lime juice, salt, black pepper, and cayenne pepper. Place the fish fillets in a lightly greased cooking basket and bake at 390 degrees F for 8 minutes.   Turn them over, add the olives, and cook an additional 4 minutes. Serve with the sautéed vegetables on the side. Bon appétit!

516. Crispy Mustardy Fish Fingers

Servings: 4   Cooking Time: 20 Minutes

Ingredients:

1 ½ pounds tilapia	1 teaspoon onion
pieces (fingers)	powder
1/2 cup all-purpose	Sea salt and ground
flour	black pepper, to taste
2 eggs	1/2 teaspoon celery
1 tablespoon yellow	powder
mustard	2 tablespoons peanut
1 cup cornmeal	oil
1 teaspoon garlic	
powder	

Directions:
Pat dry the fish fingers with a kitchen towel.   To make a breading station, place the all-purpose flour in a shallow dish. In a separate dish, whisk the eggs with mustard.   In a third bowl, mix the remaining

ingredients. Dredge the fish fingers in the flour, shaking the excess into the bowl; dip in the egg mixture and turn to coat evenly; then, dredge in the cornmeal mixture, turning a couple of times to coat evenly. Cook in the preheated Air Fryer at 390 degrees F for 5 minutes; turn them over and cook another 5 minutes. Enjoy!

517. Miso Sauce Over Grilled Salmon

Servings: 4   Cooking Time: 16 Minutes

Ingredients:

1/4 cup yellow miso paste	1 1/4 pounds skinless salmon fillets, thinly sliced
2 tablespoons mirin (Japanese rice wine)	Amaranth leaves (optional), to serve
2 teaspoons dashi powder	Shichimi togarashi, to serve
2 teaspoons superfine sugar	

Directions:

In a bowl mix well sugar, mirin, dashi powder, and miso. Thread salmon into skewers. Baste with miso glaze. Place on skewer rack in air fryer. If needed, cook in batches. For 8 minutes, cook on 360F. Halfway through cooking time, turnover and baste. Serve and enjoy.

518. Creamy Salmon

Servings: 2   Cooking Time: 20 Minutes

Ingredients:

¾ lb. salmon, cut into 6 pieces	1 tbsp. dill, chopped
¼ cup yogurt	3 tbsp. sour cream
1 tbsp. olive oil	Salt to taste

Directions:

1 Sprinkle some salt on the salmon. 2 Put the salmon slices in the Air Fryer basket and add in a drizzle of olive oil. 3 Air fry the salmon at 285°F for 10 minutes. 4 In the meantime, combine together the cream, dill, yogurt, and salt. 5 Plate up the salmon and pour the creamy sauce over it. Serve hot.

519. Mahi Mahi With Green Beans

Servings: 4   Cooking Time: 12 Minutes

Ingredients:

5 cups green beans	Salt, as required
2 tablespoons fresh dill, chopped	2 garlic cloves, minced
4 (6-ounces) Mahi Mahi fillets	2 tablespoons fresh lemon juice
1 tablespoon avocado oil	1 tablespoon olive oil

Directions:

Preheat the Air fryer to 375F and grease an Air fryer basket. Mix the green beans, avocado oil and salt in a large bowl. Arrange green beans into the Air fryer basket and cook for about 6 minutes. Combine garlic, dill, lemon juice, salt and olive oil in a bowl. Coat Mahi Mahi in this garlic mixture and place on the top of green beans. Cook for 6 more minutes and dish out to serve warm.

520. Buttered Baked Cod With Wine

Servings: 2   Cooking Time: 12 Minutes

Ingredients:

1 tablespoon butter	1-1/2 teaspoons chopped green onion
1 tablespoon butter	1/2 lemon, cut into wedges
2 tablespoons dry white wine	1/4 sleeve buttery round crackers (such as Ritz®), crushed
1/2 pound thick-cut cod loin	1/4 lemon, juiced
1-1/2 teaspoons chopped fresh parsley	

Directions:

In a small bowl, melt butter in microwave. Whisk in crackers. Lightly grease baking pan of air fryer with remaining butter. And melt for 2 minutes at 390F. In a small bowl whisk well lemon juice, white wine, parsley, and green onion. Coat cod filets in melted butter. Pour dressing. Top with butter-cracker mixture. Cook for 10 minutes at 390F. Serve and enjoy with a slice of lemon.

521. Salmon With Asparagus

Servings: 2   Cooking Time: 11 Minutes

Ingredients:

2 (6-ounces) boneless salmon fillets	1 tablespoon olive oil
1½ tablespoons fresh lemon juice	2 tablespoons fresh dill, roughly chopped
2 tablespoons fresh parsley, roughly chopped	1 bunch asparagus
	Salt and ground black pepper, as required

Directions:

In a small bowl, mix well the lemon juice, oil, herbs, salt, and black pepper. In another large bowl, mix together the salmon and ¾ of oil mixture. In a second large bowl, add the asparagus and remaining oil mixture. Mix them well. Set the temperature of air fryer to 400 degrees F. Grease an air fryer basket. Arrange asparagus into the prepared air fryer basket. Air fry for about 2-3 minutes. Now, place the salmon fillets on top of asparagus and air fry for about 8 minutes. Remove from air fryer and place the salmon fillets onto serving plates. Serve hot alongside the asparagus.

522. Cod Nuggets

Servings: 4   Cooking Time: 25 Minutes

Ingredients:

1 lb. cod fillet, cut into chunks	1 tbsp. egg and water
1 tbsp. olive oil	½ cup flour
1 cup cracker crumbs	Salt and pepper

Directions:

Place the cracker crumbs and oil in food processor and pulse together. Sprinkle the cod pieces with salt and pepper. Roll the cod pieces in the flour before dredging them in egg and coating them in the cracker crumbs. Pre-heat the Air Fryer to 350°F. Put the fish in the basket and air fry to 350°F for 15 minutes or until a light golden-brown color is achieved. Serve hot.

523. Simple Salmon Patties

Servings: 2   Cooking Time: 10 Minutes
Ingredients:

14 oz salmon	1 tsp dill
1/2 onion, diced	1/2 cup almond flour
1 egg, lightly beaten	

Directions:
Spray air fryer basket with cooking spray.   Add all ingredients into the bowl and mix until well combined.   Spray air fryer basket with cooking spray.   Make patties from salmon mixture and place into the air fryer basket.   Cook at 370 F for 5 minutes.   Turn patties to another side and cook for 5 minutes more.   Serve and enjoy.

524. Tartar Sauce 'n Crispy Cod Nuggets

Servings: 3   Cooking Time: 10 Minutes
Ingredients:

½ cup flour	1 tablespoon
½ cup non-fat mayonnaise	vegetable oil
½ teaspoon	1 teaspoon honey
Worcestershire sauce	Juice from half a
1 ½ pounds cod fillet	lemon
1 cup cracker crumbs	Salt and pepper to
1 egg, beaten	taste
1 tablespoon sweet	Zest from half of a
pickle relish	lemon

Directions:
Preheat the air fryer to 390F.   Season the cods with salt and pepper.   Dredge the fish on flour and dip in the beaten egg before dredging on the cracker crumbs. Brush with oil.   Place the fish on the double layer rack and cook for 10 minutes. Meanwhile, prepare the sauce by mixing all ingredients in a bowl.   Serve the fish with the sauce.

525. Shrimp Scampi Linguine

Servings: 4   Cooking Time: 25 Minutes
Ingredients:

1 ½ pounds shrimp, shelled and deveined	1/4 teaspoon cracked black pepper
1/2 tablespoon fresh basil leaves, chopped	1/4 cup chicken stock
2 tablespoons olive oil	2 ripe tomatoes, pureed
2 cloves garlic, minced	8 ounces linguine pasta
1/2 teaspoon fresh ginger, grated	1/2 cup parmesan cheese, preferably freshly grated
1/2 teaspoon sea salt	

Directions:

Start by preheating the Air Fryer to 395 degrees F. Place the shrimp, basil, olive oil, garlic, ginger, black pepper, salt, chicken stock, and tomatoes in the casserole dish.   Transfer the casserole dish to the cooking basket and bake for 10 minutes.   Bring a large pot of lightly salted water to a boil. Cook the linguine for 10 minutes or until al dente; drain. Divide between four serving plates. Add the shrimp sauce and top with parmesan cheese. Bon appétit!

526. Cayenne Salmon

Servings: 3   Cooking Time: 9 Minutes
Ingredients:

1-pound salmon	½ teaspoon cayenne
1 tablespoon Erythritol	pepper
1 tablespoon coconut oil, melted	1 teaspoon water
	¼ teaspoon ground nutmeg

Directions:
In the small bowl mix up Erythritol and water. Then rub the salmon with ground nutmeg and cayenne pepper. After this, brush the fish with Erythritol liquid and sprinkle with melted coconut oil. Put the salmon on the foil. Preheat the air fryer to 385F. Transfer the foil with salmon in the air fryer basket and cook for 9 minutes.

527. Soy Sauce Glazed Cod

Servings: 1   Cooking Time: 15 Minutes
Ingredients:

1 tsp olive oil	Dash of sesame oil
A pinch of sea salt	
A pinch of pepper	¼ tsp ginger powder
1 tbsp soy sauce	¼ tsp honey

Directions:
Preheat air fryer to 370 degrees. Combine olive oil, salt and pepper, and brush that mixture over the cod. Place the cod onto an aluminum sheet and then into the air fryer; cook for 6 minutes. Combine the soy sauce, ginger, honey, and sesame oil. Brush the glaze over the cod. Flip the fillet over and cook for 3 more minutes.

528. Chili Salmon Recipe

Servings: 12   Cooking Time: 25 Minutes
Ingredients:

1¼ cups coconut; shredded	1/4 cup balsamic vinegar
1 lb. salmon; cubed	A pinch of salt and
1/3 cup flour	black pepper
4 red chilies; chopped	1 egg
3 garlic cloves; minced	2 tbsp. olive oil
	1/4 cup water
	1/2 cup honey

Directions:
In a bowl; mix flour with a pinch of salt and stir.   In another bowl; mix egg with black pepper and whisk.   Put coconut in a third bowl.   Dip salmon cubes in flour, egg and coconut, put them in

your air fryer's basket, cook at 370 °F, for 8 minutes; shaking halfway and divide among plates.   Heat up a pan with the water over medium high heat, add chilies, cloves, vinegar and honey; stir very well, bring to a boil, simmer for a couple of minutes; drizzle over salmon and serve.

529.   Paprika And Cumin Shrimp

Servings: 4   Cooking Time: 10 Minutes

Ingredients:

1 teaspoon chili flakes	2 spring onions,
1 teaspoon ground	chopped
cumin	1 teaspoon apple
½ teaspoon salt	cider vinegar
½ teaspoon dried	1 tablespoon olive oil
oregano	1 teaspoon smoked
10 oz shrimps, peeled	paprika
1 green bell pepper	

Directions:
In the mixing bowl mix up chili flakes, ground cumin, salt, dried oregano, and shrimps. Shake the mixture well. After this, preheat the air fryer to 400F. Put the spring onions in the air fryer and cook it for 3 minutes. Meanwhile, slice the bell pepper. Add it in the air fryer and cook the vegetables for 2 minutes more. Then add shrimps and sprinkle the mixture with smoked paprika, olive oil, and apple cider vinegar. Shake it gently and cook for 5 minutes more. Transfer the cooked fajita in the serving plates.

530.   Delicious Prawns And Sweet Potatoes

Servings: 4   Cooking Time: 20 Minutes

Ingredients:

1 shallot, chopped	2 tablespoons dried
1 red chili pepper,	rosemary
seeded and chopped	1/3 cup olive oil,
finely	divided
12 king prawns,	4 garlic cloves,
peeled and deveined	minced
5 large sweet	Smoked paprika, to
potatoes, peeled and	taste
cut into slices	1 tablespoon honey
4 lemongrass stalks	

Directions:
Preheat the Air fryer to 355F and grease an Air fryer basket.   Mix ¼ cup of the olive oil, shallot, red chili pepper, garlic and paprika in a bowl.   Add prawns and coat evenly with the mixture.   Thread the prawns onto lemongrass stalks and refrigerate to marinate for about 3 hours.   Mix sweet potatoes, honey and rosemary in a bowl and toss to coat well. Arrange the potatoes in the Air fryer basket and cook for about 15 minutes.   Remove the sweet potatoes from the Air fryer and set the Air fryer to 390 degrees F.   Place the prawns in the Air fryer basket and cook for about 5 minutes.   Dish out in a bowl and serve with sweet potatoes.

531.   Coconut Calamari

Servings: 2   Cooking Time: 6 Minutes

Ingredients:

6 oz calamari,	1 egg, beaten
trimmed	1 teaspoon Italian
2 tablespoons	seasonings
coconut flakes	Cooking spray

Directions:
Slice the calamari into the rings and sprinkle them with Italian seasonings. Then transfer the calamari rings in the bowl with a beaten egg and stir them gently. After this, sprinkle the calamari rings with coconut flakes and shake well. Preheat the air fryer to 400F. Put the calamari rings in the air fryer basket and spray them with cooking spray. Cook the meal for 3 minutes. Then gently stir the calamari and cook them for 3 minutes more.

532.   Cajun Seasoned Salmon Filet

Servings: 1   Cooking Time: 15 Minutes

Ingredients:

1 teaspoon juice from	1 salmon fillet
lemon, freshly	A dash of Cajun
squeezed	seasoning mix
3 tablespoons extra	Salt and pepper to
virgin olive oil	taste

Directions:
Preheat the air fryer for 5 minutes.   Place all ingredients in a bowl and toss to coat.   Place the fish fillet in the air fryer basket.   Bake for 15 minutes at 325F.   Once cooked drizzle with olive oil

533.   Butter Crab Muffins

Servings: 2   Cooking Time: 20 Minutes

Ingredients:

5 oz crab meat,	½ teaspoon apple
chopped	cider vinegar
2 eggs, beaten	
2 tablespoons almond	½ teaspoon ground
flour	paprika
¼ teaspoon baking	1 tablespoon butter,
powder	softened
	Cooking spray

Directions:
Grind the chopped crab meat and put it in the bowl. Add eggs, almond flour, baking powder, apple cider vinegar, ground paprika, and butter. Stir the mixture until homogenous. Preheat the air fryer to 365F. Spray the muffin molds with cooking spray. Then pour the crab meat batter in the muffin molds and place them in the preheated air fryer. Cook the crab muffins for 20 minutes or until they are light brown. Cool the cooked muffins to the room temperature and remove from the muffin mold.

534.   Smoked And Creamed White Fish

Servings: 4   Cooking Time: 20 Minutes

Ingredients:
1/2 tablespoon yogurt
1/3 cup spring garlic, finely chopped
Fresh chopped chives, for garnish
3 eggs, beaten
1/2 teaspoon dried dill weed
1 teaspoon dried rosemary
1/3 cup scallions, chopped
1/3 cup smoked white fish, chopped
1 ½ tablespoons crème fraîche
1 teaspoon kosher salt
1 teaspoon dried marjoram
1/3 teaspoon ground black pepper, or more to taste
Cooking spray

Directions:
Firstly, spritz four oven safe ramekins with cooking spray. Then, divide smoked whitefish, spring garlic, and scallions among greased ramekins.   Crack an egg into each ramekin; add the crème, yogurt and all seasonings.   Now, air-fry approximately 13 minutes at 355 degrees F. Taste for doneness and eat warm garnished with fresh chives. Bon appétit!

---

535. Lime Cod

Servings: 4   Cooking Time: 14 Minutes
Ingredients:
4 cod fillets, boneless
1 tablespoon olive oil
Juice of 1 lime
Salt and black pepper to the taste
2 teaspoons sweet paprika

Directions:
In a bowl, mix all the ingredients, transfer the fish to your air fryer's basket and cook 350 degrees F for 7 minutes on each side. Divide the fish between plates and serve with a side salad.

---

536. Salmon Cakes

Servings: 4   Cooking Time: 15 Minutes
Ingredients:
14 oz boiled and mashed potatoes
2 oz flour
A handful of capers
A handful of chopped parsley
1 tsp olive oil
zest of 1 lemon

Directions:
Place the mashed potatoes in a large bowl and flake the salmon over. Stir in capers, parsley, and lemon zest. Shape small cakes out of the mixture. Dust them with flour and place in the fridge to set, for 1 hour. Preheat the air fryer to 350 F. Brush the olive oil over the basket's bottom and add the cakes. Cook for 7 minutes.

---

537. Cod Fillets With Lemon And Mustard

Servings: 2   Cooking Time: 20 Minutes
Ingredients:
2 medium-sized cod fillets
1/2 tablespoon fresh lemon juice
1 ½ tablespoons olive oil
1/2 tablespoon whole-grain mustard

Sea salt and ground black pepper, to savor
1/2 cup coconut flour
2 eggs

Directions:
Set your Air Fryer to cook at 355 degrees F. Thoroughly combine olive oil and coconut flour in a shallow bowl.   In another shallow bowl, whisk the egg. Drizzle each cod fillet with lemon juice and spread with mustard. Then, sprinkle each fillet with salt and ground black pepper.   Dip each fish fillet into the whisked egg; now, roll it in the olive oil/breadcrumb mix.   Place in a single layer in the Air Fryer cooking basket. Cook for 10 minutes, working in batches, turning once or twice. Serve with potato salad. Bon appétit!

---

538. Wrapped Scallops

Servings: 4   Cooking Time: 7 Minutes
Ingredients:
1 teaspoon ground coriander
½ teaspoon ground paprika
¼ teaspoon salt
16 oz scallops
4 oz bacon, sliced
1 teaspoon sesame oil

Directions:
Sprinkle the scallops with ground coriander, ground paprika, and salt. Then wrap the scallops in the bacon slices and secure with toothpicks. Sprinkle the scallops with sesame oil. Preheat the air fryer to 400F. Put the scallops in the air fryer basket and cook them for 7 minutes.

---

539. Creamy Tuna Cakes

Servings: 4   Cooking Time: 15 Minutes
Ingredients:
2 (6-ounces) cans tuna, drained
1½ tablespoon almond flour
1½ tablespoons mayonnaise
1 tablespoon fresh lemon juice
1 teaspoon dried dill
1 teaspoon garlic powder
½ teaspoon onion powder
Pinch of salt and ground black pepper

Directions:
Preheat the Air fryer to 400F and grease an Air fryer basket.   Mix the tuna, mayonnaise, almond flour, lemon juice, dill, and spices in a large bowl.   Make 4 equal-sized patties from the mixture and arrange in the Air fryer basket.   Cook for about 10 minutes and flip the sides.   Cook for 5 more minutes and dish out the tuna cakes in serving plates to serve warm.

---

540. Fried Haddock Fillets

Servings: 2   Cooking Time: 20 Minutes
Ingredients:
2 haddock fillets
1/2 cup parmesan cheese, freshly grated
1 teaspoon dried parsley flakes
1 egg, beaten
1/4 teaspoon ground black pepper
1/4 teaspoon cayenne pepper

1/2 teaspoon coarse sea salt

2 tablespoons olive oil

Directions:

Start by preheating your Air Fryer to 360 degrees F. Pat dry the haddock fillets and set aside. In a shallow bowl, thoroughly combine the parmesan and parsley flakes. Mix until everything is well incorporated. In a separate shallow bowl, whisk the egg with salt, black pepper, and cayenne pepper. Dip the haddock fillets into the egg. Then, dip the fillets into the parmesan mixture until well coated on all sides. Drizzle the olive oil all over the fish fillets. Lower the coated fillets into the lightly greased Air Fryer basket. Cook for 11 to 13 minutes. Bon appétit!

---

541. Crispy Cod Sticks

Servings: 2   Cooking Time: 7 Minutes

Ingredients:

3 (4-ounces) skinless cod fillets, cut into rectangular pieces

¾ cup flour

1 green chili, finely chopped

4 eggs

2 garlic cloves, minced

2 teaspoons light soy sauce

Salt and ground black pepper, to taste

Directions:

Preheat the Air fryer to 375F and grease an Air fryer basket. Place flour in a shallow dish and whisk the eggs, garlic, green chili, soy sauce, salt, and black pepper in a second dish. Coat the cod fillets evenly in flour and dip in the egg mixture. Arrange the cod pieces in an Air fryer basket and cook for about 7 minutes. Dish out and serve warm.

---

542. Lemon Garlic Shrimp

Servings: 2   Cooking Time: 15 Minutes

Ingredients:

½ lb. medium shrimp, shelled and deveined

½ tsp. Old Bay seasoning

1 medium lemon

2 tbsp. unsalted butter, melted

½ tsp. minced garlic

Directions:

Grate the rind of the lemon into a bowl. Cut the lemon in half and juice it over the same bowl. Toss in the shrimp, Old Bay, and butter, mixing everything to make sure the shrimp is completely covered. Transfer to a round baking dish roughly six inches wide, then place this dish in your fryer. Cook at 400°F for six minutes. The shrimp is cooked when it turns a bright pink color. Serve hot, drizzling any leftover sauce over the shrimp.

---

543. Paprika Tilapia

Servings: 4   Cooking Time: 20 Minutes

Ingredients:

4 tilapia fillets, boneless

3 tablespoons ghee, melted

A pinch of salt and black pepper

1 teaspoon garlic powder

2 tablespoons capers

½ teaspoon smoked paprika

½ teaspoon oregano, dried

2 tablespoons lemon juice

Directions:

In a bowl, mix all the ingredients except the fish and toss. Arrange the fish in a pan that fits the air fryer, pour the capers mix all over, put the pan in the air fryer and cook 360 degrees F for 20 minutes, shaking halfway. Divide between plates and serve hot.

---

544. Beer Battered Cod Filet

Servings: 2   Cooking Time: 15 Minutes

Ingredients:

½ cup all-purpose flour

¾ teaspoon baking powder

1 ¼ cup lager beer

2 cod fillets

2 eggs, beaten

Salt and pepper to taste

Directions:

Preheat the air fryer to 390F. Pat the fish fillets dry then set aside. In a bowl, combine the rest of the Ingredients to create a batter. Dip the fillets on the batter and place on the double layer rack. Cook for 15 minutes.

---

545. Creamy Shrimp

Servings: 4   Cooking Time: 8 Minutes

Ingredients:

1 lb shrimp, peeled

1 tbsp garlic, minced

1 tbsp tomato ketchup

3 tbsp mayonnaise

1/2 tsp paprika

1 tsp sriracha

1/2 tsp salt

Directions:

In a bowl, mix together mayonnaise, paprika, sriracha, garlic, ketchup, and salt. Add shrimp and stir well. Add shrimp mixture into the air fryer baking dish and place in the air fryer. Cook at 325 F for 8 minutes. Stir halfway through. Serve and enjoy.

---

546. Louisiana-style Shrimp

Servings: 4   Cooking Time: 18 Minutes

Ingredients:

1 egg, beaten

¼ cup white breadcrumbs

2 tbsp Cajun seasoning

¼ cup flour

Salt and black pepper to taste

1 lemon, cut into wedges

Directions:

Preheat your Air Fryer to 390 F. Spray the air fryer basket with cooking spray. Beat the eggs in a bowl and season with salt and black pepper. In a separate bowl, mix white breadcrumbs with Cajun seasoning. In a third bowl, pour the flour. Dip the shrimp in the flour and then in the eggs, and finally in the breadcrumb mixture. Spray with cooking spray and place in the cooking basket. Cook for 6 minutes, Slide out the fryer basket and flip; cook for 6 more minutes. Serve with lemon wedges.

547. Crispy Fish Fingers With Lemon-garlic Herbs

Servings: 1   Cooking Time: 10 Minutes
Ingredients:

¼ teaspoon baking soda	1 cup bread crumbs
½ pound fish, cut into fingers	1 teaspoon ginger garlic paste
½ teaspoon crushed black pepper	2 eggs, beaten
½ teaspoon red chili flakes	2 tablespoons lemon juice
½ teaspoon salt	2 teaspoons corn flour
½ teaspoon turmeric powder	2 teaspoons garlic powder
	Oil for brushing

Directions:
Preheat the air fryer to 390F. Season the fish fingers with salt, lemon juice, turmeric powder, chili flakes, garlic powder, black pepper, and garlic paste. Add the corn flour, eggs, and baking soda. Dredge the seasoned fish in breadcrumbs and brush with cooking oil. Place on the double layer rack. Cook for 10 minutes.

548. Garlic Shrimp Mix

Servings: 3   Cooking Time: 5 Minutes
Ingredients:

1-pound shrimps, peeled	¼ teaspoon lemon zest, grated
½ teaspoon garlic powder	½ tablespoon avocado oil
¼ teaspoon minced garlic	½ teaspoon dried parsley
1 teaspoon ground cumin	

Directions:
In the mixing bowl mix up shrimps, garlic powder, minced garlic, ground cumin, lemon zest, and dried parsley. Then add avocado oil and mix up the shrimps well. Preheat the air fryer to 400F. Put the shrimps in the preheated air fryer basket and cook for 5 minutes.

549. Spicy Cod

Servings: 2   Cooking Time: 11 Minutes
Ingredients:

2 (6-ounces) (1½-inch thick) cod fillets	1 teaspoon onion powder
1 teaspoon smoked paprika	1 teaspoon garlic powder
1 teaspoon cayenne	Salt and ground black pepper, as required

pepper
2 teaspoons olive oil
Directions:
Preheat the Air fryer to 390F and grease an Air fryer basket. Drizzle the salmon fillets with olive oil and rub with the all the spices. Arrange the salmon fillets into the Air fryer basket and cook for about 11 minutes. Dish out the salmon fillets in the serving plates and serve hot.

550. Crab Stuffed Flounder

Servings: 3   Cooking Time: 12 Minutes
Ingredients:

9 oz flounder fillets	2 spring onions, diced
4 oz crab meat, chopped	½ teaspoon dried thyme
1 tablespoon mascarpone	2 oz Parmesan, grated
½ teaspoon ground nutmeg	1 egg, beaten

Directions:
Line the air fryer baking pan with baking paper. After this, cut the flounder fillet on3 servings and transfer them in the baking pan in one layer. Sprinkle the fish fillets with ground nutmeg and dried thyme. Then top them with chopped crab meat, spring onions, and Parmesan. In the mixing bowl, mix up mascarpone and egg. Pour the liquid over the cheese. Preheat the air fryer to 385F. Place the baking pan with fish in the air fryer and cook the meal for 12 minutes.

551. Summer Fish Packets

Servings: 2   Cooking Time: 20 Minutes
Ingredients:

2 snapper fillets	1 tomato, sliced
1 shallot, peeled and sliced	1 tablespoon olive oil
2 garlic cloves, halved	1/4 teaspoon freshly ground black pepper
1 bell pepper, sliced	1/2 teaspoon paprika
1 small-sized serrano pepper, sliced	Sea salt, to taste
	2 bay leaves

Directions:
Place two parchment sheets on a working surface. Place the fish in the center of one side of the parchment paper. Top with the shallot, garlic, peppers, and tomato. Drizzle olive oil over the fish and vegetables. Season with black pepper, paprika, and salt. Add the bay leaves. Fold over the other half of the parchment. Now, fold the paper around the edges tightly and create a half moon shape, sealing the fish inside. Cook in the preheated Air Fryer at 390 degrees F for 15 minutes. Serve warm.

552. Thyme Catfish

Servings: 4   Cooking Time: 12 Minutes
Ingredients:

20 oz catfish fillet (4 oz each fillet)	½ teaspoon salt
	1 teaspoon avocado

2 eggs, beaten
1 teaspoon dried thyme
1 teaspoon apple cider vinegar

oil
¼ teaspoon cayenne pepper
1/3 cup coconut flour

Directions:
Sprinkle the catfish fillets with dried thyme, salt, apple cider vinegar, cayenne pepper, and coconut flour. Then sprinkle the fish fillets with avocado oil. Preheat the air fryer to 385F. Put the catfish fillets in the air fryer basket and cook them for 8 minutes. Then flip the fish on another side and cook for 4 minutes more.

553. Creole Crab

Servings: 6   Cooking Time: 6 Minutes

Ingredients:

1 teaspoon Creole seasonings
4 tablespoons almond flour
¼ teaspoon baking powder
1 teaspoon apple cider vinegar

¼ teaspoon onion powder
1 teaspoon dried dill
1 teaspoon ghee
13 oz crab meat, finely chopped
1 egg, beaten
Cooking spray

Directions:
In the mixing bowl mix up crab meat, egg, dried dill, ghee, onion powder, apple cider vinegar, baking powder, and Creole seasonings. Then add almond flour and stir the mixture with the help of the fork until it is homogenous. Make the small balls (hushpuppies). Preheat the air fryer to 390F. Put the hushpuppies in the air fryer basket and spray with cooking spray. Cook them for 3 minutes. Then flip them on another side and cook for 3 minutes more or until the hushpuppies are golden brown.

554. Sunday Fish With Sticky Sauce

Servings: 2   Cooking Time: 20 Minutes

Ingredients:

2 pollack fillets
Salt and black pepper, to taste
1 tablespoon olive oil
2 tablespoons light soy sauce
1 tablespoon brown sugar

1 cup chicken broth
2 tablespoons butter, melted
1 teaspoon fresh ginger, minced
1 teaspoon fresh garlic, minced
2 corn tortillas

Directions:
Pat dry the pollack fillets and season them with salt and black pepper; drizzle the sesame oil all over the fish fillets.   Preheat the Air Fryer to 380 degrees F and cook your fish for 11 minutes. Slice into bite-sized pieces.   Meanwhile, prepare the sauce. Add the broth to a large saucepan and bring to a boil. Add the soy sauce, sugar, butter, ginger, and garlic. Reduce the heat to simmer and cook until it is reduced slightly.   Add the fish pieces to the warm sauce. Serve on corn tortillas and enjoy!

555. Best Cod Ever

Servings: 2   Cooking Time: 7 Minutes

Ingredients:

2 (4-ounce) skinless codfish fillets, cut into rectangular pieces
½ cup flour
3 eggs
1 green chili, chopped finely

3 scallions, chopped finely
2 garlic cloves, minced
1 teaspoon light soy sauce
Salt and black pepper, to taste

Directions:
Preheat the Air fryer to 375F and grease an Air fryer basket.   Place the flour in a shallow dish and mix remaining ingredients in another shallow dish except cod.   Coat each fillet with the flour and then dip into the egg mixture.   Place the cod in the Air fryer basket and cook for about 7 minutes. Dish out in a platter and serve warm.

556. Stevia Cod

Servings: 4   Cooking Time: 14 Minutes

Ingredients:

2 tablespoons coconut aminos
4 cod fillets, boneless

1/3 cup stevia
A pinch of salt and black pepper

Directions:
In a pan that fits the air fryer, combine all the ingredients and toss gently. Introduce the pan in the fryer and cook at 350 degrees F for 14 minutes, flipping the fish halfway. Divide everything between plates and serve.

557. Chili Sea Bass Mix

Servings: 4   Cooking Time: 15 Minutes

Ingredients:

4 sea bass fillets, boneless
4 garlic cloves, minced
Juice of 1 lime
1 cup veggie stock
A pinch of salt and black pepper

1 tablespoon black peppercorns, crushed
1-inch ginger, grated
4 lemongrass, chopped
4 small chilies, minced
1 bunch coriander, chopped

Directions:
In a blender, combine all the ingredients except the fish and pulse well. Pour the mix in a pan that fits the air fryer, add the fish, toss, introduce in the fryer and cook at 380 degrees F for 15 minutes. Divide between plates and serve.

558. Cajun Fish Cakes With Cheese

Servings: 4   Cooking Time: 30 Minutes

Ingredients:

2 catfish fillets
1 cup all-purpose flour
1 teaspoon baking

3 ounces butter
1/2 cup buttermilk
1 teaspoon Cajun seasoning

powder
1 teaspoon baking soda

1 cup Swiss cheese, shredded

Directions:
Bring a pot of salted water to a boil. Boil the fish fillets for 5 minutes or until it is opaque. Flake the fish into small pieces. Mix the remaining ingredients in a bowl; add the fish and mix until well combined. Shape the fish mixture into 12 patties. Cook in the preheated Air Fryer at 380 degrees F for 15 minutes. Work in batches. Enjoy!

559. Grilled Shrimp With Chipotle-orange Seasoning

Servings: 2   Cooking Time: 24 Minutes

Ingredients:

3 tablespoons minced chipotles in adobo sauce
salt

½-pound large shrimps
juice of 1/2 orange
1/4 cup barbecue sauce

Directions:
In a small shallow dish, mix well all Ingredients except for shrimp. Save ¼ of the mixture for basting. Add shrimp in dish and toss well to coat. Marinate for at least 10 minutes.   Thread shrimps in skewers. Place on skewer rack in air fryer.   For 12 minutes, cook on 360F. Halfway through cooking time, turnover skewers and baste with sauce. If needed, cook in batches.   Serve and enjoy.

560. Grilled Salmon Fillets

Servings: 2   Cooking Time: 20 Minutes

Ingredients:

2 salmon fillets
⅓ cup of water
⅓ cup of light soy sauce
⅓ cup sugar

2 tbsp. olive oil
Black pepper and salt to taste
Garlic powder [optional]

Directions:
1 Sprinkle some salt and pepper on top of the salmon fillets. Season with some garlic powder if desired. 2 In a medium bowl, mix together the remaining ingredients with a whisk and use this mixture to coat the salmon fillets. Leave to marinate for 2 hours. 3 Pre-heat the Air Fryer at 355°F.   4 Remove any excess liquid from the salmon fillets and transfer to the fryer. Cook for 8 minutes before serving warm.

561. Tuna Steaks With Pearl Onions

Servings: 4   Cooking Time: 20 Minutes

Ingredients:

4 tuna steaks
1 pound pearl onions
4 teaspoons olive oil
1 teaspoon dried rosemary

1 tablespoon cayenne pepper
1/2 teaspoon sea salt
1/2 teaspoon black pepper, preferably

1 teaspoon dried marjoram

freshly cracked
1 lemon, sliced

Directions:
Place the tuna steaks in the lightly greased cooking basket. Top with the pearl onions; add the olive oil, rosemary, marjoram, cayenne pepper, salt, and black pepper.   Bake in the preheated Air Fryer at 400 degrees F for 9 to 10 minutes. Work in two batches.   Serve warm with lemon slices and enjoy!

562. Shrimp Magic

Servings: 3   Cooking Time: 5 Minutes

Ingredients:

1½ pounds shrimps, peeled and deveined
4 garlic cloves, minced
1 red chili pepper, seeded and chopped

Lemongrass stalks
2 tablespoons olive oil
½ teaspoon smoked paprika

Directions:
Preheat the Air fryer to 390F and grease an Air fryer basket.   Mix all the ingredients in a large bowl and refrigerate to marinate for about 2 hours.   Thread the shrimps onto lemongrass stalks and transfer into the Air fryer basket.   Cook for about 5 minutes and dish out to serve warm.

563. Mediterranean Salad

Servings: 2   Cooking Time: 15 Minutes

Ingredients:

1 red bell pepper, chopped
2 prosciutto slices, chopped
¼ cup chopped kalamata olives
½ cup crumbled feta cheese

1 cup cooked quinoa
1 tsp. olive oil
1 tsp. dried oregano
6 cherry tomatoes, halved
Salt and pepper, to taste

Directions:
1 Pre-heat your Air Fryer to 350°F.   2 Drizzle the inside of the fryer with the olive oil. Place the red bell pepper inside and allow to cook for roughly 2 minutes. Put the prosciutto slices in the fryer and cook for an additional 3 minutes.   3 Put the ham and pepper in an oven-proof bowl and remove any excess grease. Combine with the remaining ingredients, save for the tomatoes.   4 Finally, stir in the cherry tomato halves.

564. Old Bay Calamari

Servings: 3   Cooking Time: 20 Minutes + Marinating Time

Ingredients:

1 cup beer
1 pound squid, cleaned and cut into rings
1 cup all-purpose flour
2 eggs

1/2 cup cornstarch
Sea salt, to taste
1/2 teaspoon ground black pepper
1 tablespoon Old Bay seasoning

Directions:
Add the beer and squid in a glass bowl, cover and let it sit in your refrigerator for 1 hour. Preheat your Air Fryer to 390 degrees F. Rinse the squid and pat it dry. Place the flour in a shallow bowl. In another bowl, whisk the eggs. Add the cornstarch and seasonings to a third shallow bowl. Dredge the calamari in the flour. Then, dip them into the egg mixture; finally, coat them with the cornstarch on all sided. Arrange them in the cooking basket. Spritz with cooking oil and cook for 9 to 12 minutes, depending on the desired level of doneness. Work in batches. Serve warm with your favorite dipping sauce. Enjoy!

565.	**Breaded Scallops**

Servings: 6   Cooking Time: 5 Minutes
Ingredients:

3 tbsp flour	1 egg, lightly beaten
4 salt and black pepper	1 cup breadcrumbs
	Cooking spray

Directions:
Coat the scallops with flour. Dip into the egg, then into the breadcrumbs. Spray them with olive oil and arrange them in the air fryer. Cook for 6 minutes at 360 F, turning once halfway through cooking.

566.	**Lemony-sage On Grilled Swordfish**

Servings: 2   Cooking Time: 16 Minutes
Ingredients:

½ lemon, sliced thinly in rounds	1/2-pound swordfish, sliced into 2-inch chunks
1 tbsp lemon juice	
1 tsp parsley	2 tbsp olive oil
1 zucchini, peeled and then thinly sliced in lengths	6-8 sage leaves
	salt and pepper to taste

Directions:
In a shallow dish, mix well lemon juice, parsley, and sliced swordfish. Toss well to coat and generously season with pepper and salt. Marinate for at least 10 minutes. Place one length of zucchini on a flat surface. Add one piece of fish and sage leaf. Roll zucchini and then thread into a skewer. Repeat process to remaining Ingredients. Brush with oil and place on skewer rack in air fryer. For 8 minutes, cook on 390F. If needed, cook in batches. Serve and enjoy with lemon slices.

567.	**Tuna Cake Burgers With Beer Cheese Sauce**

Servings: 4   Cooking Time: 2 Hours 20 Minutes
Ingredients:

1 pound canned tuna, drained	1 egg, whisked
1 garlic clove, minced	1 tablespoon sesame oil
2 tablespoons shallots, minced	Beer Cheese Sauce:
1 cup fresh	1 tablespoon butter
	1 cup beer

breadcrumbs	1 tablespoon rice flour
Sea salt and ground black pepper, to taste	2 tablespoons Colby cheese, grated

Directions:
In a mixing bowl, thoroughly combine the tuna, egg, garlic, shallots, breadcrumbs, salt, and black pepper. Shape the tuna mixture into four patties and place in your refrigerator for 2 hours. Brush the patties with sesame oil on both sides. Cook in the preheated Air Fryer at 360 degrees F for 14 minutes. In the meantime, melt the butter in a pan over a moderate heat. Add the beer and flour and whisk until it starts bubbling. Now, stir in the grated cheese and cook for 3 to 4 minutes longer or until the cheese has melted. Spoon the sauce over the fish cake burgers and serve immediately.

568.	**Sesame Prawns With Firecracker Sauce**

Servings: 4   Cooking Time: 20 Minutes
Ingredients:

Salt and black pepper to taste	Firecracker sauce
1 egg	⅓ cup sour cream
½ cup flour	2 tbsp buffalo sauce
¼ cup sesame seeds	¼ cup spicy ketchup
¾ cup seasoned breadcrumbs	1 green onion, chopped

Directions:
Preheat your Air Fryer to 390 F. Spray the air fryer basket with cooking spray. Beat the eggs in a bowl with salt. In a separate bowl, mix seasoned breadcrumbs with sesame seeds. In a third bowl, pour the flour mixed with black pepper. Dip prawns in the flour and then in the eggs, and finally in the breadcrumb mixture. Spray with cooking spray and add to the cooking basket. Cook for 10 minutes, flipping halfway through. Meanwhile, mix well all the sauce ingredients, except for the green onion in a bowl. Serve the prawns with firecracker sauce.

569.	**Cheesy Crab Dip**

Servings: 4   Cooking Time: 7 Minutes
Ingredients:

1 cup crabmeat, cooked	2 cups Jalapeno jack cheese, grated
2 tbsp fresh parsley, chopped	1/2 cup green onions, sliced
2 tbsp fresh lemon juice	1/4 cup mayonnaise
2 tbsp hot sauce	1 tsp pepper
	1/2 tsp salt

Directions:
Add all ingredients except parsley and lemon juice in air fryer baking dish and stir well. Place dish in the air fryer basket and cook at 400 F for 7 minutes. Add parsley and lemon juice. Mix well. Serve and enjoy.

570. Full Baked Trout En Papillote With Herbs

Servings: 2   Cooking Time: 30 Minutes

Ingredients:
- ¼ bulb fennel, sliced
- ½ brown onion, sliced
- 3 tbsp chopped parsley
- 3 tbsp chopped dill
- 2 tbsp olive oil
- 1 lemon, sliced
- Salt and pepper to taste

Directions:
In a bowl, add the onion, parsley, dill, fennel, and garlic. Mix and drizzle the olive oil over. Preheat the air fryer to 350 F. Open the cavity of the fish and fill with the fennel mixture.   Wrap the fish completely in parchment paper and then in foil. Place the fish in the fryer basket and cook for 10 minutes. Remove the paper and foil, and top with lemon slices. Serve with cooked mushrooms.

571. Leamony-parsley Linguine With Grilled Tuna

Servings: 2   Cooking Time: 20 Minutes

Ingredients:
- 1 tablespoon capers, chopped
- 1 tablespoon olive oil
- 12 ounces linguine, cooked according to package Directions:
- 1-pound fresh tuna fillets
- 2 cups parsley leaves, chopped
- Juice from 1 lemon
- Salt and pepper to taste

Directions:
Preheat the air fryer to 390F.   Place the grill pan accessory in the air fryer.   Season the tuna with salt and pepper. Brush with oil.   Grill for 20 minutes.   Once the tuna is cooked, shred using forks and place on top of cooked linguine. Add parsley and capers. Season with salt and pepper and add lemon juice.

572. Paprika Cod And Endives

Servings: 4   Cooking Time: 20 Minutes

Ingredients:
- 2 endives, shredded
- 2 tablespoons olive oil
- Salt and back pepper to the taste
- 4 salmon fillets, boneless
- ½ teaspoon sweet paprika

Directions:
In a pan that fits the air fryer, combine the fish with the rest of the ingredients, toss, introduce in the fryer and cook at 350 degrees F for 20 minutes, flipping the fish halfway. Divide between plates and serve right away.

573. Herbed Calamari Rings

Servings: 4   Cooking Time: 4 Minutes

Ingredients:
- 1 chili pepper, chopped
- ¼ teaspoon salt
- 10 oz calamari
- ½ teaspoon dried cilantro
- ½ teaspoon dried parsley
- 1 teaspoon apple cider vinegar
- 1 teaspoon butter, melted
- ¼ teaspoon ground coriander
- 1 teaspoon sesame oil

Directions:
Trimmed and wash the calamari. Then slice it into rings and sprinkle with salt, dried cilantro, ground coriander, and apple cider vinegar. Add sesame oil and stir the calamari rings. Preheat the air fryer to 400F. Put the calamari rings in the air fryer basket and cook them for 2 minutes. When the time is finished, shake them well and cook for 2 minutes more. Transfer the calamari rings in the big bowl and sprinkle with butter.

574. Crispy Coconut Covered Shrimps

Servings: 6   Cooking Time: 6 Minutes

Ingredients:
- ½ cup almond flour
- 1 cup dried coconut
- 12 large shrimps, peeled and deveined
- 1 cup egg white
- 4 tablespoons butter
- Salt and pepper to taste

Directions:
Season the shrimps with salt and pepper.   Place all ingredients in a Ziploc bag and shake until well combined.   Place the ingredients in the air fryer basket.   Close and cook for 6 minutes 400F.

575. Citrusy Branzini On The Grill

Servings: 2   Cooking Time: 15 Minutes

Ingredients:
- Salt and pepper to taste
- 3 lemons, juice freshly squeezed
- 2 branzini fillets
- 2 oranges, juice freshly squeezed

Directions:
Place all ingredients in a Ziploc bag. Allow to marinate in the fridge for 2 hours.   Preheat the air fryer at 390F.   Place the grill pan accessory in the air fryer.   Place the fish on the grill pan and cook for 15 minutes until the fish is flaky.

576. Salmon And Blackberry Sauce

Servings: 2   Cooking Time: 12 Minutes

Ingredients:
- 2 salmon fillets, boneless
- 1 tablespoon honey
- 1 tablespoon olive oil
- ½ cup blackberries
- Juice of ½ lemon
- Salt and black pepper to taste

Directions:
In a blender, mix the blackberries with the honey, oil, lemon juice, salt, and pepper; pulse well.   Spread the blackberry mixture over the salmon, and then place the fish in your air fryer's basket.   Cook at

380 degrees F for 12 minutes, flipping the fish halfway.   Serve hot, and enjoy!

577.   Coconut Shrimp With Orange Sauce

Servings: 3   Cooking Time: 1 Hour 30 Minutes
Ingredients:

1 pound shrimp, cleaned and deveined	1 lemon, cut into wedges
Sea salt and white pepper, to taste	Dipping Sauce:
1/2 cup all-purpose flour	2 tablespoons butter
1 egg	1/2 cup orange juice
1/4 cup shredded coconut, unsweetened	2 tablespoons soy sauce
	A pinch of salt
3/2 cup fresh bread crumbs	1/2 teaspoon tapioca starch
2 tablespoons olive oil	2 tablespoons fresh parsley, minced

Directions:
Pat dry the shrimp and season them with salt and white pepper.   Place the flour on a large tray; then, whisk the egg in a shallow bowl. In a third shallow bowl, place the shredded coconut and breadcrumbs. Dip the shrimp in the flour, then, dip in the egg. Lastly, coat the shrimp with the shredded coconut and bread crumbs. Refrigerate for 1 hour.   Then, transfer to the cooking basket. Drizzle with olive oil and cook in the preheated Air Fryer at 370 degrees F for 6 minutes. Work in batches.   Meanwhile, melt the butter in a small saucepan over medium-high heat; add the orange juice and bring it to a boil; reduce the heat and allow it to simmer approximately 7 minutes.   Add the soy sauce, salt, and tapioca; continue simmering until the sauce has thickened and reduced. Spoon the sauce over the shrimp and garnish with lemon wedges and parsley. Serve immediately.

578.   Salmon Patties

Servings: 4   Cooking Time: 20 Minutes
Ingredients:

1 egg	4 tbsp. onion, minced
14 oz. canned salmon, drained	1/2 tsp. garlic powder
4 tbsp. flour	2 tbsp. mayonnaise
4 tbsp. cup cornmeal	Salt and pepper to taste

Directions:
Flake apart the salmon with a fork.   Put the flakes in a bowl and combine with the garlic powder, mayonnaise, flour, cornmeal, egg, onion, pepper, and salt.   Use your hands to shape equal portions of the mixture into small patties and put each one in the Air Fryer basket.   Air fry the salmon patties at 350°F for 15 minutes. Serve hot.

579.   Snapper Fillets And Veggies Recipe

Servings: 2   Cooking Time: 24 Minutes
Ingredients:

2 red snapper fillets; boneless	1 tbsp. olive oil
	1 tsp. tarragon; dried
1/2 cup red bell pepper; chopped.	A splash of white wine
1/2 cup green bell pepper; chopped	Salt and black pepper to the taste
1/2 cup leeks; chopped.	

Directions:
In a heat proof dish that fits your air fryer; mix fish fillets with salt, pepper, oil, green bell pepper, red bell pepper, leeks, tarragon and wine; toss well everything, introduce in preheated air fryer at 350 °F and cook for 14 minutes; flipping fish fillets halfway. Divide fish and veggies on plates and serve warm.

580.   Perfect Salmon Fillets

Servings: 2   Cooking Time: 15 Minutes
Ingredients:

2 salmon fillets	1 tbsp fresh dill, chopped
1/2 tsp garlic powder	
1/4 cup plain yogurt	1 lemon, sliced
1 tsp fresh lemon juice	Pepper
	Salt

Directions:
Place lemon slices into the air fryer basket. Season salmon with pepper and salt and place on top of lemon slices into the air fryer basket.   Cook salmon at 330 F for 15 minutes.   Meanwhile, in a bowl, mix together yogurt, garlic powder, lemon juice, dill, pepper, and salt.   Place salmon on serving plate and top with yogurt mixture.   Serve and enjoy.

581.   Filipino Bistek

Servings: 4   Cooking Time: 10 Minutes + Marinating Time
Ingredients:

2 milkfish bellies, deboned and sliced into 4 portions	2 tbsp. calamansi juice
3/4 tsp. salt	1/2 cup tamari sauce
1/4 tsp. ground black pepper	2 tbsp. fish sauce [Patis]
1/4 tsp. cumin powder	2 tbsp. sugar
2 lemongrass, trimmed and cut crosswise into small pieces	1 tsp. garlic powder
	1/2 cup chicken broth
	2 tbsp. olive oil

Directions:
Dry the fish using some paper towels.   Put the fish in a large bowl and coat with the rest of the ingredients. Allow to marinate for 3 hours in the refrigerator.   Cook the fish steaks on an Air Fryer grill basket at 340°F for 5 minutes.   Turn the

steaks over and allow to grill for an additional 4 minutes. Cook until medium brown.   Serve with steamed white rice.

582.   Wild Alaskan Salmon With Parsley Sauce

Servings: 4   Cooking Time: 20 Minutes

Ingredients:

4 Alaskan wild salmon fillets, 6 oz each	½ cup heavy cream
2 tsp olive oil	½ cup milk
A pinch of salt	A pinch of salt
For Dill Sauce	2 tbsp chopped parsley

Directions:
Preheat air fryer to 380 F. In a bowl, add salmon and drizzle 1 tsp of oil. Season with salt and pepper. Place the salmon in your air fryer's cooking basket and cook for 15 minutes, until tender and crispy. In a bowl, mix milk, chopped parsley, salt, and whipped cream. Serve the salmon with the sauce.

583.   Grilled Shellfish With Vegetables

Servings: 8   Cooking Time: 30 Minutes

Ingredients:

1 bunch broccolini	16 small oysters, scrubbed
8 asparagus spears	
8 small carrots, peeled and sliced	16 littleneck clams, scrubbed
4 tomatoes, halved	24 large mussels, scrubbed
1 red onion, wedged	
2 tablespoons olive oil	2 tablespoons lemon juice
Salt and pepper to taste	4 basil sprigs

Directions:
Preheat the air fryer at 390F.   Place the grill pan accessory in the air fryer.   Place all vegetables in a bowl and drizzle with oil. Season with salt and pepper then toss to coat the vegetables with the seasoning.   Place on the grill pan and grill for 15 minutes or until the edges of the vegetables are charred. Set aside   On a large foil, place all the shellfish and season with salt, lemon juice, and basil. Fold the foil and crimp the edges.   Place the foil packet on the grill pan and cook for another 15 minutes or until the shellfish have opened.   Serve the shellfish with the charred vegetables.

584.   Parmesan And Garlic Trout

Servings: 4   Cooking Time: 15 Minutes

Ingredients:

2 tablespoons olive oil	4 trout fillets, boneless
2 garlic cloves, minced	¾ cup parmesan, grated
½ cup chicken stock	

Salt and black pepper to the taste	¼ cup tarragon, chopped

Directions:
In a pan that fits your air fryer, mix all the ingredients except the fish and the parmesan and whisk. Add the fish and grease it well with this mix. Sprinkle the parmesan on top, put the pan in the air fryer and cook at 380 degrees F for 15 minutes. Divide everything between plates and serve.

585.   Honey-ginger Soy Sauce Over Grilled Tuna

Servings: 3   Cooking Time: 20 Minutes

Ingredients:

1 ½ pounds tuna, thick slices	2 tablespoons peanut oil
1 serrano chili, seeded and minced	2 tablespoons rice vinegar
2 tablespoons grated fresh ginger	2 tablespoons soy sauce
2 tablespoons honey	

Directions:
Place all ingredients in a Ziploc bag.   Allow to marinate in the fridge for at least 2 hours.   Preheat the air fryer to 390F.   Place the grill pan accessory in the air fryer.   Grill the fish for 15 to 20 minutes. Flip the fish halfway through the cooking time. Meanwhile, pour the marinade in a saucepan and allow to simmer for 10 minutes until the sauce thickens.   Brush the tuna with the sauce before serving.

586.   Shrimp Scampi Dip With Cheese

Servings: 8   Cooking Time: 25 Minutes

Ingredients:

2 teaspoons butter, melted	1/2 teaspoon red pepper flakes
8 ounces shrimp, peeled and deveined	4 ounces cream cheese, at room temperature
2 garlic cloves, minced	1/2 cup sour cream
1/4 cup chicken stock	4 tablespoons mayonnaise
2 tablespoons fresh lemon juice	1/4 cup mozzarella cheese, shredded
Salt and ground black pepper, to taste	

Directions:
Start by preheating the Air Fryer to 395 degrees F. Grease the sides and bottom of a baking dish with the melted butter.   Place the shrimp, garlic, chicken stock, lemon juice, salt, black pepper, and red pepper flakes in the baking dish.   Transfer the baking dish to the cooking basket and bake for 10 minutes. Add the mixture to your food processor; pulse until the coarsely is chopped.   Add the cream cheese, sour cream, and mayonnaise. Top with the mozzarella cheese and bake in the preheated Air Fryer at 360 degrees F for 6 to 7

minutes or until the cheese is bubbling. Serve immediately with breadsticks if desired. Bon appétit!

587. Pistachio Crusted Salmon

Servings: 1   Cooking Time: 15 Minutes

Ingredients:

1 tsp mustard	A pinch of sea salt
3 tbsp pistachios	1 tsp lemon juice
A pinch of garlic powder	1 tsp grated Parmesan cheese
A pinch of black pepper	1 tsp olive oil

Directions:

Preheat the air fryer to 350 F, and whisk mustard and lemon juice together. Season the salmon with salt, pepper, and garlic powder. Brush the olive oil on all sides. Brush the mustard mixture onto salmon. Chop the pistachios finely and combine them with the Parmesan cheese; sprinkle on top of the salmon. Place the salmon in the air fryer basket with the skin side down. Cook for 12 minutes, or to your liking.

588. Cajun Fish Fritters

Servings: 4   Cooking Time: 30 Minutes

Ingredients:

2 catfish fillets	3 ounces butter
1 cup parmesan cheese	1/2 cup buttermilk
1 teaspoon baking powder	1 teaspoon Cajun seasoning
1 teaspoon baking soda	1 cup Swiss cheese, shredded

Directions:

Bring a pot of salted water to a boil. Boil the fish fillets for 5 minutes or until it is opaque. Flake the fish into small pieces. Mix the remaining ingredients in a bowl; add the fish and mix until well combined. Shape the fish mixture into 12 patties. Cook in the preheated Air Fryer at 380 degrees F for 15 minutes. Work in batches. Enjoy!

589. Celery Leaves 'n Garlic-oil Grilled Turbot

Servings: 2   Cooking Time: 20 Minutes

Ingredients:

½ cup chopped celery leaves	2 whole turbot, scaled and head removed
1 clove of garlic, minced	Salt and pepper to taste
2 tablespoons olive oil	

Directions:

Preheat the air fryer to 390F. Place the grill pan accessory in the air fryer. Season the turbot with salt, pepper, garlic, and celery leaves. Brush with oil. Place on the grill pan and cook for 20 minutes until the fish becomes flaky.

590. Delicious Snapper En Papillote

Servings: 2   Cooking Time: 20 Minutes

Ingredients:

2 snapper fillets	1 tomato, sliced
1 shallot, peeled and sliced	1 tablespoon olive oil
2 garlic cloves, halved	1/4 teaspoon freshly ground black pepper
1 bell pepper, sliced	1/2 teaspoon paprika
1 small-sized serrano pepper, sliced	Sea salt, to taste
	2 bay leaves

Directions:

Place two parchment sheets on a working surface. Place the fish in the center of one side of the parchment paper. Top with the shallot, garlic, peppers, and tomato. Drizzle olive oil over the fish and vegetables. Season with black pepper, paprika, and salt. Add the bay leaves. Fold over the other half of the parchment. Now, fold the paper around the edges tightly and create a half moon shape, sealing the fish inside. Cook in the preheated Air Fryer at 390 degrees F for 15 minutes. Serve warm.

591. Char-grilled 'n Herbed Sea Scallops

Servings: 3   Cooking Time: 10 Minutes

Ingredients:

1-pound sea scallops, meat only	1 teaspoon dried sage
3 tablespoons olive oil, divided	1 cup grape tomatoes, halved
Salt and pepper to taste	1/3 cup basil leaves, shredded

Directions:

Preheat the air fryer at 390F. Place the grill pan accessory in the air fryer. Season the scallops with half of the olive oil, sage, salt and pepper. Toss into the air fryer and grill for 10 minutes. Once cooked, serve with tomatoes and basil leaves. Drizzle the remaining olive oil and season with more salt and pepper to taste.

592. Favorite Shrimp Fritatta

Servings: 4   Cooking Time: 25 Minutes

Ingredients:

Pinch salt	½ cup baby spinach
½ cup rice, cooked	
½ cup Monterey Jack cheese, grated	½ cup shrimp, chopped and cooked

Directions:

Preheat air fryer to 320 F. In a bowl, add eggs, salt, and basil; stir until frothy. Spray baking pan with cooking spray. Add in rice, spinach and shrimp. Pour egg mixture over and top with cheese. Place the pan in the air fryer's basket and cook for 14 minutes until the frittata is puffed and golden brown. Serve.

593. Minty Trout And Pine Nuts

Servings: 4   Cooking Time: 16 Minutes

114

Ingredients:

4 rainbow trout
1 cup olive oil + 3 tablespoons
Juice of 1 lemon
A pinch of salt and black pepper
1 cup parsley, chopped

3 garlic cloves, minced
½ cup mint, chopped
Zest of 1 lemon
1/3 pine nuts
1 avocado, peeled, pitted and roughly chopped

Directions:

Pat dry the trout, season with salt and pepper and rub with 3 tablespoons oil. Put the fish in your air fryer's basket and cook for 8 minutes on each side. Divide the fish between plates and drizzle half of the lemon juice all over. In a blender, combine the rest of the oil with the remaining lemon juice, parsley, garlic, mint, lemon zest, pine nuts and the avocado and pulse well. Spread this over the trout and serve.

594. Coriander Cod And Green Beans

Servings: 4   Cooking Time: 15 Minutes

Ingredients:

½ cup green beans, trimmed and halved
1 tablespoon avocado oil

12 oz cod fillet
1 teaspoon salt
1 teaspoon ground coriander

Directions:

Cut the cod fillet on 4 servings and sprinkle every serving with salt and ground coriander. After this, place the fish on 4 foil squares. Top them with green beans and avocado oil and wrap them into parcels. Preheat the air fryer to 400F. Place the cod parcels in the air fryer and cook them for 15 minutes.

595. Salad Niçoise With Peppery Halibut

Servings: 6   Cooking Time: 15 Minutes

Ingredients:

1 ½ pounds halibut fillets
1 cup cherry tomatoes, halved
2 pounds mixed vegetables
2 tablespoons olive oil

4 cups torn lettuce leaves
4 large hard-boiled eggs, peeled and sliced
Salt and pepper to taste

Directions:

Preheat the air fryer to 390F.   Place the grill pan accessory in the air fryer.   Rub the halibut with salt and pepper. Brush the fish with oil.   Place on the grill.   Surround the fish fillet with the mixed vegetables and cook for 15 minutes.   Assemble the salad by serving the fish fillet with grilled mixed vegetables, lettuce, cherry tomatoes, and hard-boiled eggs.

596. Lemon And Oregano Tilapia Mix

Servings: 4   Cooking Time: 20 Minutes

Ingredients:

4 tilapia fillets, boneless and halved
Salt and black pepper to the taste
1 cup roasted peppers, chopped
¼ cup keto tomato sauce
1 cup tomatoes, cubed

1 tablespoon lemon juice
2 tablespoons olive oil
1 teaspoon garlic powder
1 teaspoon oregano, dried

Directions:

In a baking dish that fits your air fryer, mix the fish with all the other ingredients, toss, introduce in your air fryer and cook at 380 degrees F for 20 minutes. Divide into bowls and serve.

597. Drunken Skewered Shrimp, Tomatoes 'n Sausages

Servings: 6   Cooking Time: 20 Minutes

Ingredients:

1/2 teaspoon dried crushed red pepper
1/2 teaspoon freshly ground black pepper
12 1-inch-long pieces andouille or other fully cooked smoked sausage
12 2-layer sections of red onion wedges
12 uncooked extra-large shrimp (13 to 15 per pound), peeled, deveined

12 cherry tomatoes
2 tablespoons chopped fresh thyme
3/4 cup olive oil
3/4 teaspoon salt
4 large garlic cloves, pressed
4 teaspoons Sherry wine vinegar
5 teaspoons smoked paprika*
Nonstick vegetable oil spray

Directions:

In medium bowl, mix well red pepper, black pepper, salt, wine vinegar, smoked paprika, thyme, garlic, and oil. Transfer half to a small bowl for dipping. Thread alternately sausage and shrimp in skewers. Place on skewer rack on air fryer and baste with the paprika glaze. Cook in batches.   For 10 minutes, cook on 360F. Halfway through cooking time, baste and turnover skewers.   Serve and enjoy with the reserved dip on the side.

598. Cheese Crust Salmon

Servings: 5   Cooking Time: 20 Minutes

Ingredients:

2 lb. salmon fillet
2 garlic cloves, minced
¼ cup fresh parsley, chopped

½ cup parmesan cheese, grated
Salt and pepper to taste

Directions:

Pre-heat the Air Fryer to 350°F. Lay the salmon, skin-side-down, on a sheet of aluminum foil. Place another sheet of foil on top. Transfer the salmon to the fryer and cook for 10 minutes. Remove the salmon from the fryer. Take off the top layer of foil and add the minced garlic, parmesan cheese, pepper, salt and parsley on top of the fish. Return the salmon to the Air Fryer and resume cooking for another minute.

---

599. Creamed Trout Salad

Servings: 2   Cooking Time: 20 Minutes

Ingredients:
- 1/2 pound trout fillets, skinless
- 2 tablespoons horseradish, prepared, drained
- 1/4 cup mayonnaise
- 1 tablespoon fresh lemon juice
- 1 teaspoon mustard
- Salt and ground white pepper, to taste
- 6 ounces chickpeas, canned and drained
- 1 red onion, thinly sliced
- 1 cup Iceberg lettuce, torn into pieces

Directions:

Spritz the Air Fryer basket with cooking spray. Cook the trout fillets in the preheated Air Fryer at 395 degrees F for 10 minutes or until opaque. Make sure to turn them halfway through the cooking time. Break the fish into bite-sized chunks and place in the refrigerator to cool. Toss your fish with the remaining ingredients. Bon appétit!

---

600. Lime, Oil 'n Leeks On Grilled Swordfish

Servings: 4   Cooking Time: 20 Minutes

Ingredients:
- 2 tablespoons olive oil
- 3 tablespoons lime juice
- 4 swordfish steaks
- 4 medium leeks, cut into an inch long
- Salt and pepper to taste

Directions:

Preheat the air fryer to 390F. Place the grill pan accessory in the air fryer. Season the swordfish with salt, pepper and lime juice. Brush the fish with olive oil Place fish fillets on grill pan and top with leeks. Grill for 20 minutes.

Vegan & Vegetarian Recipes

601. Crispy Shawarma Broccoli

Servings: 4   Cooking Time: 25 Minutes

Ingredients:

1 pound broccoli, steamed and drained
2 tablespoons canola oil
1 teaspoon sea salt
1 teaspoon cayenne pepper
1 tablespoon Shawarma spice blend

Directions:

Toss all ingredients in a mixing bowl.   Roast in the preheated Air Fryer at 380 degrees F for 10 minutes, shaking the basket halfway through the cooking time.   Work in batches. Bon appétit!

602. Hearty Celery Croquettes With Chive Mayo

Servings: 4   Cooking Time: 15 Minutes

Ingredients:

2 medium-sized celery stalks, trimmed and grated
1/2 cup of leek, finely chopped
1 tablespoon garlic paste
1/4 cup freshly cracked black pepper
1 teaspoon fine sea salt
1 tablespoon fresh dill, finely chopped
1 egg, lightly whisked
1/4 cup almond flour
1/2 cup parmesan cheese, freshly grated
1/4 teaspoon baking powder
2 tablespoons fresh chives, chopped
4 tablespoons mayonnaise

Directions:

Place the celery on a paper towel and squeeze them to remove excess liquid.   Combine the vegetables with the other ingredients, except the chives and mayo. Shape the balls using 1 tablespoon of the vegetable mixture.   Then, gently flatten each ball with your palm or a wide spatula. Spritz the croquettes with a non - stick cooking oil.   Air-fry the vegetable croquettes in a single layer for 6 minutes at 360 degrees F.   Meanwhile, mix fresh chives and mayonnaise. Serve warm croquettes with chive mayo. Bon appétit!

603. Radish And Mozzarella Salad With Balsamic Vinaigrette

Servings: 4   Cooking Time: 30 Minutes

Ingredients:

1½ pounds radishes, trimmed and halved
½ pound fresh mozzarella, sliced
3 tablespoons olive oil
Salt and freshly ground black pepper, to taste
1 teaspoon honey
1 tablespoon balsamic vinegar

Directions:

Preheat the Air fryer to 350F and grease an Air fryer basket.   Mix radishes, salt, black pepper and 2 tablespoons of olive oil in a bowl and toss to coat well. Arrange the radishes in the Air fryer basket and cook for about 30 minutes, flipping twice in between. Dish out in a bowl and top with the remaining ingredients to serve.

604. Easy Vegan "chicken"

Servings: 4   Cooking Time: 20 Minutes

Ingredients:

8 ounces soy chunks
1/4 cup all-purpose flour
1 teaspoon cayenne pepper
1/2 teaspoon mustard powder
1/2 cup cornmeal
1 teaspoon celery seeds
Sea salt and ground black pepper, to taste

Directions:

Boil the soya chunks in lots of water in a saucepan over medium-high heat. Remove from the heat and let them soak for 10 minutes.   Drain, rinse, and squeeze off the excess water.   Mix the remaining ingredients in a bowl. Roll the soy chunks over the breading mixture, pressing to adhere.   Arrange the soy chunks in the lightly greased Air Fryer basket. Cook in the preheated Air Fryer at 390 degrees for 10 minutes, turning them over halfway through the cooking time; work in batches. Bon appétit!

605. Baked Potato Topped With Cream Cheese 'n Olives

Servings: 1   Cooking Time: 40 Minutes

Ingredients:

¼ teaspoon onion powder
1 medium russet potato, scrubbed and peeled
1 tablespoon chives, chopped
1 teaspoon olive oil
1 tablespoon Kalamata olives
1/8 teaspoon salt
a dollop of vegan butter
a dollop of vegan cream cheese

Directions:

Place inside the air fryer basket and cook for 40 minutes. Be sure to turn the potatoes once halfway. Place the potatoes in a mixing bowl and pour in olive oil, onion powder, salt, and vegan butter.   Preheat the air fryer to 400F.   Serve the potatoes with vegan cream cheese, Kalamata olives, chives, and other vegan toppings that you want.

606. Easy Roast Winter Vegetable Delight

Servings: 2   Cooking Time: 30 Minutes

Ingredients:

1 cup chopped butternut squash
1 tbsp chopped fresh thyme

2 small red onions, cut in wedges
1 cup chopped celery
Salt and pepper to taste
2 tsp olive oil

Directions:
Preheat the air fryer to 200 F, and in a bowl, add turnip, squash, red onions, celery, thyme, pepper, salt, and olive oil; mix well. Pour the vegetables into the fryer's basket and cook for 16 minutes, tossing once halfway through.

---

607. Cauliflower, Broccoli And Chickpea Salad

Servings: 4   Cooking Time: 20 Minutes + Chilling Time

Ingredients:

1/2 pound cauliflower florets
1/2 pound broccoli florets
1/2 teaspoon red pepper flakes
2 tablespoons soy sauce
2 tablespoons cider vinegar
1 teaspoon Dijon mustard
2 tablespoons extra-virgin olive oil
Sea salt, to taste
1 cup canned or cooked chickpeas, drained
1 avocado, pitted, peeled and sliced
1 small sized onion, peeled and sliced
1 garlic clove, minced
2 cups arugula
2 tablespoons sesame seeds, lightly toasted

Directions:
Start by preheating your Air Fryer to 400 degrees F. Brush the cauliflower and broccoli florets with cooking spray.   Cook for 12 minutes, shaking the cooking basket halfway through the cooking time. Season with salt and red pepper.   In a mixing dish, whisk the soy sauce, cider vinegar, Dijon mustard, and olive oil. Dress the salad. Add the chickpeas, avocado, onion, garlic, and arugula. Top with sesame seeds.   Bon appétit!

---

608. Keto Cauliflower Hash Browns

Servings: 6   Cooking Time: 23 Minutes

Ingredients:

1/2 cup Cheddar cheese, shredded
1 tablespoon soft cheese, at room temperature
1/3 cup almond meal
1 ½ yellow or white medium-sized onion, chopped
5 ounces condensed cream of celery soup
1 tablespoon fresh cilantro, finely minced
1/3 cup sour cream
3 cloves garlic, peeled and finely minced
2 cups cauliflower, grated
1 1/2 tablespoons margarine, melted
Sea salt and freshly ground black pepper, to your liking
Crushed red pepper flakes, to your liking

Directions:

Grab a large-sized bowl and whisk the celery soup, sour cream, soft cheese, red pepper, salt, and black pepper. Stir in the cauliflower, onion, garlic, cilantro, and Cheddar cheese. Mix until everything is thoroughly combined.   Scrape the mixture into a baking dish that is previously lightly greased.   In another mixing bowl, combine together the almond meal and melted margarine. Spread the mixture evenly over the top of the hash brown mixture. Bake for 17 minutes at 290 degrees F. Eat warm, garnished with some extra sour cream if desired.

---

609. Corn Cakes

Servings: 8   Cooking Time: 25 Minutes

Ingredients:

2 eggs, lightly beaten
⅓ cup finely chopped green onions
1 cup flour
¼ cup roughly chopped parsley
½ tsp baking powder
Salt and black pepper

Directions:
In a bowl, add corn, eggs, parsley and green onions, and season with salt and pepper; mix well to combine. Sift flour and baking powder into the bowl and stir. Line the air fryer's basket with baking paper and spoon batter dollops, making sure they are separated by at least an inch. Cook for 10 minutes at 400 F, turning once halfway through. Serve with sour cream.

---

610. Sesame Seeds Bok Choy(2)

Servings: 4   Cooking Time: 6 Minutes

Ingredients:

4 bunches spinach leaves
2 teaspoons sesame seeds
Salt, to taste
1 teaspoon garlic powder
1 teaspoon ginger powder

Directions:
Preheat the Air fryer to 325F and grease an Air fryer basket.   Arrange the spinach leaves into the Air fryer basket and season with salt, garlic powder and ginger powder.   Cook for about 6 minutes, shaking once in between and dish out onto serving plates.   Top with sesame seeds and serve hot.

---

611. Parsnip & Potato Bake

Servings: 8   Cooking Time: 30 Minutes

Ingredients:

3 tbsp pine nuts
28 oz parsnips, chopped
1 ¾ oz coarsely chopped Parmesan cheese
6 ¾ oz crème fraiche
1 slice bread
2 tbsp sage
4 tbsp butter
4 tsp mustard

Directions:
Preheat air fryer to 360 F. Put salted water in a pot over medium heat. Add potatoes and parsnips. Bring to a boil for 15 minutes.   In a bowl, mix

mustard, crème fraiche, sage, salt and pepper. Drain the potatoes and parsnips and mash them with butter using a potato masher. Add mustard mixture, bread, cheese, and nuts to the mash and mix. Add the batter to your air fryer's basket and cook for 15 minutes, shaking once. Serve.

612. Black Bean Burger With Garlic-chipotle

Servings: 3   Cooking Time: 20 Minutes
Ingredients:

½ cup corn kernels	¾ cup salsa
½ teaspoon chipotle powder	1 ½ cup rolled oats
½ teaspoon garlic powder	1 can black beans, rinsed and drained
1 ¼ teaspoon chili powder	1 tablespoon soy sauce

Directions:
In a mixing bowl, combine all Ingredients and mix using your hands.   Form small patties using your hands and set aside.   Brush patties with oil if desired.   Place the grill pan in the air fryer and place the patties on the grill pan accessory.   Close the lid and cook for 20 minutes on each side at 330F. Halfway through the cooking time, flip the patties to brown the other side evenly

613. Hearty Carrots

Servings: 4   Cooking Time: 25 Minutes
Ingredients:

2 shallots, chopped	2 garlic cloves, minced
3 carrots, sliced	
Salt to taste	3 tbsp parsley, chopped
¼ cup yogurt	

Directions:
Preheat air fryer to 370 F. In a bowl, mix carrots, salt, garlic, shallots, parsley and yogurt. Sprinkle with oil. Place the veggies in air fryer basket and cook for 15 minutes. Serve with basil and garlic mayo.

614. Open-faced Vegan Flatbread-wich

Servings: 4   Cooking Time: 25 Minutes
Ingredients:

1 can chickpeas, drained and rinsed	2 ripe avocados, mashed
1 medium-sized head of cauliflower, cut into florets	2 tablespoons lemon juice
1 tablespoon extra-virgin olive oil	4 flatbreads, toasted
	salt and pepper to taste

Directions:
Preheat the air fryer to 425F.   In a mixing bowl, combine the cauliflower, chickpeas, olive oil, and lemon juice. Season with salt and pepper to taste. Place inside the air fryer basket and cook for 25 minutes.   Once cooked, place on half of the flatbread and add avocado mash.   Season with

more salt and pepper to taste.   Serve with hot sauce.

615. Eggplant Cheeseburger

Servings: 1   Cooking Time: 10 Minutes
Ingredients:

2-inch eggplant slice, cut along the round axis	1 mozzarella slice
	1 lettuce leaf
	½ tbsp tomato sauce
1 red onion cut into 3 rings	1 pickle, sliced

Directions:
Preheat the air fryer to 330 F. Place the eggplant to roast for 6 minutes. Top with the mozzarella slice and cook for 30 more seconds. Spread the tomato sauce on one half of the bun. Place the lettuce leaf on top of the sauce along with cheesy eggplant, onion rings and pickles. Finish with the other bun half.

616. Eggplant Gratin With Mozzarella Crust

Servings: 2   Cooking Time: 30 Minutes
Ingredients:

¼ cup chopped red pepper	¼ cup chopped onion
¼ cup chopped green pepper	1 tsp capers
⅓ cup chopped tomatoes	¼ tsp dried basil
1 clove garlic, minced	¼ tsp dried marjoram
1 tbsp sliced pimiento-stuffed olives	Salt and pepper to taste
	Cooking spray
	¼ cup grated mozzarella cheese
	1 tbsp breadcrumbs

Directions:
Preheat the air fryer to 300 F, and in a bowl, add the eggplant, green pepper, red pepper, onion, tomatoes, olives, garlic, basil marjoram, capers, salt, and pepper. Lightly grease a baking dish with the olive oil cooking spray.   Ladle the eggplant mixture into the baking dish and level it using the vessel. Sprinkle the mozzarella cheese on top and cover with the breadcrumbs. Place the dish in the air fryer and cook for 20 minutes.

617. Crispy Green Beans With Pecorino Romano

Servings: 3   Cooking Time: 15 Minutes
Ingredients:

2 tablespoons buttermilk	1 egg
4 tablespoons almond meal	Coarse salt and crushed black pepper, to taste
4 tablespoons golden flaxseed meal	1 teaspoon smoked paprika
4 tablespoons	

Pecorino Romano cheese, finely grated | 6 ounces green beans, trimmed

Directions:

In a shallow bowl, whisk together the buttermilk and egg. In a separate bowl, combine the almond meal, golden flaxseed meal, Pecorino Romano cheese, salt, black pepper, and paprika. Dip the green beans in the egg mixture, then, in the cheese mixture. Place the green beans in the lightly greased cooking basket. Cook in the preheated Air Fryer at 390 degrees F for 4 minutes. Shake the basket and cook for a further 3 minutes. Taste, adjust the seasonings, and serve with the dipping sauce if desired. Bon appétit!

618. Vegetable Kabobs With Simple Peanut Sauce

Servings: 4   Cooking Time: 30 Minutes

Ingredients:

8 whole baby potatoes, diced into 1-inch pieces
2 bell peppers, diced into 1-inch pieces
8 pearl onions, halved
8 small button mushrooms, cleaned
2 tablespoons extra-virgin olive oil
Sea salt and ground black pepper, to taste

1 teaspoon red pepper flakes, crushed
1 teaspoon dried rosemary, crushed
1/3 teaspoon granulated garlic
Peanut Sauce:
2 tablespoons peanut butter
1 tablespoon balsamic vinegar
1 tablespoon soy sauce
1/2 teaspoon garlic salt

Directions:

Soak the wooden skewers in water for 15 minutes. Thread the vegetables on skewers; drizzle the olive oil all over the vegetable skewers; sprinkle with spices. Cook in the preheated Air Fryer at 400 degrees F for 13 minutes. Meanwhile, in a small dish, whisk the peanut butter with the balsamic vinegar, soy sauce, and garlic salt. Serve your kabobs with the peanut sauce on the side. Enjoy!

619. Ultra-crispy Tofu

Servings: 4   Cooking Time: 30 Minutes

Ingredients:

1 teaspoon chicken bouillon granules
12-ounce extra-firm tofu, drained and cubed into 1-inch size

1 teaspoon butter
2 tablespoons low-sodium soy sauce
2 tablespoons fish sauce
1 teaspoon sesame oil

Directions:

Preheat the Air fryer to 355F and grease an Air fryer basket. Mix soy sauce, fish sauce, sesame oil and chicken granules in a bowl and toss to coat well. Stir in the tofu cubes and mix until well combined. Keep aside to marinate for about 30 minutes and

then transfer into Air fryer basket. Cook for about 30 minutes, flipping every 10 minutes and serve hot.

620. Broccoli With Olives

Servings: 4   Cooking Time: 19 Minutes

Ingredients:

2 pounds broccoli, stemmed and cut into 1-inch florets
¼ cup Parmesan cheese, grated
2 tablespoons olive oil

1/3 cup Kalamata olives, halved and pitted
Salt and ground black pepper, as required
2 teaspoons fresh lemon zest, grated

Directions:

Preheat the Air fryer to 400F and grease an Air fryer basket. Boil the broccoli for about 4 minutes and drain well. Mix broccoli, oil, salt, and black pepper in a bowl and toss to coat well. Arrange broccoli into the Air fryer basket and cook for about 15 minutes. Stir in the olives, lemon zest and cheese and dish out to serve.

621. Herby Zucchini 'n Eggplant Bake

Servings: 4   Cooking Time: 25 Minutes

Ingredients:

½ lemon, juiced
1 fennel bulb, sliced crosswise
1 sprig flat-leaf parsley
1 sprig mint
1 sprig of basil
1 tablespoon coriander powder
1 teaspoon capers
2 eggplants, sliced crosswise
2 red peppers, sliced crosswise

2 red onions, chopped
2 teaspoons herb de Provence
3 large zucchinis, sliced crosswise
4 cloves of garlic, minced
4 large tomatoes, chopped
5 tablespoons olive oil
salt and pepper to taste

Directions:

In a blender, combine basil, parsley, mint, coriander, capers and lemon juice. Season with salt and pepper to taste. Pulse until well combined. Preheat the air fryer to 400F. Toss the eggplant, onions, garlic, peppers, fennel, and zucchini with olive oil. In a baking dish that can fit in the air fryer, arrange the vegetables and pour over the tomatoes and the herb puree. Season with more salt and pepper and sprinkle with herbs de Provence. Place inside the air fryer and cook for 25 minutes.

622. Baked Polenta With Chili-cheese

Servings: 3   Cooking Time: 10 Minutes

Ingredients:

1 commercial polenta roll, sliced
1 cup cheddar cheese sauce

1 tablespoon chili powder

Directions:
Place the baking dish accessory in the air fryer. Arrange the polenta slices in the baking dish. Add the chili powder and cheddar cheese sauce. Close the air fryer and cook for 10 minutes at 390F.

623. Shallots 'n Almonds On French Green Beans

Servings: 4   Cooking Time: 10 Minutes

Ingredients:

¼ cup slivered almonds, toasted	1 ½ pound French green beans, stems removed and blanched
½ pounds shallots, peeled and cut into quarters	
½ teaspoon ground white pepper	1 tablespoon salt
	2 tablespoon olive oil

Directions:
Preheat the air fryer to 400F. Mix all ingredients in a mixing bowl. Toss until well combined. Place inside the air fryer basket and cook for 10 minutes or until lightly browned.

624. Oatmeal Stuffed Bell Peppers

Servings: 2   Cooking Time: 16 Minutes

Ingredients:

2 large red bell peppers, halved lengthwise and seeded	2 cups cooked oatmeal
4 tablespoons canned red kidney beans, rinsed and drained	¼ teaspoon ground cumin
4 tablespoons coconut yogurt	¼ teaspoon smoked paprika
	Salt and ground black pepper, as required

Directions:
Set the temperature of air fryer to 355 degrees F. Grease an air fryer basket. Arrange bell peppers into the prepared air fryer basket, cut-side down. Air fry for about 8 minutes. Remove from the air fryer and set aside to cool. Meanwhile, in a bowl, mix well oatmeal, beans, coconut yogurt, and spices. Stuff each bell pepper half with the oatmeal mixture. Now, set the air fryer to 355 degrees F. Arrange bell peppers into the air fryer basket and air fry for about 8 minutes. Remove from air fryer and transfer the bell peppers onto a serving platter. Set aside to cool slightly. Serve warm.

625. Vegetable Spring Rolls

Servings: 4   Cooking Time: 15 Minutes

Ingredients:

2 carrots, grated	1 tsp sesame seeds
1 tsp minced ginger	½ tsp salt
1 tsp minced garlic	1 tsp olive oil
1 tsp sesame oil	1 package spring roll wrappers
1 tsp soy sauce	

Directions:
Preheat the air fryer to 370 F, and combine all ingredients in a large bowl. Divide the mixture between the spring roll sheets, and roll them up; arrange on the baking mat. Cook in the air fryer for 5 minutes.

626. Air-fried Falafel

Servings: 6   Cooking Time: 25 Minutes

Ingredients:

½ cup chickpea flour	1 onion, chopped
1 cup fresh parsley, chopped	2 tsp ground cumin
Juice of 1 lemon	2 tsp ground coriander
4 garlic cloves, chopped	1 tsp chili powder
	Salt and black pepper

Directions:
In a blender, add chickpeas, flour, parsley, lemon juice, garlic, onion, cumin, coriander, chili, turmeric, salt and pepper, and blend until well-combined but not too battery; there should be some lumps. Shape the mixture into 15 balls and press them with hands, making sure they are still around. Spray with oil and arrange them in a paper-lined air fryer basket; work in batches if needed. Cook at 360 F for 14 minutes, turning once halfway through. They should be crunchy and golden.

627. Salted Beet Chips

Servings: 2   Cooking Time: 6 Minutes

Ingredients:

1 tablespoon cooking oil	Salt and pepper to taste
1-pound beets, peeled and sliced	

Directions:
Place all Ingredients in a bowl and toss to coat everything. Place the sliced beets in the double layer rack. Place the rack with the beets in the air fryer. Close the air fryer and cook for 6 minutes at 390F.

628. Air-fried Veggie Sushi

Servings: 4   Cooking Time: 60 Minutes

Ingredients:

4 nori sheets	1 tbsp rice wine vinegar
1 carrot, sliced lengthways	1 cup panko crumbs
1 red bell pepper, seeds removed, sliced	2 tbsp sesame seeds
1 avocado, sliced	Soy sauce, wasabi and pickled ginger to serve
1 tbsp olive oil mixed with	

Directions:
Prepare a clean working board, a small bowl of lukewarm water and a sushi mat. Wet hands, and lay a nori sheet onto sushi mat and spread half cup sushi rice, leaving a half-inch of nori clear, so you can seal the roll. Place carrot, pepper and avocado sideways to the rice. Roll sushi tightly and rub warm water along the clean nori strip to seal. In a bowl, mix

oil and rice vinegar. In another bowl, mix crumbs and sesame seeds. Roll each sushi log in the vinegar mixture and then straight to the sesame bowl to coat. Arrange sushi onto air fryer and cook for 14 minutes at 360 F, turning once. Slice and serve with soy sauce, pickled ginger and wasabi.

629. Surprising Quinoa Eggplant Rolls

Servings: 3   Cooking Time: 15 Minutes
Ingredients:

Marinara sauce for dipping	2 tbsp milk
½ cup cheese, grated	1 whole egg, beaten
	2 cups breadcrumbs

Directions:
Preheat air fryer to 400 F. In a bowl, mix beaten egg and milk. In another bowl, mix crumbs and cheese until crumbly. Place eggplant slices in the egg mixture, followed by a dip in the crumb mixture. Place eggplant slices in the cooking basket and cook for 5 minutes. Serve with marinara sauce.

630. Polenta Fries

Servings: 4   Cooking Time: 80 Minutes
Ingredients:

2 cups milk	Cooking spray
1 cup instant polenta	fresh thyme, chopped
Salt and black pepper	

Directions:
Line a tray with paper. Pour water and milk into a saucepan and let it simmer. Keep whisking as you pour in the polenta. Continue to whisk until polenta thickens and bubbles; season to taste.   Add polenta into the lined tray and spread out. Refrigerate for 45 minutes. Slice the cold, set polenta into batons and spray with oil. Arrange polenta chips into the air fryer basket and cook for 16 minutes at 380 F, turning once halfway through. Make sure the fries are golden and crispy.

631. Garlic Broccoli

Servings: 3   Cooking Time: 20 Minutes
Ingredients:

1 tablespoon butter	3 garlic cloves, sliced
2 teaspoons vegetable bouillon granules	½ teaspoon fresh lemon zest, finely grated
1 large head broccoli, cut into bite-sized pieces	½ teaspoon red pepper flakes, crushed
1 tablespoon fresh lemon juice	

Directions:
Preheat the Air fryer to 355F and grease an Air fryer pan.   Mix the butter, bouillon granules, and lemon juice in the Air fryer pan.   Cook for about 1½ minutes and stir in the garlic.   Cook for about 30 seconds and add broccoli, lemon zest, and red pepper flakes.   Cook for about 18 minutes and dish out in a bowl to serve hot.

632. Tomato Sandwiches With Feta And Pesto

Servings: 2   Cooking Time: 60 Minutes
Ingredients:

1 (4- oz) block Feta cheese	Salt to taste
1 small red onion, thinly sliced	1 ½ tbsp toasted pine nuts
1 clove garlic	¼ cup chopped parsley
2 tsp + ¼ cup olive oil	¼ cup grated Parmesan cheese
	¼ cup chopped basil

Directions:
Add basil, pine nuts, garlic and salt to a food processor. Process while adding the ¼ cup of olive oil slowly. Once the oil is finished, pour the basil pesto into a bowl and refrigerate for 30 minutes. Preheat the air fryer to 390 F. Slice the feta cheese and tomato into ½ inch circular slices. Use a kitchen towel to pat the tomatoes dry. Remove the pesto from the fridge and use a tablespoon to spread some pesto on each slice of tomato. Top with a slice of feta cheese. Add the onion and remaining olive oil in a bowl and toss. Spoon on top of feta cheese.   Place the tomato in the fryer's basket and cook for 12 minutes. Remove to a serving platter, sprinkle lightly with salt and top with the remaining pesto. Serve with a side of rice or lean meat.

633. Garlic-roasted Brussels Sprouts With Mustard

Servings: 3   Cooking Time: 20 Minutes
Ingredients:

1 pound Brussels sprouts, halved	Sea salt and freshly ground black pepper, to taste
2 tablespoons olive oil	1 tablespoon Dijon mustard
2 garlic cloves, minced	

Directions:
Toss the Brussels sprouts with the olive oil, salt, black pepper, and garlic.   Roast in the preheated Air Fryer at 380 degrees F for 15 minutes, shaking the basket occasionally.   Serve with Dijon mustard and enjoy!

634. Banana Pepper Stuffed With Tofu 'n Spices

Servings: 8   Cooking Time: 10 Minutes
Ingredients:

½ teaspoon red chili powder	1 teaspoon coriander powder
½ teaspoon turmeric powder	3 tablespoons coconut oil
1 onion, finely chopped	8 banana peppers, top end sliced and

1 package firm tofu, seeded
crumbled Salt to taste

Directions:
Preheat the air fryer for 5 minutes. In a mixing bowl, combine the tofu, onion, coconut oil, turmeric powder, red chili powder, coriander power, and salt. Mix until well-combined. Scoop the tofu mixture into the hollows of the banana peppers. Place the stuffed peppers in the air fryer. Close and cook for 10 minutes at 325F.

635. Cheesy Muffins

Servings: 3   Cooking Time: 8 Minutes

Ingredients:

1 cup cheddar cheese, smoked and shredded	1 tomato, chopped
1 mashed avocado	1 sweet onion, chopped
¼ cup ranch-style salad dressing	¼ cup sesame seeds, toasted
1 cup alfalfa sprouts	

Directions:
Arrange the muffins open-faced in the air fryer's basket. Spread the mashed avocado on each half of the muffin. Place the halves close to each other. Cover the muffins with the sprouts, tomatoes, onion, dressing, sesame seeds and the cheese. Cook for 7-8 minutes at 350 F.

636. Vegetable Tortilla Pizza

Servings: 1   Cooking Time: 15 Minutes

Ingredients:

¼ cup grated cheddar cheese	4 red onion rings
¼ cup grated mozzarella cheese	½ green bell pepper, chopped
1 tbsp cooked sweet corn	3 cherry tomatoes, quartered
4 zucchini slices	1 tortilla
4 eggplant slices	¼ tsp basil
	¼ tsp oregano

Directions:
Preheat the air fryer to 350 F. Spread the tomato paste on the tortilla. Arrange the zucchini and eggplant slices first, then green peppers, and onion rings. Arrange the cherry tomatoes and sprinkle the sweet corn over. Sprinkle with oregano and basil and top with cheddar and mozzarella. Place in the fryer and cook for 10 minutes.

637. Vegetable Bake With Cheese And Olives

Servings: 3   Cooking Time: 25 Minutes

Ingredients:

1/2 pound cauliflower, cut into 1-inch florets	1 cup dry white wine
1/4 pound zucchini, cut into 1-inch	Sea salt and freshly cracked black pepper, to taste
	1/2 teaspoon dried

chunks
1 red onion, sliced
2 bell peppers, cut into 1-inch chunks
2 tablespoons extra-virgin olive oil
1 teaspoon dried rosemary

basil
1/2 cup tomato, pureed
1/2 cup cheddar cheese, grated
1 ounce Kalamata olives, pitted and halved

Directions:
Toss the vegetables with the olive oil, wine, rosemary, salt, black pepper, and basil until well coated. Add the pureed tomatoes to a lightly greased baking dish; spread to cover the bottom of the baking dish. Add the vegetables and top with grated cheese. Scatter the Kalamata olives over the top. Bake in the preheated Air Fryer at 390 degrees F for 20 minutes, rotating the dish halfway through the cooking time. Serve warm and enjoy!

638. Baked Zucchini Recipe From Mexico

Servings: 4   Cooking Time: 30 Minutes

Ingredients:

1 tablespoon olive oil	1/2 teaspoon cayenne pepper, or to taste
1-1/2 pounds zucchini, cubed	1/2 cup cooked long-grain rice
1/2 cup chopped onion	1/2 cup cooked pinto beans
1/2 teaspoon garlic salt	1-1/4 cups salsa
1/2 teaspoon paprika	3/4 cup shredded Cheddar cheese
1/2 teaspoon dried oregano	

Directions:
Lightly grease baking pan of air fryer with olive oil. Add onions and zucchini and for 10 minutes, cook on 360F. Halfway through cooking time, stir. Season with cayenne, oregano, paprika, and garlic salt. Mix well. Stir in salsa, beans, and rice. Cook for 5 minutes. Stir in cheddar cheese and mix well. Cover pan with foil. Cook for 15 minutes at 390F until bubbly. Serve and enjoy.

639. Crispy Brussels Sprout Chips

Servings: 2   Cooking Time: 20 Minutes

Ingredients:

10 Brussels sprouts, separated into leaves	1 teaspoon coarse sea salt
1 teaspoon canola oil	1 teaspoon paprika

Directions:
Toss all ingredients in the lightly greased Air Fryer basket. Bake at 380 degrees F for 15 minutes, shaking the basket halfway through the cooking time to ensure even cooking. Serve and enjoy!

640. Baby Portabellas With Romano Cheese

Servings: 4   Cooking Time: 15 Minutes

Ingredients:

1 pound baby portabellas
1/2 cup almond meal
2 eggs
2 tablespoons milk
1 cup Romano cheese, grated
Sea salt and ground black pepper

1/2 teaspoon shallot powder
1 teaspoon garlic powder
1/2 teaspoon cumin powder
1/2 teaspoon cayenne pepper

Directions:
Pat the mushrooms dry with a paper towel. To begin, set up your breading station. Place the almond meal in a shallow dish. In a separate dish, whisk the eggs with milk. Finally, place grated Romano cheese and seasonings in the third dish. Start by dredging the baby portabellas in the almond meal mixture; then, dip them into the egg wash. Press the baby portabellas into Romano cheese, coating evenly. Spritz the Air Fryer basket with cooking oil. Add the baby portabellas and cook at 400 degrees F for 6 minutes, flipping them halfway through the cooking time. Bon appétit!

641.   Zoodles With Cheese

Servings: 4   Cooking Time: 30 Minutes
Ingredients:

12 ounces zucchini noodles
2 garlic cloves, minced
1/3 cup butter
2 tablespoons milk
1/2 teaspoon curry powder
1/2 teaspoon mustard powder

1/2 teaspoon celery seeds
Sea salt and white pepper, to taste
1 cup cheddar cheese, grated
1 heaping tablespoon Italian parsley, roughly chopped

Directions:
Place zucchini noodles in a colander and salt generously. Let them sit for 15 minutes to remove any excess water. Cook in the preheated Air Fryer at 425 degrees F and fry for 20 minutes or until they have softened. In a mixing dish, thoroughly combine the remaining ingredients. Toss the cheese mixture with your zoodles and serve immediately. Bon appétit!

642.   Spicy Tofu

Servings: 3   Cooking Time: 13 Minutes
Ingredients:

1 (14-ounces) block extra-firm tofu, pressed and cut into ¾-inch cubes
3 teaspoons cornstarch
1½ tablespoons avocado oil

1½ teaspoons paprika
1 teaspoon onion powder
1 teaspoon garlic powder
Salt and black pepper, to taste

Directions:
Preheat the Air fryer to 390F and grease an Air fryer basket. Mix the tofu, oil, cornstarch, and spices in

a bowl and toss to coat well. Arrange the tofu pieces in the Air fryer basket and cook for about 13 minutes, tossing twice in between. Dish out the tofu onto serving plates and serve hot.

643.   Broccoli With Cauliflower

Servings: 4   Cooking Time: 20 Minutes
Ingredients:

1½ cups broccoli, cut into 1-inch pieces
1 tablespoon olive oil

1½ cups cauliflower, cut into 1-inch pieces
Salt, as required

Directions:
Preheat the Air fryer to 375F and grease an Air fryer basket. Mix the vegetables, olive oil, and salt in a bowl and toss to coat well. Arrange the veggie mixture in the Air fryer basket and cook for about 20 minutes, tossing once in between. Dish out in a bowl and serve hot.

644.   Tofu With Peanut Butter Sauce

Servings: 3   Cooking Time: 15 Minutes
Ingredients:

For Tofu
1 (14-ounces) block tofu, pressed and cut into strips
6 bamboo skewers, presoaked and halved
For Tofu
2 tablespoons fresh lime juice
2 tablespoons soy sauce
1 tablespoon maple syrup
1 teaspoon Sriracha sauce
2 teaspoons fresh ginger, peeled

2 garlic cloves, peeled
For Sauce
1 (2-inches) piece fresh ginger, peeled
2 garlic cloves, peeled
½ cup creamy peanut butter
1 tablespoon soy sauce
1 tablespoon fresh lime juice
1-2 teaspoons Sriracha sauce
6 tablespoons of water

Directions:
Preheat the Air fryer to 370F and grease an Air fryer basket. Put all the ingredients except tofu in a food processor and pulse until smooth. Transfer the mixture into a bowl and marinate tofu in it. Thread one tofu strip onto each little bamboo stick and arrange them in the Air fryer basket. Cook for about 15 minutes and dish out onto serving plates. Mix all the ingredients for the sauce in a food processor and pulse until smooth. Drizzle the sauce over tofu and serve warm.

645.   Three Veg Bake

Servings: 3   Cooking Time: 30 Minutes
Ingredients:

1 large red onion, cut into rings
1 large zucchini, sliced

2 cloves garlic, crushed
1 bay leaf, cut in 6 pieces

Salt and pepper to taste

1 tbsp olive oil
Cooking spray

Directions:
Place the turnips, onion, and zucchini in a bowl. Toss with olive oil and season with salt and pepper. Preheat the air fryer to 330 F, and place the veggies into a baking pan that fits in the air fryer. Slip the bay leaves in the different parts of the slices and tuck the garlic cloves in between the slices. Insert the pan in the air fryer's basket and cook for 15 minutes. Serve warm with salad.

646.   Tofu With Veggies

Servings: 3   Cooking Time: 22 Minutes
Ingredients:

½ (14-ounces) block firm tofu, pressed and crumbled
1 cup carrot, peeled and chopped
3 cups cauliflower rice
½ cup broccoli, finely chopped
4 tablespoons low-sodium soy sauce, divided

½ cup frozen peas
1 teaspoon ground turmeric
1 tablespoon fresh ginger, minced
2 garlic cloves, minced
1 tablespoon rice vinegar
1½ teaspoons sesame oil, toasted

Directions:
Preheat the Air fryer to 370F and grease an Air fryer pan.   Mix the tofu, carrot, onion, 2 tablespoons of soy sauce, and turmeric in a bowl.   Transfer the tofu mixture into the Air fryer basket and cook for about 10 minutes.   Meanwhile, mix the cauliflower rice, broccoli, peas, ginger, garlic, vinegar, sesame oil, and remaining soy sauce in a bowl.   Stir in the cauliflower rice into the Air fryer pan and cook for about 12 minutes.   Dish out the tofu mixture onto serving plates and serve hot.

647.   Barbecue Tofu With Green Beans

Servings: 3   Cooking Time: 1 Hour
Ingredients:

12 ounces super firm tofu, pressed and cubed
1/4 cup ketchup
1 tablespoon white vinegar
1 tablespoon coconut sugar
1 tablespoon mustard
1/4 teaspoon ground black pepper

1/2 teaspoon sea salt
1/4 teaspoon smoked paprika
1/2 teaspoon freshly grated ginger
2 cloves garlic, minced
2 tablespoons olive oil
1 pound green beans

Directions:
Toss the tofu with the ketchup, white vinegar, coconut sugar, mustard, black pepper, sea salt, paprika, ginger, garlic, and olive oil. Let it marinate for 30 minutes.   Cook at 360 degrees F for 10 minutes; turn them over and cook for 12 minutes more. Reserve.   Place the green beans in the lightly greased Air Fryer basket. Roast at 400 degrees F for 5 minutes. Bon appétit!

648.   Grilled 'n Glazed Strawberries

Servings: 2   Cooking Time: 20 Minutes
Ingredients:

1 tbsp honey
1 tsp lemon zest
1-lb large strawberries

3 tbsp melted butter
Lemon wedges
Pinch kosher salt

Directions:
Thread strawberries in 4 skewers.   In a small bowl, mix well remaining Ingredients except for lemon wedges. Brush all over strawberries.   Place skewer on air fryer skewer rack.   For 10 minutes, cook on 360F. Halfway through cooking time, brush with honey mixture and turnover skewer.   Serve and enjoy with a squeeze of lemon.

649.   Crispy Vegie Tempura Style

Servings: 3   Cooking Time: 15 Minutes
Ingredients:

1/4 teaspoon salt
3/4 cup club soda
1 1/2 cups panko break crumbs
1 cup broccoli florets
1 egg, beaten
1 small sweet potato, peeled and cut into thick slices

1 red bell pepper, cut into strips
1 small zucchini, cut into thick slices
1/3 cup all-purpose flour
2/3 cup cornstarch
Non-stick cooking spray

Directions:
Dredge the vegetables in a cornstarch and all-purpose flour mixture.   Once all vegetables are dusted with flour, dip each vegetable in a mixture of egg and club soda before dredging in bread crumbs. Place the vegetables on the double layer rack accessory and spray with cooking oil.   Place inside the air fryer.   Close and cook for 20 minutes at 330F.

650.   Air Fried Vegetables With Garlic

Servings: 6   Cooking Time: 25 Minutes
Ingredients:

3/4 lb tomatoes
1 medium onion
1 tbsp lemon juice
1 tbsp olive oil

½ tbsp salt
1 tbsp coriander powder

Directions:
Preheat air fryer to 360 F. Place peppers, tomatoes, and onion in the basket. Cook for 5 minutes, then flip and cook for 5 more minutes. Remove and peel the skin. Place the vegetables in a blender and sprinkle with the salt and coriander powder. Blend to smooth and season with salt and olive oil.

651. Sautéed Bacon With Spinach

Servings: 2   Cooking Time: 9 Minutes
Ingredients:

3 meatless bacon slices, chopped
1 onion, chopped
4-ounce fresh spinach

2 tablespoons olive oil
1 garlic clove, minced

Directions:
Preheat the Air fryer to 340F and grease an Air fryer pan.   Put olive oil and garlic in the Air fryer pan and place in the Air fryer basket.   Cook for about 2 minutes and add bacon and onions.   Cook for about 3 minutes and stir in the spinach.   Cook for about 4 minutes and dish out in a bowl to serve.

652. Cinnamon Pear Chips

Servings: 1   Cooking Time: 25 Minutes
Ingredients:

2 tablespoons cinnamon & sugar mixture

1 medium pear, cored and thinly sliced

Directions:
Toss the pear slices with the cinnamon & sugar mixture. Transfer them to the lightly greased Air Fryer basket.   Bake in the preheated Air Fryer at 380 degrees F for 8 minutes, turning them over halfway through the cooking time.   Transfer to wire rack to cool. Bon appétit!

653. Easy Fry Portobello Mushroom

Servings: 2   Cooking Time: 10 Minutes
Ingredients:

1 tablespoon cooking oil
1-pound Portobello mushroom, sliced

Salt and pepper to taste

Directions:
Place the grill pan accessory in the air fryer.   In a bowl, place all Ingredients and toss to coat and season the mushrooms.   Place in the grill pan. Close the air fryer and cook for 10 minutes at 330F.

654. Mushrooms With Tahini Sauce

Servings: 5   Cooking Time: 22 Minutes
Ingredients:

1/2 teaspoon turmeric powder
1/3 teaspoon cayenne pepper
2 tablespoons lemon juice, freshly squeezed
1 teaspoon kosher salt

1/2 cup tahini
1/3 teaspoon freshly cracked black pepper
1 1/2 tablespoons vermouth
1 ½ tablespoons olive oil
1 ½ pounds Cremini mushrooms

Directions:

Grab a mixing dish and toss the mushrooms with the olive oil, turmeric powder, salt, black pepper, and cayenne pepper.   Cook them in your air fryer for 9 minutes at 355 degrees F.   Pause your Air Fryer, give it a good stir and cook for 10 minutes longer. Meanwhile, thoroughly combine lemon juice, vermouth, and tahini. Serve warm mushrooms with tahini sauce. Bon appétit!

655. Prawn Toast

Servings: 2   Cooking Time: 12 Minutes
Ingredients:

1 large spring onion, finely sliced
3 white bread slices
½ cup sweet corn

1 egg white, whisked
1 tbsp black sesame seeds

Directions:
In a bowl, place prawns, corn, spring onion and the sesame seeds. Add the whisked egg and mix the ingredients. Spread the mixture over the bread slices. Place in the prawns in the air fryer's basket and sprinkle oil. Fry the prawns until golden, for 8-10 minutes at 370 F. Serve with ketchup or chili sauce.

656. Rice & Beans Stuffed Bell Peppers

Servings: 5   Cooking Time: 15 Minutes
Ingredients:

½ small bell pepper, seeded and chopped
1 (15-ounces) can diced tomatoes with juice
1 (15-ounces) can red kidney beans, rinsed and drained
1 cup cooked rice

1½ teaspoons Italian seasoning
5 large bell peppers, tops removed and seeded
½ cup mozzarella cheese, shredded
1 tablespoon Parmesan cheese, grated

Directions:
In a bowl, mix well chopped bell pepper, tomatoes with juice, beans, rice, and Italian seasoning. Stuff each bell pepper evenly with the rice mixture. Set the temperature of air fryer to 360 degrees F. Grease an air fryer basket.   Arrange bell peppers into the air fryer basket in a single layer.   Air fry for about 12 minutes.   Meanwhile, in a bowl, mix together the mozzarella and Parmesan cheese. Remove the air fryer basket and top each bell pepper with cheese mixture.   Air fry for 3 more minutes. Remove from air fryer and transfer the bell peppers onto a serving platter.   Set aside to cool slightly. Serve warm.

657. Delightful Mushrooms

Servings: 4   Cooking Time: 22 Minutes
Ingredients:

2 cups mushrooms, sliced
2 tablespoons

1 tablespoon fresh chives, chopped

cheddar cheese, shredded · 2 tablespoons olive oil

Directions:
Preheat the Air fryer to 355F and grease an Air fryer basket. Coat the mushrooms with olive oil and arrange into the Air fryer basket. Cook for about 20 minutes and dish out in a platter. Top with chives and cheddar cheese and cook for 2 more minutes. Dish out and serve warm.

---

658. Jalapeno Stuffed With Bacon 'n Cheeses

Servings: 8   Cooking Time: 15 Minutes

Ingredients:
- ¼ cup cheddar cheese, shredded
- 16 fresh jalapenos, sliced lengthwise and seeded
- 1 teaspoon paprika
- 16 strips of uncured bacon, cut into half
- 4-ounce cream cheese
- Salt to taste

Directions:
In a mixing bowl, mix together the cream cheese, cheddar cheese, salt, and paprika until well-combined. Scoop half a teaspoon onto each half of jalapeno peppers. Use a thin strip of bacon and wrap it around the cheese-filled jalapeno half. Wear gloves when doing this step because jalapeno is very spicy. Place in the air fryer basket and cook for 15 minutes in a 350F preheated air fryer.

---

659. Rosemary Olive-oil Over Shrooms N Asparagus

Servings: 6   Cooking Time: 15 Minutes

Ingredients:
- ½ pound fresh mushroom, quartered
- 1 bunch fresh asparagus, trimmed and cleaned
- 2 sprigs of fresh rosemary, minced
- 2 teaspoon olive oil
- salt and pepper to taste

Directions:
Preheat the air fryer to 400F. Place the asparagus and mushrooms in a bowl and pour the rest of the ingredients. Toss to coat the asparagus and mushrooms. Place inside the air fryer and cook for 15 minutes.

---

660. Rainbow Roasted Vegetables

Servings: 4   Cooking Time: 25 Minutes

Ingredients:
- 1 red bell pepper, seeded and cut into 1/2-inch chunks
- 1 cup squash, peeled and cut into 1/2-inch chunks
- 1 yellow bell pepper, seeded and cut into 1/2-inch chunks
- 1 green bell pepper, seeded and cut into 1/2-inch chunks
- 1 cup broccoli, broken into 1/2-inch florets
- 2 parsnips, trimmed and cut into 1/2-inch chunks
- 1 yellow onion, quartered
- 2 garlic cloves, minced
- Pink Himalayan salt and ground black pepper, to taste
- 1/2 teaspoon marjoram
- 1/2 teaspoon dried oregano
- 1/4 cup dry white wine
- 1/4 cup vegetable broth
- 1/2 cup Kalamata olives, pitted and sliced

Directions:
Arrange your vegetables in a single layer in the baking pan in the order of the rainbow (red, orange, yellow, and green). Scatter the minced garlic around the vegetables. Season with salt, black pepper, marjoram, and oregano. Drizzle the white wine and vegetable broth over the vegetables. Roast in the preheated Air Fryer at 390 degrees F for 15 minutes, rotating the pan once or twice. Scatter the Kalamata olives all over your vegetables and serve warm. Bon appétit!

---

661. Classic Vegan Chili

Servings: 3   Cooking Time: 40 Minutes

Ingredients:
- 1 tablespoon olive oil
- 1/2 yellow onion, chopped
- 2 garlic cloves, minced
- 2 red bell peppers, seeded and chopped
- 1 red chili pepper, seeded and minced
- Sea salt and ground black pepper, to taste
- 1 teaspoon ground cumin
- 1 teaspoon cayenne pepper
- 1 teaspoon Mexican oregano
- 1/2 teaspoon mustard seeds
- 1/2 teaspoon celery seeds
- 1 can (28-ounces) diced tomatoes with juice
- 1 cup vegetable broth
- 1 (15-ounce) can black beans, rinsed and drained
- 1 bay leaf
- 1 teaspoon cider vinegar
- 1 avocado, sliced

Directions:
Start by preheating your Air Fryer to 365 degrees F. Heat the olive oil in a baking pan until sizzling. Then, sauté the onion, garlic, and peppers in the baking pan. Cook for 4 to 6 minutes. Now, add the salt, black pepper, cumin, cayenne pepper, oregano, mustard seeds, celery seeds, tomatoes, and broth. Cook for 20 minutes, stirring every 4 minutes. Stir in the canned beans, bay leaf, cider vinegar; let it cook for a further 8 minutes, stirring halfway through the cooking time. Serve in individual bowls garnished with the avocado slices. Enjoy!

---

662. Pesto Tomatoes

Servings: 4   Cooking Time: 16 Minutes

Ingredients:
- For Pesto:
- ½ cup plus 1 tablespoon olive oil, divided
- 3 tablespoons pine
- Salt, to taste
- For Tomatoes:
- 2 heirloom tomatoes, cut into ½ inch thick slices

nuts
½ cup fresh basil, chopped
½ cup fresh parsley, chopped
1 garlic clove, chopped
½ cup Parmesan cheese, grated

8 ounces feta cheese, cut into ½ inch thick slices.
½ cup red onions, thinly sliced
1 tablespoon olive oil
Salt, to taste

Directions:
Set the temperature of air fryer to 390 degrees F. Grease an air fryer basket.   In a bowl, mix together one tablespoon of oil, pine nuts and pinch of salt. Arrange pine nuts into the prepared air fryer basket. Air fry for about 1-2 minutes.   Remove from air fryer and transfer the pine nuts onto a paper towel-lined plate.   In a food processor, add the toasted pine nuts, fresh herbs, garlic, Parmesan, and salt and pulse until just combined.   While motor is running, slowly add the remaining oil and pulse until smooth.   Transfer into a bowl, covered and refrigerate until serving.   Spread about one tablespoon of pesto onto each tomato slice.   Top each tomato slice with one feta and onion slice and drizzle with oil.   Arrange tomato slices into the prepared air fryer basket in a single layer.   Air fry for about 12-14 minutes.   Remove from air fryer and transfer the tomato slices onto serving plates. Sprinkle with a little salt and serve with the remaining pesto.

663.   The Best Avocado Fries Ever

Servings: 4   Cooking Time: 50 Minutes
Ingredients:
1/2 head garlic (6-7 cloves)
1/2 cup almond meal
Sea salt and ground black pepper, to taste
1/2 cup parmesan cheese, grated

2 eggs
2 avocados, cut into wedges
Sauce:
1/2 cup mayonnaise
1 teaspoon lemon juice
1 teaspoon mustard

Directions:
Place the garlic on a piece of aluminum foil and spritz with cooking spray. Wrap the garlic in the foil. Cook in the preheated Air Fryer at 400 degrees for 12 minutes. Check the garlic, open the top of the foil and continue to cook for 10 minutes more.   Let it cool for 10 to 15 minutes; remove the cloves by squeezing them out of the skins; mash the garlic and reserve.   In a shallow bowl, combine the almond meal, salt, and black pepper. In another shallow dish, whisk the eggs until frothy.   Place the parmesan cheese in a third shallow dish. Dredge the avocado wedges in the almond meal mixture, shaking off the excess. Then, dip in the egg mixture; lastly, dredge in parmesan cheese.   Spritz the avocado wedges with cooking oil on all sides.   Cook in the preheated Air Fryer at 395 degrees F approximately 8 minutes, turning them over halfway through the cooking time.   Meanwhile, combine the sauce

ingredients with the smashed roasted garlic. To serve, divide the avocado fries between plates and top with the sauce. Enjoy!

664.   Tender Butternut Squash Fry

Servings: 2   Cooking Time: 10 Minutes
Ingredients:
1 tablespoon cooking oil
Salt and pepper to taste

1-pound butternut squash, seeded and sliced

Directions:
Place the grill pan accessory in the air fryer.   In a bowl, place all Ingredients and toss to coat and season the squash.   Place in the grill pan.   Close the air fryer and cook for 10 minutes at 330F.

665.   Quinoa & Veggie Stuffed Peppers

Servings: 1   Cooking Time: 16 Minutes
Ingredients:
1 bell pepper
½ tbsp diced onion
½ diced tomato, plus one tomato slice
¼ tsp smoked paprika

Salt and pepper, to taste
1 tsp olive oil
¼ tsp dried basil

Directions:
Preheat the air fryer to 350 F, core and clean the bell pepper to prepare it for stuffing. Brush the pepper with half of the olive oil on the outside. In a small bowl, combine all of the other ingredients, except the tomato slice and reserved half-teaspoon of olive oil.   Stuff the pepper with the filling and top with the tomato slice. Brush the tomato slice with the remaining half-teaspoon of olive oil and sprinkle with basil. Air fry for 10 minutes, until thoroughly cooked.

666.   Greek-style Roasted Vegetables

Servings: 3   Cooking Time: 25 Minutes
Ingredients:
1/2 pound butternut squash, peeled and cut into 1-inch chunks
1/2 pound cauliflower, cut into 1-inch florets
1/2 pound zucchini, cut into 1-inch chunks
2 bell peppers, cut into 1-inch chunks
2 tablespoons extra-virgin olive oil

1 red onion, sliced
1 cup dry white wine
1 teaspoon dried rosemary
Sea salt and freshly cracked black pepper, to taste
1/2 teaspoon dried basil
1 (28-ounce) canned diced tomatoes with juice
1/2 cup Kalamata olives, pitted

Directions:
Toss the vegetables with the olive oil, wine, rosemary, salt, black pepper, and basil until well

coated. Pour 1/2 of the canned diced tomatoes into a lightly greased baking dish; spread to cover the bottom of the baking dish. Add the vegetables and top with the remaining diced tomatoes. Scatter the Kalamata olives over the top. Bake in the preheated Air Fryer at 390 degrees F for 20 minutes, rotating the dish halfway through the cooking time. Serve warm and enjoy!

667. Caramelized Carrots

Servings: 3   Cooking Time: 15 Minutes
Ingredients:

1 small bag baby carrots	½ cup butter, melted
	½ cup brown sugar

Directions:
Preheat the Air fryer to 400F and grease an Air fryer basket. Mix the butter and brown sugar in a bowl. Add the carrots and toss to coat well. Arrange the carrots in the Air fryer basket and cook for about 15 minutes. Dish out and serve warm.

668. The Best Falafel Ever

Servings: 2   Cooking Time: 20 Minutes
Ingredients:

1 cup dried chickpeas, soaked overnight	1 tablespoon flour
1 small-sized onion, chopped	1/2 teaspoon baking powder
2 cloves garlic, minced	1 teaspoon cumin powder
2 tablespoons fresh cilantro leaves, chopped	A pinch of ground cardamom
	Sea salt and ground black pepper, to taste

Directions:
Pulse all the ingredients in your food processor until the chickpeas are ground. Form the falafel mixture into balls and place them in the lightly greased Air Fryer basket. Cook at 380 degrees F for about 15 minutes, shaking the basket occasionally to ensure even cooking. Serve in pita bread with toppings of your choice. Enjoy!

669. Rich Asparagus And Mushroom Patties

Servings: 4   Cooking Time: 15 Minutes
Ingredients:

3/4 pound asparagus spears	1 teaspoon paprika
1 tablespoon canola oil	1 cup button mushrooms, chopped
Sea salt and freshly ground black pepper, to taste	1/2 cup parmesan cheese, grated
1 teaspoon garlic powder	2 tablespoons flax seeds
3 tablespoons scallions, chopped	2 eggs, beaten
	4 tablespoons sour cream, for garnish

Directions:

Place the asparagus spears in the lightly greased cooking basket. Toss the asparagus with the canola oil, paprika, salt, and black pepper. Cook in the preheated Air Fryer at 400 degrees F for 5 minutes. Chop the asparagus spears and add the garlic powder, scallions, mushrooms, parmesan, flax seeds, and eggs. Mix until everything is well incorporated and form the asparagus mixture into patties. Cook in the preheated Air Fryer at 400 degrees F for 5 minutes, flipping halfway through the cooking time. Serve with well-chilled sour cream. Bon appétit!

670. Vegetable Skewers With Asian-style Peanut Sauce

Servings: 4   Cooking Time: 30 Minutes
Ingredients:

2 bell peppers, diced into 1-inch pieces	1 teaspoon dried rosemary, crushed
4 pearl onions, halved	1/3 teaspoon granulated garlic
8 small button mushrooms, cleaned	Peanut Sauce:
2 tablespoons extra-virgin olive oil	2 tablespoons peanut butter
Sea salt and ground black pepper, to taste	1 tablespoon balsamic vinegar
1 teaspoon red pepper flakes, crushed	1 tablespoon soy sauce
	1/2 teaspoon garlic salt

Directions:
Soak the wooden skewers in water for 15 minutes. Thread the vegetables on skewers; drizzle the olive oil all over the vegetable skewers; sprinkle with spices. Cook in the preheated Air Fryer at 400 degrees F for 13 minutes. Meanwhile, in a small dish, whisk the peanut butter with the balsamic vinegar, soy sauce, and garlic salt. Serve your skewers with the peanut sauce on the side. Enjoy!

671. Dad's Roasted Pepper Salad

Servings: 4   Cooking Time: 25 Minutes + Chilling Time
Ingredients:

2 yellow bell peppers	1 Serrano pepper
2 red bell peppers	Sea salt, to taste
2 green bell peppers	1/2 teaspoon mixed peppercorns, freshly crushed
4 tablespoons olive oil	
2 tablespoons cider vinegar	1/2 cup pine nuts
2 garlic cloves, peeled and pressed	1/4 cup loosely packed fresh Italian parsley leaves, roughly chopped
1 teaspoon cayenne pepper	

Directions:
Start by preheating your Air Fryer to 400 degrees F. Brush the Air Fryer basket lightly with cooking oil. Then, roast the peppers for 5 minutes. Give the peppers a half turn; place them back in the cooking

basket and roast for another 5 minutes. Turn them one more time and roast until the skin is charred and soft or 5 more minutes. Peel the peppers and let them cool to room temperature. In a small mixing dish, whisk the olive oil, vinegar, garlic, cayenne pepper, salt, and crushed peppercorns. Dress the salad and set aside. Add the pine nuts to the cooking basket. Roast at 360 degrees F for 4 minutes; give the nuts a good toss. Put the cooking basket back again and roast for a further 3 to 4 minutes. Scatter the toasted nuts over the peppers and garnish with parsley. Bon appétit!

672. Healthy Apple-licious Chips

Servings: 1   Cooking Time: 6 Minutes

Ingredients:

½ teaspoon ground cumin	1 apple, cored and sliced thinly
1 tablespoon sugar	A pinch of salt

Directions:

Place all ingredients in a bowl and toss to coat everything. Put the grill pan accessory in the air fryer and place the sliced apples on the grill pan. Close the air fryer and cook for 6 minutes at 390F.

673. Warm Farro Salad With Roasted Tomatoes

Servings: 2   Cooking Time: 40 Minutes

Ingredients:

3/4 cup farro	2 tablespoons champagne vinegar
3 cups water	
1 tablespoon sea salt	2 tablespoons white wine
1 pound cherry tomatoes	
2 spring onions, chopped	2 tablespoons extra-virgin olive oil
2 carrots, grated	1 teaspoon red pepper flakes
2 heaping tablespoons fresh parsley leaves	

Directions:

Place the farro, water, and salt in a saucepan and bring it to a rapid boil. Turn the heat down to medium-low, and simmer, covered, for 30 minutes or until the farro has softened. Drain well and transfer to an air fryer-safe pan. Meanwhile, place the cherry tomatoes in the lightly greased Air Fryer basket. Roast at 400 degrees F for 4 minutes. Add the roasted tomatoes to the pan with the cooked farro, Toss the salad ingredients with the spring onions, carrots, parsley, vinegar, white wine, and olive oil. Bake at 360 degrees F an additional 5 minutes. Serve garnished with red pepper flakes and enjoy!

674. Grilled 'n Spiced Tomatoes On Garden Salad

Servings: 4   Cooking Time: 20 Minutes

Ingredients:

¼ cup golden raisins	½ cup chopped chives
¼ cup hazelnuts, toasted and chopped	2 tablespoons white balsamic vinegar
¼ cup pistachios, toasted and chopped	3 large green tomatoes
¾ cup cilantro leaves, chopped	4 leaves iceberg lettuce
¾ cup fresh parsley, chopped	5 tablespoons olive oil
1 clove of garlic, minced	Salt and pepper to taste

Directions:

Preheat the air fryer to 330F. Place the grill pan accessory in the air fryer. In a mixing bowl, season the tomatoes with garlic, oil, salt and pepper to taste. Place on the grill pan and grill for 20 minutes. Once the tomatoes are done, toss in a salad bowl together with the rest of the Ingredients.

675. Traditional Indian Bhaji

Servings: 4   Cooking Time: 40 Minutes

Ingredients:

2 eggs, beaten	1 teaspoon cumin seed
1/2 cup almond meal	
1/2 cup coconut flour	Salt and black pepper, to your liking
1/2 teaspoon baking powder	
	2 red onions, chopped
1 teaspoon curry paste	1 Indian green chili, pureed
1 teaspoon minced fresh ginger root	Non-stick cooking spray

Directions:

Whisk the eggs, almond meal, coconut flour and baking powder in a mixing dish to make a thick batter; add in the cold water if needed. Add in curry paste, cumin seeds, ginger root, salt, and black pepper. Now, add onions and chili pepper; mix until everything is well incorporated. Shape the balls and slightly press them to make the patties. Spritz the patties with cooking oil on all sides. Place a sheet of aluminum foil in the Air Fryer food basket. Place the fritters on foil. Then, air-fry them at 360 degrees F for 15 minutes; flip them over, press the power button and cook for another 20 minutes. Serve right away!

676. Cottage Cheese And Potatoes

Servings: 5   Cooking Time: 30 Minutes

Ingredients:

1 bunch asparagus, trimmed	¼ cup fresh cream
¼ cup cottage cheese, cubed	1 tbsp whole-grain mustard

Directions:

Preheat the air fryer to 400 F and place the potatoes in the basket; cook for 25 minutes. Boil salted water in a pot over medium heat. Add asparagus and cook for 3 minutes until tender. In a bowl, mix cooked potatoes, cottage cheese, cream, asparagus and mustard. Toss well and season with salt and black pepper. Transfer the mixture to the potato skin shells and serve.

677. Refreshingly Zesty Broccoli

Servings: 4   Cooking Time: 15 Minutes

Ingredients:

1 large head broccoli, cut into bite-sized pieces	1 tablespoon butter
	3 garlic cloves, chopped
1 tablespoon white sesame seeds	½ teaspoon fresh lemon zest, grated finely
2 tablespoons vegetable stock	
1 tablespoon fresh lemon juice	½ teaspoon red pepper flakes, crushed

Directions:

Preheat the Air fryer to 355F and grease an Air fryer pan.   Mix butter, vegetable stock and lemon juice in the Air fryer pan.   Transfer into the Air fryer and cook for about 2 minutes.   Stir in garlic and broccoli and cook for about 14 minutes.   Add sesame seeds, lemon zest and red pepper flakes and cook for 5 minutes.   Dish out and serve warm.

678. Spiced Soy Curls

Servings: 2   Cooking Time: 10 Minutes

Ingredients:

3 cups boiling water	2 teaspoons Cajun seasoning
4 ounces soy curls	
¼ cup nutritional yeast	1 teaspoon poultry seasoning
¼ cup fine ground cornmeal	Salt and ground white pepper, as required

Directions:

In a heatproof bowl, add the boiling water and soak the soy curls for about 10 minutes.   Through a strainer, drain the soy curls and then with a large spoon, press to release the extra water.   In a bowl, mix well nutritional yeast, cornmeal, seasonings, salt, and white pepper.   Add the soy curls and generously coat with the mixture.   Set the temperature of air fryer to 380 degrees F. Grease an air fryer basket.   Arrange soy curls into the prepared air fryer basket in a single layer.   Air fry for about 10 minutes, shaking once halfway through. Remove from air fryer and transfer the soy curls onto serving plates.   Serve warm.

679. Fried Broccoli Recipe From India

Servings: 6   Cooking Time: 15 Minutes

Ingredients:

¼ teaspoon turmeric powder	1 teaspoon garam masala
½ pounds broccoli, cut into florets	2 tablespoons coconut milk

1 tablespoon almond flour	Salt and pepper to taste

Directions:

Preheat the air fryer for 5 minutes.   In a bowl, combine all ingredients until the broccoli florets are coated with the other ingredients.   Place in a fryer basket and cook for 15 minutes until crispy.

680. Almond Asparagus

Servings: 3   Cooking Time: 6 Minutes

Ingredients:

1 pound asparagus	2 tablespoons balsamic vinegar
1/3 cup almonds, sliced	
2 tablespoons olive oil	Salt and black pepper, to taste

Directions:

Preheat the Air fryer to 400F and grease an Air fryer basket.   Mix asparagus, oil, vinegar, salt, and black pepper in a bowl and toss to coat well. Arrange asparagus into the Air fryer basket and sprinkle with the almond slices.   Cook for about 6 minutes and dish out to serve hot.

681. Curly Vegan Fries

Servings: 2   Cooking Time: 20 Minutes

Ingredients:

1 tbsp tomato ketchup	2 tbsp olive oil
	2 tbsp coconut oil
Salt and pepper to taste	

Directions:

Preheat your air fryer to 360 F and use a spiralizer to spiralize the potatoes. In a bowl, mix oil, coconut oil, salt and pepper. Cover the potatoes with the oil mixture. Place the potatoes in the cooking basket and cook for 15 minutes. Serve with ketchup and enjoy!

682. Curried Cauliflower Florets

Servings: 4   Cooking Time: 34 Minutes

Ingredients:

Salt to taste	½ cup olive oil
1 ½ tbsp curry powder	1/3 cup fried pine nuts

Directions:

Preheat the air fryer to 390 F, and mix the pine nuts and 1 tsp of olive oil, in a medium bowl. Pour them in the air fryer's basket and cook for 2 minutes; remove to cool.   Place the cauliflower on a cutting board. Use a knife to cut them into 1-inch florets. Place them in a large mixing bowl. Add the curry powder, salt, and the remaining olive oil; mix well. Place the cauliflower florets in the fryer's basket in 2 batches, and cook each batch for 10 minutes. Remove the curried florets onto a serving platter, sprinkle with the pine nuts, and toss. Serve the florets with tomato sauce or as a side to a meat dish.

131

683. Eggplant Salad

Servings: 2   Cooking Time: 15 Minutes

Ingredients:

1 eggplant, cut into ½-inch-thick slices crosswise	For Dressing
	1 tablespoon red wine vinegar
1 avocado, peeled, pitted and chopped	1 tablespoon honey
2 tablespoons canola oil	1 tablespoon fresh oregano leaves, chopped
Salt and ground black pepper, as required	1 teaspoon fresh lemon zest, grated
1 teaspoon fresh lemon juice	1 teaspoon Dijon mustard
1 tablespoon extra-virgin olive oil	Salt and ground black pepper, as required

Directions:

Preheat the Air fryer to 400F and grease an Air fryer basket.   Mix eggplant, oil, salt, and black pepper in a bowl and toss to coat well.   Arrange the eggplants pieces in the Air fryer basket and cook for about 15 minutes, flipping twice in between.   Dish out the Brussel sprouts in a serving bowl and keep aside to cool.   Add avocado and lemon juice and mix well.   Mix all the ingredients for dressing in a bowl and pour over the salad.   Toss to coat well and serve immediately.

684. Ricotta Cauliflower Fritters

Servings: 4   Cooking Time: 30 Minutes

Ingredients:

1 tablespoon olive oil	1/4 cup almond flour
1/2 pound cauliflower	1/2 onion, chopped
1/2 cup Ricotta cheese	1 garlic clove, minced
1/4 cup ground flaxseed meal	Sea salt and ground black pepper, to your liking
1/2 teaspoon baking powder	1 cup parmesan cheese, grated

Directions:

Start by preheating your Air Fryer to 400 degrees F. Drizzle the olive oil all over the cauliflower. Place the cauliflower in the Air Fryer basket and cook approximately 15 minutes, shaking the basket periodically.   Then, mash the cauliflower and combine with the other ingredients. Form the mixture into patties.   Bake in the preheated Air Fryer at 380 degrees F for 14 minutes, flipping them halfway through the cooking time to ensure even cooking. Bon appétit!

685. Easy Glazed Carrots

Servings: 4   Cooking Time: 12 Minutes

Ingredients:

3 cups carrots, peeled and cut into large chunks	1 tablespoon olive oil
1 tablespoon honey	Salt and black pepper, to taste

Directions:

Preheat the Air fryer to 390F and grease an Air fryer basket.   Mix all the ingredients in a bowl and toss to coat well.   Transfer into the Air fryer basket and cook for about 12 minutes.   Dish out and serve hot.

686. Herbed Potatoes

Servings: 4   Cooking Time: 15 Minutes

Ingredients:

6 small potatoes, chopped	2 teaspoons mixed dried herbs
2 tablespoons fresh parsley, chopped	Salt and black pepper, to taste
3 tablespoons olive oil	

Directions:

Preheat the Air fryer to 360F and grease an Air fryer basket.   Mix the potatoes, oil, herbs, salt and black pepper in a bowl.   Arrange the chopped potatoes into the Air fryer basket and cook for about 15 minutes, tossing once in between.   Dish out the potatoes onto serving plates and serve garnished with parsley.

687. Tofu With Capers Sauce

Servings: 4   Cooking Time: 27 Minutes

Ingredients:

4 tablespoons fresh parsley, divided	2 teaspoons cornstarch
1 (14-ounces) block extra-firm tofu, pressed and cut into 8 rectangular cutlets	1 cup vegetable broth
	½ cup lemon juice
	2 garlic cloves, peeled
1 cup panko breadcrumbs	½ cup mayonnaise
2 tablespoons capers	Salt and black pepper, to taste

Directions:

Preheat the Air fryer to 375F and grease an Air fryer basket.   Put half of lemon juice, 2 tablespoons parsley, 2 garlic cloves, salt and black pepper in a food processor and pulse until smooth.   Transfer the mixture into a bowl and marinate tofu in it. Place the mayonnaise in a shallow bowl and put the panko breadcrumbs in another bowl.   Coat the tofu pieces with mayonnaise and then, roll into the breadcrumbs.   Arrange the tofu pieces in the Air fryer pan and cook for about 20 minutes.   Mix broth, remaining lemon juice, remaining garlic, remaining parsley, cornstarch, salt and black pepper in a food processor and pulse until smooth. Transfer the sauce into a small pan and stir in the capers.   Boil the sauce over medium heat and allow to simmer for about 7 minutes.   Dish out the tofu onto serving plates and drizzle with the caper sauce to serve.

688. Crispy Bacon-wrapped Asparagus Bundles

Servings: 4   Cooking Time: 8 Minutes

Ingredients:

1 pound asparagus
4 bacon slices
½ tablespoon sesame seeds, toasted
1 garlic clove, minced

1½ tablespoons brown sugar
1½ tablespoons olive oil
½ tablespoon sesame oil, toasted

Directions:
Preheat the Air fryer to 355F and grease an Air fryer basket.   Mix garlic, brown sugar, olive oil and sesame oil in a bowl till sugar is dissolved.   Divide asparagus into 4 equal bunches and wrap a bacon slice around each bunch.   Rub the asparagus bunch with garlic mixture and arrange in the Air fryer basket.   Sprinkle with sesame seeds and cook for about 8 minutes.   Dish out and serve hot.

689.   Radish Salad

Servings: 4   Cooking Time: 30 Minutes
Ingredients:
1½ pounds radishes, trimmed and halved
½ pound fresh mozzarella, sliced
6 cups fresh salad greens
1 teaspoon honey

3 tablespoons olive oil
1 tablespoon balsamic vinegar
Salt and black pepper, to taste

Directions:
Preheat the Air fryer to 350F and grease an Air fryer basket.   Mix the radishes, salt, black pepper, and olive oil in a bowl and toss to coat well.   Arrange the radishes in the Air fryer basket and cook for about 30 minutes, flipping twice in between.   Dish out the radishes in a serving bowl and keep aside to cool.   Add mozzarella cheese and greens and mix well.   Mix honey, oil, vinegar, salt, and black pepper in a bowl and pour over the salad.   Toss to coat well and serve immediately.

690.   Your Traditional Mac 'n Cheese

Servings: 3   Cooking Time: 32 Minutes
Ingredients:
1/2 pinch ground nutmeg
1/2 teaspoon Dijon mustard
1/4 cup panko bread crumbs
1/8 teaspoon cayenne pepper
1/8 teaspoon dried thyme
1/8 teaspoon white pepper
1/8 teaspoon Worcestershire sauce

1/2 teaspoon salt
1-1/2 cups milk
1-1/2 cups shredded sharp Cheddar cheese, divided
1-1/2 teaspoons butter, melted
2 tablespoons all-purpose flour
2 tablespoons butter
8-ounce elbow macaroni, cooked according to package
Directions:

Directions:
Melt 2 tbsp butter in baking pan of air fryer for 2 minutes at 360F. Stir in flour and cook for 3 minutes,

stirring every now and then. Stir in white pepper, cayenne pepper, and thyme. Cook for 2 minutes. Stir in a cup of milk and whisk well. Cook for 5 minutes while mixing constantly.   Mix in salt, Worcestershire sauce, and nutmeg . Mix well. Cook for 5 minutes or until thickened while stirring frequently.   Add cheese and mix well. Cook for 3 minutes or until melted and thoroughly mixed. Stir in Dijon mustard and mix well. Add macaroni and toss well to coat. Sprinkle remaining cheese on top.   In a small bowl mix well 1 ½ tsp butter and panko. Sprinkle on top of cheese.   Cook for 15 minutes at 390F until tops are lightly browned. Serve and enjoy.

691.   Two-cheese Vegetable Frittata

Servings: 2   Cooking Time: 35 Minutes
Ingredients:
⅓ cup sliced mushrooms
1 large zucchini, sliced with a 1-inch thickness
1 small red onion, sliced
¼ cup chopped chives
¼ lb asparagus, trimmed and sliced thinly

2 tsp olive oil
4 eggs, cracked into a bowl
⅓ cup milk
Salt and pepper to taste
⅓ cup grated Cheddar cheese
⅓ cup crumbled Feta cheese

Directions:
Preheat the air fryer to 380 F. Line a baking dish with parchment paper; set aside. In the egg bowl, add milk, salt, and pepper; beat evenly. Place a skillet over medium heat on a stovetop, and heat olive oil.   Add the asparagus, zucchini, onion, mushrooms, and baby spinach; stir-fry for 5 minutes. Pour the veggies into the baking dish and top with the egg mixture. Sprinkle feta and cheddar cheese over and place in the air fryer. Cook for 15 minutes. Remove the baking dish and garnish with fresh chives.

692.   Kurkuri Bhindi (indian Fried Okra)

Servings: 4   Cooking Time: 20 Minutes
Ingredients:
2 tbsp garam masala
1 cup cornmeal
¼ cup flour
Salt to taste

½ pound okra, trimmed and halved lengthwise
1 egg

Directions:
Preheat the Air Fryer to 380 F.   In a bowl, mix cornmeal, flour, chili powder, garam masala, salt, and pepper. In another bowl, whisk the egg; season with salt and pepper. Dip the okra in the egg and then coat in cornmeal mixture. Spray okra with cooking spray and place in the air fryer basket in a single layer. Cook for 6 minutes. Slide out the basket

and shake; cook for another 6 minutes until golden brown. Serve with your favorite dip.

693. Sweet & Spicy Parsnips

Servings: 6   Cooking Time: 44 Minutes
Ingredients:

2 pounds parsnip, peeled and cut into 1-inch chunks	1 tablespoon butter, melted
2 tablespoons honey	¼ teaspoon red pepper flakes, crushed
1 tablespoon dried parsley flakes, crushed	Salt and ground black pepper, as required

Directions:
Set the temperature of air fryer to 355 degrees F. Grease an air fryer basket.   In a large bowl, mix together the parsnips and butter.   Arrange parsnip chunks into the prepared air fryer basket in a single layer.   Air fry for about 40 minutes. Meanwhile, in another large bowl, mix well remaining ingredients.   After 40 minutes, transfer parsnips into the bowl of honey mixture and toss to coat well.   Again, arrange the parsnip chunks into air fryer basket in a single layer.   Air fry for 3-4 more minutes.   Remove from air fryer and transfer the parsnip chunks onto serving plates. Serve hot.

694. Lemony Green Beans

Servings: 3   Cooking Time: 12 Minutes
Ingredients:

1 pound green beans, trimmed and halved	1 tablespoon fresh lemon juice
1 teaspoon butter, melted	¼ teaspoon garlic powder

Directions:
Preheat the Air fryer to 400F and grease an Air fryer basket.   Mix all the ingredients in a bowl and toss to coat well.   Arrange the green beans into the Air fryer basket and cook for about 12 minutes.   Dish out in a serving plate and serve hot.

695. Air Fried Halloumi With Veggies

Servings: 2   Cooking Time: 15 Minutes
Ingredients:

2 zucchinis, cut into even chunks	1 large carrot, cut into chunks
1 large eggplant, peeled, cut into chunks	1 tsp dried mixed herbs
2 tsp olive oil	Salt and black pepper

Directions:
In a bowl, add halloumi, zucchini, carrot, eggplant, olive oil, herbs, salt and pepper. Sprinkle with oil, salt and pepper. Arrange halloumi and veggies on the air fryer basket and drizzle with olive oil. Cook for 14 minutes at 340 F, shaking once. Sprinkle with mixed herbs to serve.

696. Avocado Rolls

Servings: 5   Cooking Time: 15 Minutes
Ingredients:

10 egg roll wrappers	¼ tsp pepper
1 tomato, diced	½ tsp salt

Directions:
Place all filling ingredients in a bowl; mash with a fork until somewhat smooth. There should be chunks left. Divide the feeling between the egg wrappers. Wet your finger and brush along the edges, so the wrappers can seal well. Roll and seal the wrappers.   Arrange them on a baking sheet lined dish, and place in the air fryer. Cook at 350 F for 5 minutes. Serve with sweet chili dipping and enjoy.

697. Classic Baked Banana

Servings: 2   Cooking Time: 20 Minutes
Ingredients:

2 just-ripe bananas	2 tablespoons honey
2 teaspoons lime juice	1/2 teaspoon ground cinnamon
1/4 teaspoon grated nutmeg	A pinch of salt

Directions:
Toss the banana with all ingredients until well coated. Transfer your bananas to the parchment-lined cooking basket.   Bake in the preheated Air Fryer at 370 degrees F for 12 minutes, turning them over halfway through the cooking time. Enjoy!

698. Mediterranean-style Potato Chips With Vegveeta Dip

Servings: 4   Cooking Time: 1 Hour
Ingredients:

1 large potato, cut into 1/8 inch thick slices	Sea salt, to taste
1 tablespoon olive oil	1/2 teaspoon fresh basil
1/2 teaspoon red pepper flakes, crushed	Dipping Sauce:
1 teaspoon fresh rosemary	1/3 cup raw cashews
1/2 teaspoon fresh sage	1 tablespoon tahini
	1 ½ tablespoons olive oil
	1/4 cup raw almonds
	1/4 teaspoon prepared yellow mustard

Directions:
Soak the potatoes in a large bowl of cold water for 20 to 30 minutes. Drain the potatoes and pat them dry with a kitchen towel.   Toss with olive oil and seasonings.   Place in the lightly greased cooking basket and cook at 380 degrees F for 30 minutes. Work in batches.   Meanwhile, puree the sauce ingredients in your food processor until smooth. Serve the potato chips with the Vegveeta sauce for dipping. Bon appétit!

699. Baked Spicy Tortilla Chips

Servings: 3   Cooking Time: 20 Minutes

Ingredients:

- 6 (6-inch) corn tortillas
- 1 teaspoon canola oil
- 1/4 teaspoon ground white pepper
- 1 teaspoon salt
- 1/2 teaspoon ground cumin
- 1/2 teaspoon ancho chili powder

Directions:

Slice the tortillas into quarters. Brush the tortilla pieces with the canola oil until well coated.   Toss with the spices and transfer to the Air Fryer basket. Bake at 360 degrees F for 8 minutes or until lightly golden. Work in batches. Bon appétit!

700. Mozzarella Cabbage With Blue Cheese

Servings: 4   Cooking Time: 25 Minutes

Ingredients:

- 2 cups Parmesan cheese, chopped
- Salt and pepper to taste
- 4 tbsp melted butter
- ½ cup blue cheese sauce

Directions:

Preheat your air fryer to 380 F, and cover cabbage wedges with melted butter; coat with mozzarella. Place the coated cabbage in the cooking basket and cook for 20 minutes. Serve with blue cheese.

Other Air Fryer Recipes

701. Spring Chocolate Doughnuts

Servings: 6   Cooking Time: 20 Minutes

Ingredients:

1 can (16-ounce can buttermilk biscuits	Chocolate Glaze:
	1 cup powdered sugar
4 tablespoons unsweetened baking cocoa	2 tablespoon butter, melted
	2 tablespoons milk

Directions:

Bake your biscuits in the preheated Air Fryer at 350 degrees F for 8 minutes, flipping them halfway through the cooking time.   While the biscuits are baking, make the glaze.   Beat the ingredients with whisk until smooth, adding enough milk for the desired consistency; set aside.   Dip your doughnuts into the chocolate glaze and transfer to a cooling rack to set. Bon appétit!

702. Frittata With Porcini Mushrooms

Servings: 4   Cooking Time: 40 Minutes

Ingredients:

3 cups Porcini mushrooms, thinly sliced	1/3 teaspoon table salt
	8 eggs
1 tablespoon melted butter	1/2 teaspoon ground black pepper, preferably freshly ground
1 shallot, peeled and slice into thin rounds	
1 garlic cloves, peeled and finely minced	1 teaspoon cumin powder
1 lemon grass, cut into 1-inch pieces	1/3 teaspoon dried or fresh dill weed
	1/2 cup goat cheese, crumbled

Directions:

Melt the butter in a nonstick skillet that is placed over medium heat. Sauté the shallot, garlic, thinly sliced Porcini mushrooms, and lemon grass over a moderate heat until they have softened. Now, reserve the sautéed mixture.   Preheat your Air Fryer to 335 degrees F. Then, in a mixing bowl, beat the eggs until frothy. Now, add the seasonings and mix to combine well.   Coat the sides and bottom of a baking dish with a thin layer of vegetable spray. Pour the egg/seasoning mixture into the baking dish; throw in the onion/mushroom sauté. Top with the crumbled goat cheese.   Place the baking dish in the Air Fryer cooking basket. Cook for about 32 minutes or until your frittata is set. Enjoy!

703. Zesty Broccoli Bites With Hot Sauce

Servings: 6   Cooking Time: 20 Minutes

Ingredients:

For the Broccoli Bites:	1/2 teaspoon granulated garlic
1 medium-sized head broccoli, broken into florets	1/3 teaspoon celery seeds
1/2 teaspoon lemon zest, freshly grated	1 ½ tablespoons olive oil
1/3 teaspoon fine sea salt	For the Hot Sauce:
1/2 teaspoon hot paprika	1/2 cup tomato sauce
1 teaspoon shallot powder	3 tablespoons brown sugar
1 teaspoon porcini powder	1 tablespoon balsamic vinegar
	½ teaspoon ground allspice

Directions:

Toss all the ingredients for the broccoli bites in a mixing bowl, covering the broccoli florets on all sides.   Cook them in the preheated Air Fryer at 360 degrees for 13 to 15 minutes. In the meantime, mix all ingredients for the hot sauce.   Pause your Air Fryer, mix the broccoli with the prepared sauce and cook for further 3 minutes. Bon appétit!

704. Wine-braised Turkey Breasts

Servings: 4   Cooking Time: 30 Minutes + Marinating Time

Ingredients:

1/3 cup dry white wine	1/2 tablespoon honey
1½ tablespoon sesame oil	1/2 cup plain flour
	2 tablespoons oyster sauce
1/2 pound turkey breasts, boneless, skinless and sliced	Sea salt flakes and cracked black peppercorns, to taste

Directions:

Set the air fryer to cook at 385 degrees. Pat the turkey slices dry and season with the sea salt flakes and the cracked peppercorns.   In a bowl, mix the other ingredients together, minus the flour; rub your turkey with this mixture. Set aside to marinate for at least 55 minutes.   Coat each turkey slice with the plain flour. Cook for 27 minutes; make sure to flip once or twice and work in batches. Bon appétit!

705. Homemade Pork Scratchings

Servings: 10   Cooking Time: 50 Minutes

Ingredients:

1 pound pork rind raw, scored by the butcher	1 tablespoon sea salt
	2 tablespoon smoked paprika

Directions:

Sprinkle and rub salt on the skin side of the pork rind. Allow it to sit for 30 minutes.   Roast at 380 degrees F for 8 minutes; turn them over and cook for a further 8 minutes or until blistered.   Sprinkle the smoked paprika all over the pork scratchings and serve. Bon appétit!

706. Baked Apples With Crisp Topping

Servings: 3   Cooking Time: 25 Minutes

Ingredients:

3 Granny Smith apples, cored
2/3 cup rolled oats
1 tablespoon fresh orange juice
1/2 teaspoon ground cardamom
1/2 teaspoon ground cinnamon
3 tablespoons honey
1/4 teaspoon ground cloves
1/4 teaspoon ground star anise
2 tablespoons butter, cut in pieces
3 tablespoons cranberries

Directions:

Use a paring knife to remove the stem and seeds from the apples, making deep holes.   In a mixing bowl, combine together the rolled oats, honey, orange juice, cardamom, cinnamon, cloves, anise, butter, and cranberries.   Pour enough water into an Air Fryer safe dish. Place the apples in the dish. Bake at 340 degrees F for 16 to 18 minutes. Serve at room temperature. Bon appétit!

707. Cornbread With Pulled Pork

Servings: 2   Cooking Time: 24 Minutes

Ingredients:

2 ½ cups pulled pork, leftover works well too
1 teaspoon dried rosemary
1/2 teaspoon chili powder
1/2 recipe cornbread
3 cloves garlic, peeled and pressed
1/2 tablespoon brown sugar
1/3 cup scallions, thinly sliced
1 teaspoon sea salt

Directions:

Preheat a large-sized nonstick skillet over medium heat; now, cook the scallions together with the garlic and pulled pork.   Next, add the sugar, chili powder, rosemary, and salt. Cook, stirring occasionally, until the mixture is thickened.   Preheat your air fryer to 335 degrees F. Now, coat two mini loaf pans with a cooking spray. Add the pulled pork mixture and spread over the bottom using a spatula.   Spread the previously prepared cornbread batter over top of the spiced pulled pork mixture.   Bake this cornbread in the preheated air fryer until a tester inserted into the center of it comes out clean, or for 18 minutes. Bon appétit!

708. Double Cheese Mushroom Balls

Servings: 4   Cooking Time: 30 Minutes

Ingredients:

1 ½ tablespoons olive oil
4 ounces cauliflower florets
3 garlic cloves, peeled
2 cups white mushrooms, finely chopped
Sea salt and ground black pepper, or more
to taste
1/2 yellow onion, finely chopped
1 small-sized red chili pepper, seeded and minced
1/2 cup roasted vegetable stock
1/2 cup Swiss cheese, grated
1/4 cup pork rinds
1 egg, beaten
1/4 cup Romano cheese, grated

Directions:

Blitz the cauliflower florets in your food processor until they're crumbled (it is the size of rice).   Heat a saucepan over a moderate heat; now, heat the oil and sweat the cauliflower. garlic, onions, and chili pepper until tender.   Throw in the mushrooms and fry until they are fragrant and the liquid has almost evaporated.   Add the vegetable stock and boil for 18 minutes. Now, add the salt, black pepper, Swiss cheese pork rinds, and beaten egg; mix to combine.   Allow the mixture to cool completely. Shape the mixture into balls. Dip the balls in the grated Romano cheese. Air-fry the balls for 7 minutes at 400 degrees F. Bon appétit!

709. Rosemary Roasted Mixed Nuts

Servings: 6   Cooking Time: 20 Minutes

Ingredients:

2 tablespoons butter, at room temperature
1 tablespoon dried rosemary
1/2 teaspoon paprika
1 teaspoon coarse sea salt
1/2 cup pine nuts
1 cup pecans
1/2 cup hazelnuts

Directions:

Toss all the ingredients in the mixing bowl.   Line the Air Fryer basket with baking parchment. Spread out the coated nuts in a single layer in the basket. Roast at 350 degrees F for 6 to 8 minutes, shaking the basket once or twice. Work in batches. Enjoy!

710. Creamed Asparagus And Egg Salad

Servings: 4   Cooking Time: 25 Minutes + Chilling Time

Ingredients:

2 eggs
1 pound asparagus, chopped
2 cup baby spinach
1/2 cup mayonnaise
1 teaspoon mustard
1 teaspoon fresh lemon juice
Sea salt and ground black pepper, to taste

Directions:

Place the wire rack in the Air Fryer basket; lower the eggs onto the wire rack.   Cook at 270 degrees F for 15 minutes.   Transfer them to an ice-cold water bath to stop the cooking. Peel the eggs under cold running water; coarsely chop the hard-boiled eggs and set aside.   Increase the temperature to 400 degrees F. Place your asparagus in the lightly greased Air Fryer basket.   Cook for 5 minutes or until tender. Place in a nice salad bowl. Add the baby spinach. In a mixing dish, thoroughly combine the remaining ingredients. Drizzle this dressing over the asparagus in the salad bowl and top with the chopped eggs. Bon appétit!

711. Delicious Hot Fruit Bake

Servings: 4   Cooking Time: 40 Minutes
Ingredients:

2 cups blueberries	2 cups raspberries
1 tablespoon cornstarch	A pinch of freshly grated nutmeg
3 tablespoons maple syrup	A pinch of salt
	1 cinnamon stick
2 tablespoons coconut oil, melted	1 vanilla bean

Directions:
Place your berries in a lightly greased baking dish. Sprinkle the cornstarch onto the fruit. Whisk the maple syrup, coconut oil, nutmeg, and salt in a mixing dish; add this mixture to the berries and gently stir to combine. Add the cinnamon and vanilla. Bake in the preheated Air Fryer at 370 degrees F for 35 minutes. Serve warm or at room temperature. Enjoy!

712. Gorgonzola Stuffed Mushrooms With Horseradish Mayo

Servings: 5   Cooking Time: 15 Minutes
Ingredients:

1/2 cup of breadcrumbs	1 ½ tablespoons olive oil
2 cloves garlic, pressed	1/2 cup Gorgonzola cheese, grated
2 tablespoons fresh coriander, chopped	1/4 cup low-fat mayonnaise
1/3 teaspoon kosher salt	1 teaspoon prepared horseradish, well-drained
1/2 teaspoon crushed red pepper flakes	1 tablespoon fresh parsley, finely chopped
20 medium-sized mushrooms, cut off the stems	

Directions:
Mix the breadcrumbs together with the garlic, coriander, salt, red pepper, and the olive oil; mix to combine well. Stuff the mushroom caps with the breadcrumb filling. Top with grated Gorgonzola. Place the mushrooms in the Air Fryer grill pan and slide them into the machine. Grill them at 380 degrees F for 8 to 12 minutes or until the stuffing is warmed through. Meanwhile, prepare the horseradish mayo by mixing the mayonnaise, horseradish and parsley. Serve with the warm fried mushrooms. Enjoy!

713. Scrambled Egg Muffins With Cheese

Servings: 6   Cooking Time: 20 Minutes
Ingredients:

6 ounces smoked turkey sausage, chopped	6 eggs, lightly beaten
2 tablespoons shallots, finely chopped	2 garlic cloves, minced
	1 teaspoon cayenne pepper
Sea salt and ground black pepper, to taste	6 ounces Monterey Jack cheese, shredded

Directions:
Simply combine the sausage, eggs, shallots, garlic, salt, black pepper, and cayenne pepper in a mixing dish. Mix to combine well. Spoon the mixture into 6 standard-size muffin cups with paper liners. Bake in the preheated Air Fryer at 340 degrees F for 8 minutes. Top with the cheese and bake an additional 8 minutes. Enjoy!

714. French Toast With Blueberries And Honey

Servings: 6   Cooking Time: 20 Minutes
Ingredients:

1/4 cup milk	2 eggs
2 tablespoons butter, melted	1 teaspoon vanilla extract
1/2 teaspoon ground cinnamon	6 slices day-old French baguette
1/4 teaspoon ground cloves	2 tablespoons honey
	1/2 cup blueberries

Directions:
In a mixing bowl, whisk the milk eggs, butter, cinnamon, cloves, and vanilla extract. Dip each piece of the baguette into the egg mixture and place in the parchment-lined Air Fryer basket. Cook in the preheated Air Fryer at 360 degrees F for 6 to 7 minutes, turning them over halfway through the cooking time to ensure even cooking. Serve garnished with honey and blueberries. Enjoy!

715. Vegetarian Tofu Scramble

Servings: 2   Cooking Time: 15 Minutes
Ingredients:

1/2 teaspoon fresh lemon juice	1 tablespoon butter, melted
1 teaspoon coarse salt	1/3 cup fresh basil, roughly chopped
1 teaspoon coarse ground black pepper	1/2 teaspoon fresh lemon juice
4 ounces fresh spinach, chopped	13 ounces soft silken tofu, drained

Directions:
Add the tofu and olive oil to a baking dish. Cook for 9 minutes at 272 degrees F. Add the other ingredients and cook another 5 minutes. Serve warm.

716. Breakfast Eggs With Swiss Chard And Ham

Servings: 2   Cooking Time: 20 Minutes
Ingredients:

1/4 teaspoon dried or fresh marjoram
2 teaspoons chili powder
1/3 teaspoon kosher salt
1/2 cup steamed Swiss Chard

2 eggs
1/4 teaspoon dried or fresh rosemary
4 pork ham slices
1/3 teaspoon ground black pepper, or more to taste

Directions:
Divide the Swiss Chard and ham among 2 ramekins; crack an egg into each ramekin. Sprinkle with seasonings. Cook for 15 minutes at 335 degrees F or until your eggs reach desired texture. Serve warm with spicy tomato ketchup and pickles. Bon appétit!

717. Baked Eggs With Linguica Sausage

Servings: 2   Cooking Time: 18 Minutes
Ingredients:

1/2 cup Cheddar cheese, shredded
4 eggs
2 ounces Linguica (Portuguese pork sausage), chopped
1/2 onion, peeled and chopped
2 tablespoons olive oil

1/2 teaspoon rosemary, chopped
½ teaspoon marjoram
1/4 cup sour cream
Sea salt and freshly ground black pepper, to taste
½ teaspoon fresh sage, chopped

Directions:
Lightly grease 2 oven safe ramekins with olive oil. Now, divide the sausage and onions among these ramekins. Crack an egg into each ramekin; add the remaining items, minus the cheese. Air-fry at 355 degrees F approximately 13 minutes. Immediately top with Cheddar cheese, serve, and enjoy.

718. Steak Fingers With Mushrooms And Swiss Cheese

Servings: 4   Cooking Time: 25 Minutes
Ingredients:

2 eggs, beaten
4 tablespoons yogurt
1 cup parmesan cheese, grated
1 teaspoon dry mesquite flavored seasoning mix
Coarse salt and ground black pepper, to taste

1/2 teaspoon onion powder
1 pound cube steak, cut into 3 inch long strips
1 pound button mushrooms
1 cup Swiss cheese, shredded

Directions:
In a shallow bowl, beat the eggs and yogurt. In a resealable bag, mix the parmesan cheese, mesquite seasoning, salt, pepper, and onion powder. Dip the steak pieces in the egg mixture; then, place in the bag, and shake to coat on all sides. Cook at 400 degrees F for 14 minutes, flipping halfway through the cooking time. Add the mushrooms to the lightly greased cooking basket. Top with shredded Swiss cheese. Bake in the preheated Air Fryer at 400 degrees F for 5 minutes. Serve with the beef nuggets. Bon appétit!

719. Japanese Fried Rice With Eggs

Servings: 2   Cooking Time: 30 Minutes
Ingredients:

2 cups cauliflower rice
2 teaspoons sesame oil
Sea salt and freshly ground black pepper, to your liking
2 eggs, beaten

2 scallions, white and green parts separated, chopped
1 tablespoon Shoyu sauce
1 tablespoon sake
2 tablespoons Kewpie Japanese mayonnaise

Directions:
Thoroughly combine the cauliflower rice, sesame oil, salt, and pepper in a baking dish. Cook at 340 degrees F about 13 minutes, stirring halfway through the cooking time. Pour the eggs over the cauliflower rice and continue to cook about 5 minutes. Next, add the scallions and stir to combine. Continue to cook 2 to 3 minutes longer or until everything is heated through. Meanwhile, make the sauce by whisking the Shoyu sauce, sake, and Japanese mayonnaise in a mixing bowl. Divide the fried cauliflower rice between individual bowls and serve with the prepared sauce. Enjoy!

720. Eggs Florentine With Spinach

Servings: 2   Cooking Time: 20 Minutes
Ingredients:

2 tablespoons ghee, melted
2 cups baby spinach, torn into small pieces
2 tablespoons shallots, chopped

1/4 teaspoon red pepper flakes
Salt, to taste
1 tablespoon fresh thyme leaves, roughly chopped
4 eggs

Directions:
Start by preheating your Air Fryer to 350 degrees F. Brush the sides and bottom of a gratin dish with the melted ghee. Put the spinach and shallots into the bottom of the gratin dish. Season with red pepper, salt, and fresh thyme. Make four indents for the eggs; crack one egg into each indent. Bake for 12 minutes, rotating the pan once or twice to ensure even cooking. Enjoy!

721. Party Pancake Kabobs

Servings: 4   Cooking Time: 40 Minutes
Ingredients:

Pancakes:
1 cup all-purpose flour
1 teaspoon baking powder

1/2 cup milk
2 tablespoons unsalted butter, melted
Kabobs:

1 tablespoon sugar
1/4 teaspoon salt
1 large egg, beaten
1/2 teaspoon vanilla extract

1 banana, diced
1 Granny Smith apples, diced
1/4 cup maple syrup, for serving

Directions:

Mix all ingredients for the pancakes until creamy and fluffy. Let it stand for 20 minutes. Spritz the Air Fryer baking pan with cooking spray. Drop the pancake batter on the pan with a small spoon. Cook at 230 degrees F for 4 minutes or until golden brown. Repeat with the remaining batter. Tread the mini pancakes and the fruit onto bamboo skewers, alternating between the mini pancakes and fruit. Drizzle maple syrup all over the kabobs and serve immediately.

722. Savory Italian Crespelle

Servings: 3   Cooking Time: 35 Minutes

Ingredients:

3/4 cup all-purpose flour
2 eggs, beaten
1/4 teaspoon allspice
1/2 teaspoon salt
3/4 cup milk

1 cup ricotta cheese
1/2 cup Parmigiano-Reggiano cheese, preferably freshly grated
1 cup marinara sauce

Directions:

Mix the flour, eggs, allspice, and salt in a large bowl. Gradually add the milk, whisking continuously, until well combined. Let it stand for 20 minutes. Spritz the Air Fryer baking pan with cooking spray. Pour the batter into the prepared pan. Cook at 230 degrees F for 3 minutes. Flip and cook until browned in spots, 2 to 3 minutes longer. Repeat with the remaining batter. Serve with the cheese and marinara sauce. Bon appétit!

723. Country-style Pork Meatloaf

Servings: 4   Cooking Time: 25 Minutes

Ingredients:

1/2 pound lean minced pork
1/3 cup breadcrumbs
1/2 tablespoons minced green garlic
1½ tablespoon fresh cilantro, minced
1/2 tablespoon fish sauce

1/3 teaspoon dried basil
2 leeks, chopped
2 tablespoons tomato puree
1/2 teaspoons dried thyme
Salt and ground black pepper, to taste

Directions:

Add all ingredients, except for breadcrumbs, to a large-sized mixing dish and combine everything using your hands. Lastly, add the breadcrumbs to form a meatloaf. Bake for 23 minutes at 365 degrees F. Afterward, allow your meatloaf to rest for 10 minutes before slicing and serving. Bon appétit!

724. Easy Fried Button Mushrooms

Servings: 4   Cooking Time: 15 Minutes

Ingredients:

1 pound button mushrooms
1 cup cornstarch
1 cup all-purpose flour
1/2 teaspoon baking powder

2 eggs, whisked
2 cups seasoned breadcrumbs
1/2 teaspoon salt
2 tablespoons fresh parsley leaves, roughly chopped

Directions:

Pat the mushrooms dry with a paper towel. To begin, set up your breading station. Mix the cornstarch, flour, and baking powder in a shallow dish. In a separate dish, whisk the eggs. Finally, place your breadcrumbs and salt in a third dish. Start by dredging the mushrooms in the flour mixture; then, dip them into the eggs. Press your mushrooms into the breadcrumbs, coating evenly. Spritz the Air Fryer basket with cooking oil. Add the mushrooms and cook at 400 degrees F for 6 minutes, flipping them halfway through the cooking time. Serve garnished with fresh parsley leaves. Bon appétit!

725. Cheese Sticks With Ketchup

Servings: 4   Cooking Time: 15 Minutes

Ingredients:

1/4 cup coconut flour
1/4 cup almond flour
1/2 cup parmesan cheese, grated
1 tablespoon Cajun seasonings

2 eggs
8 cheese sticks, kid-friendly
1/4 cup ketchup, low-carb

Directions:

To begin, set up your breading station. Place the flour in a shallow dish. In a separate dish, whisk the eggs. Finally, mix the parmesan cheese and Cajun seasoning in a third dish. Start by dredging the cheese sticks in the flour; then, dip them into the egg. Press the cheese sticks into the parmesan mixture, coating evenly. Place the breaded cheese sticks in the lightly greased Air Fryer basket. Cook at 380 degrees F for 6 minutes. Serve with ketchup and enjoy!

726. Oatmeal Pizza Cups

Servings: 4   Cooking Time: 30 Minutes

Ingredients:

1 cup rolled oats
1 teaspoon baking powder
1/4 teaspoon ground black pepper
2 tablespoons butter, melted

Salt, to taste
1 cup milk
4 slices smoked ham, chopped
4 ounces mozzarella cheese, shredded
4 tablespoons ketchup

Directions:

Start by preheating your Air Fryer to 350 degrees F. Now, lightly grease a muffin tin with nonstick spray. Pulse the rolled oats, baking powder, pepper, and salt in your food processor until the mixture looks like coarse meal.   Add the remaining ingredients and stir to combine well. Spoon the mixture into the prepared muffin tin.   Bake in the preheated Air Fryer for 20 minutes until a toothpick inserted comes out clean. Bon appétit!

727.   Keto Rolls With Halibut And Eggs

Servings: 4   Cooking Time: 25 Minutes
Ingredients:

4 keto rolls	4 eggs
1 pound smoked halibut, chopped	1 teaspoon dried basil
1 teaspoon dried thyme	Salt and black pepper, to taste

Directions:
Cut off the top of each keto roll; then, scoop out the insides to make the shells.   Lay the prepared keto roll shells in the lightly greased cooking basket. Spritz with cooking oil; add the halibut. Crack an egg into each keto roll shell; sprinkle with thyme, basil, salt, and black pepper.   Bake in the preheated Air Fryer at 325 degrees F for 20 minutes. Bon appétit!

728.   Easy Roasted Hot Dogs

Servings: 6   Cooking Time: 25 Minutes
Ingredients:

6 hot dogs	6 tablespoons ketchup
6 hot dog buns	6 lettuce leaves
1 tablespoon mustard	

Directions:
Place the hot dogs in the lightly greased Air Fryer basket.   Bake at 380 degrees F for 15 minutes, turning them over halfway through the cooking time to promote even cooking.   Place on the bun and add the mustard, ketchup, and lettuce leaves. Enjoy!

729.   Hearty Southwestern Cheeseburger Frittata

Servings: 2   Cooking Time: 30 Minutes
Ingredients:

3 tablespoons goat cheese, crumbled	2 eggs
2 cups lean ground beef	½ onion, peeled and chopped
1 ½ tablespoons olive oil	½ teaspoon paprika
½ teaspoon dried marjoram	½ teaspoon kosher salt
	1 teaspoon ground black pepper

Directions:
Set your air fryer to cook at 345 degrees F.   Melt the oil in a skillet over a moderate flame; then, sweat the onion until it has softened. Add ground beef and cook until browned; crumble with a fork and set aside, keeping it warm.   Whisk the eggs with all the seasonings.   Spritz the inside of a baking dish with a pan spray. Pour the beaten egg mixture into the baking dish, followed by the reserved beef/onion

mixture. Top with the crumbled goat cheese. Bake for about 27 minutes or until a tester comes out clean and dry when stuck in the center of the frittata. Bon appétit!

730.   Sweet Mini Monkey Rolls

Servings: 6   Cooking Time: 25 Minutes
Ingredients:

3/4 cup brown sugar	1/4 teaspoon ground cardamom
1 stick butter, melted	1 (16-ounce) can refrigerated buttermilk biscuit dough
1/4 cup granulated sugar	
1 teaspoon ground cinnamon	

Directions:
Spritz 6 standard-size muffin cups with nonstick spray. Mix the brown sugar and butter; divide the mixture between muffin cups.   Mix the granulated sugar with cinnamon and cardamom. Separate the dough into 16 biscuits; cut each in 6 pieces. Roll the pieces over the cinnamon sugar mixture to coat. Divide between muffin cups.   Bake at 340 degrees F for about 20 minutes or until golden brown. Turn upside down and serve.

731. Potato And Kale Croquettes

Servings: 6   Cooking Time: 9 Minutes
Ingredients:

4 eggs, slightly beaten	1 cup kale, steamed
⅓ cup flour	⅓ cup breadcrumbs
⅓ cup goat cheese, crumbled	1/3 teaspoon red pepper flakes
1 ½ teaspoons fine sea salt	3 potatoes, peeled and quartered
4 garlic cloves, minced	1/3 teaspoon dried dill weed

Directions:
Firstly, boil the potatoes in salted water. Once the potatoes are cooked, mash them; add the kale, goat cheese, minced garlic, sea salt, red pepper flakes, dill and one egg; stir to combine well.   Now, roll the mixture to form small croquettes.   Grab three shallow bowls. Place the flour in the first shallow bowl.   Beat the remaining 3 eggs in the second bowl. After that, throw the breadcrumbs into the third shallow bowl.   Dip each croquette in the flour; then, dip them in the eggs bowl; lastly, roll each croquette in the breadcrumbs.   Air fry at 335 degrees F for 7 minutes or until golden. Tate, adjust for seasonings and serve warm.

732.   Easiest Vegan Burrito Ever

Servings: 6   Cooking Time: 35 Minutes
Ingredients:

2 tablespoons olive oil	Sea salt and ground black pepper, to taste
1 small onion, chopped	10 ounces cooked pinto beans
2 sweet peppers,	12 ounces canned

seeded and chopped
1 chili pepper, seeded and minced
1 teaspoon red pepper flakes, crushed
1 teaspoon dried parsley flakes

sweet corn, drained
6 large corn tortillas
1/2 cup vegan sour cream

Directions:
Begin by preheating your Air Frye to 400 degrees F. Heat the olive oil in a baking pan. Once hot, cook the onion and peppers until they are tender and fragrant, about 15 minutes. Stir in the salt, black pepper, red pepper, parsley, beans, and sweet corn; stir to combine well. Divide the bean mixture between the corn tortillas. Roll up your tortillas and place them on the parchment-lined Air Fryer basket. Bake in the preheated Air Fryer at 350 degrees F for 15 minutes. Serve garnished with sour cream. Bon appétit!

---

733. Hanukkah Latkes

Servings: 4   Cooking Time: 20 Minutes
Ingredients:

6 potatoes
4 onions
Sea salt and ground black pepper, to taste

2 eggs, beaten
1/2 teaspoon smoked paprika
1/2 cup all-purpose flour

Directions:
Pulse the potatoes and onions in your food processor until smooth. Drain the mixture well and stir in the other ingredients. Mix to combine well. Drop the pancake batter on the baking pan with a small spoon. Flatten them slightly so the center can cook. Cook at 370 degrees for 5 minutes; turn over and cook for a further 5 minutes. Repeat with the additional batter. Serve with sour cream if desired.

---

734. Mozzarella Stick Nachos

Servings: 4   Cooking Time: 40 Minutes
Ingredients:

1 (16-ounce) package mozzarella cheese sticks
2 eggs
1/2 cup flour
1/2 (7 12-ounce bag multigrain tortilla chips, crushed

1 teaspoon garlic powder
1 teaspoon dried oregano
1/2 cup salsa, preferably homemade

Directions:
Set up your breading station. Put the flour into a shallow bowl; beat the eggs in another shallow bowl; in a third bowl, mix the crushed tortilla chips, garlic powder, and oregano. Coat the mozzarella sticks lightly with flour, followed by the egg, and then the tortilla chips mixture. Place in your freezer for 30 minutes. Place the breaded cheese sticks in the lightly greased Air Fryer basket. Cook at 380 degrees

F for 6 minutes. Serve with salsa on the side and enjoy!

---

735. Rum Roasted Cherries

Servings: 3   Cooking Time: 40 Minutes
Ingredients:

9 ounces dark sweet cherries
2 tablespoons brown sugar
1 tablespoon honey
A pinch of grated nutmeg

3 tablespoons rum
1/4 teaspoon ground cloves
1/4 teaspoon ground cardamom
1 teaspoon vanilla

Directions:
Place the cherries in a lightly greased baking dish. Whisk the remaining ingredients until everything is well combined; add this mixture to the baking dish and gently stir to combine. Bake in the preheated Air Fryer at 370 degrees F for 35 minutes. Serve at room temperature. Bon appétit!

---

736. The Best Sweet Potato Fries Ever

Servings: 4   Cooking Time: 20 Minutes
Ingredients:

1 1/2 tablespoons olive oil
1/2 teaspoon smoked cayenne pepper
3 sweet potatoes, peeled and cut into 1/4-inch long slices

1/2 teaspoon shallot powder
1/3 teaspoon freshly ground black pepper, or more to taste
3/4 teaspoon garlic salt

Directions:
Firstly, preheat your air fryer to 360 degrees F. Then, add the sweet potatoes to a mixing dish; toss them with the other ingredients. Cook the sweet potatoes approximately 14 minutes. Serve with a dipping sauce of choice.

---

737. Super Easy Sage And Lime Wings

Servings: 4   Cooking Time: 30 Minutes + Marinating Time
Ingredients:

1 teaspoon onion powder
1/3 cup fresh lime juice
1/2 tablespoon corn flour
1/2 heaping tablespoon fresh chopped parsley
1/2 pound turkey wings, cut into smaller pieces

1/3 teaspoon mustard powder
2 heaping tablespoons fresh chopped sage
1/2 teaspoon garlic powder
1/2 teaspoon seasoned salt
1 teaspoon freshly cracked black or white peppercorns

Directions:
Simply dump all of the above ingredients into a mixing dish; cover and let it marinate for about 1

hours in your refrigerator. Air-fry turkey wings for 28 minutes at 355 degrees F. Bon appétit!

738. Egg Salad With Asparagus And Spinach

Servings: 4   Cooking Time: 25 Minutes + Chilling Time

Ingredients:

4 eggs	1 teaspoon fresh
1 pound asparagus,	lemon juice
chopped	Sea salt and ground
2 cup baby spinach	black pepper, to taste
1/2 cup mayonnaise	
1 teaspoon mustard	

Directions:
Place the wire rack in the Air Fryer basket; lower the eggs onto the wire rack.   Cook at 270 degrees F for 15 minutes.   Transfer them to an ice-cold water bath to stop the cooking. Peel the eggs under cold running water; coarsely chop the hard-boiled eggs and set aside.   Increase the temperature to 400 degrees F. Place your asparagus in the lightly greased Air Fryer basket.   Cook for 5 minutes or until tender. Place in a nice salad bowl. Add the baby spinach.   In a mixing dish, thoroughly combine the remaining ingredients. Drizzle this dressing over the asparagus in the salad bowl and top with the chopped eggs. Bon appétit!

739. Traditional Onion Bhaji

Servings: 3   Cooking Time: 40 Minutes

Ingredients:

1 egg, beaten	1 ounce all-purpose
2 tablespoons olive	flour
oil	Salt and black
2 onions, sliced	pepper, to taste
1 green chili,	1 teaspoon cumin
deseeded and finely	seeds
chopped	1/2 teaspoon ground
2 ounces chickpea	turmeric
flour	

Directions:
Place all ingredients, except for the onions, in a mixing dish; mix to combine well, adding a little water to the mixture.   Once you've got a thick batter, add the onions; stir to coat well.   Cook in the preheated Air Fryer at 370 degrees F for 20 minutes flipping them halfway through the cooking time.   Work in batches and transfer to a serving platter. Enjoy!

740. Dijon And Curry Turkey Cutlets

Servings: 4   Cooking Time: 30 Minutes + Marinating Time

Ingredients:

1/2 tablespoon Dijon	1/3 pound turkey
mustard	cutlets
1/2 teaspoon curry	1/2 cup fresh lemon
powder	juice

Sea salt flakes and	1/2 tablespoons
freshly cracked black	tamari sauce
peppercorns, to savor	

Directions:
Set the air fryer to cook at 375 degrees. Then, put the turkey cutlets into a mixing dish; add fresh lemon juice, tamari, and mustard; let it marinate at least 2 hours.   Coat each turkey cutlet with the curry powder, salt, and freshly cracked black peppercorns; roast for 28 minutes; work in batches. Bon appétit!

741. Snapper With Gruyere Cheese

Servings: 4   Cooking Time: 25 Minutes

Ingredients:

2 tablespoons olive	Sea salt and ground
oil	black pepper, to taste
1 shallot, thinly sliced	1/2 teaspoon dried
2 garlic cloves,	basil
minced	1/2 cup tomato puree
1 ½ pounds snapper	1/2 cup white wine
fillets	1 cup Gruyere cheese,
1 teaspoon cayenne	shredded
pepper	

Directions:
Heat 1 tablespoon of olive oil in a saucepan over medium-high heat. Now, cook the shallot and garlic until tender and aromatic.   Preheat your Air Fryer to 370 degrees F.   Grease a casserole dish with 1 tablespoon of olive oil. Place the snapper fillet in the casserole dish. Season with salt, black pepper, and cayenne pepper. Add the sautéed shallot mixture. Add the basil, tomato puree and wine to the casserole dish. Cook for 10 minutes in the preheated Air Fryer.   Top with the shredded cheese and cook an additional 7 minutes. Serve immediately.

742. Fingerling Potatoes With Cashew Sauce

Servings: 4   Cooking Time: 20 Minutes

Ingredients:

1 pound fingerling	1/2 cup raw cashews
potatoes	1 teaspoon cayenne
1 tablespoon butter,	pepper
melted	3 tablespoons
Sea salt and ground	nutritional yeast
black pepper, to your	2 teaspoons white
liking	vinegar
1 teaspoon shallot	4 tablespoons water
powder	1/4 teaspoon dried
1 teaspoon garlic	rosemary
powder	1/4 teaspoon dried
Cashew Sauce:	dill

Directions:
Toss the potatoes with the butter, salt, black pepper, shallot powder, and garlic powder.   Place the fingerling potatoes in the lightly greased Air Fryer basket and cook at 400 degrees F for 6 minutes; shake the basket and cook for a further 6 minutes. Meanwhile, make the sauce by mixing all ingredients in your food processor or high-speed

blender. Drizzle the cashew sauce over the potato wedges. Bake at 400 degrees F for 2 more minutes or until everything is heated through. Enjoy!

743. Mother's Day Pudding

Servings: 6   Cooking Time: 45 Minutes

Ingredients:

1 pound French baguette bread, cubed	2 cups whole milk
4 eggs, beaten	1/2 cup heavy cream
1/4 cup chocolate liqueur	1 teaspoon vanilla extract
1 cup granulated sugar	1/4 teaspoon ground cloves
2 tablespoons honey	2 ounces milk chocolate chips

Directions:

Place the bread cubes in a lightly greased baking dish. In a mixing bowl, thoroughly combine the eggs, chocolate liqueur, sugar, honey, milk, heavy cream, vanilla, and ground cloves. Pour the custard over the bread cubes. Scatter the milk chocolate chips over the top of your bread pudding. Let stand for 30 minutes, occasionally pressing with a wide spatula to submerge. Cook in the preheated Air Fryer at 370 degrees F degrees for 7 minutes; check to ensure even cooking and cook an additional 5 to 6 minutes. Bon appétit!

744. Scrambled Eggs With Sausage

Servings: 6   Cooking Time: 25 Minutes

Ingredients:

1 teaspoon lard	1 scallion, chopped
1/2 pound turkey sausage	1 chili pepper, seeded and chopped
6 eggs	Sea salt and ground black pepper, to taste
1 garlic clove, minced	1/2 cup Swiss cheese, shredded
1 sweet pepper, seeded and chopped	

Directions:

Start by preheating your Air Fryer to 330 degrees F. Now, spritz 6 silicone molds with cooking spray. Melt the lard in a saucepan over medium-high heat. Now, cook the sausage for 5 minutes or until no longer pink. Coarsely chop the sausage; add the eggs, scallions, garlic, peppers, salt, and black pepper. Divide the egg mixture between the silicone molds. Top with the shredded cheese. Bake in the preheated Air Fryer at 340 degrees F for 15 minutes, checking halfway through the cooking time to ensure even cooking. Enjoy!

745. Quinoa With Baked Eggs And Bacon

Servings: 4   Cooking Time: 40 Minutes

Ingredients:

1/2 cup quinoa	1 tablespoon butter, melted
1/2 pound potatoes, diced	Sea salt and ground
1 onion, diced	
6 slices bacon, precooked	black pepper, to taste
	6 eggs

Directions:

Rinse the quinoa under cold running water. Place the rinsed quinoa in a pan and add 1 cup of water. Bring it to the boil. Turn the heat down and let it simmer for 13 to 15 minutes or until tender; reserve. Place the diced potatoes and onion in a lightly greased casserole dish. Add the bacon and the reserved quinoa. Drizzle the melted butter over the quinoa and sprinkle with salt and pepper. Bake in the preheated Air Fryer at 390 degrees F for 10 minutes. Turn the temperature down to 350 degrees F. Make six indents for the eggs; crack one egg into each indent. Bake for 12 minutes, rotating the pan once or twice to ensure even cooking. Enjoy!

746. Italian Creamy Frittata With Kale

Servings: 3   Cooking Time: 20 Minutes

Ingredients:

1 yellow onion, finely chopped	1/4 cup double cream
6 ounces wild mushrooms, sliced	1 tablespoon butter, melted
6 eggs	2 tablespoons fresh Italian parsley, chopped
1/2 teaspoon cayenne pepper	2 cups kale, chopped
Sea salt and ground black pepper, to taste	1/2 cup mozzarella, shredded

Directions:

Begin by preheating the Air Fryer to 360 degrees F. Spritz the sides and bottom of a baking pan with cooking oil. Add the onions and wild mushrooms, and cook in the preheated Air Fryer at 360 degrees F for 4 to 5 minutes. In a mixing dish, whisk the eggs and double cream until pale. Add the spices, butter, parsley, and kale; stir until everything is well incorporated. Pour the mixture into the baking pan with the mushrooms. Top with the cheese. Cook in the preheated Air Fryer for 10 minutes. Serve immediately and enjoy!

747. Roasted Turkey Sausage With Potatoes

Servings: 6   Cooking Time: 40 Minutes

Ingredients:

1/2 teaspoon onion salt	1/2 pound red potatoes, peeled and diced
1/2 teaspoon dried sage	
1/2 pound ground turkey	1 ½ tablespoons olive oil
1/3 teaspoon ginger, ground	1/2 teaspoon paprika
1 sprig rosemary, chopped	2 sprigs thyme, chopped
	1 teaspoon ground black pepper

Directions:

In a bowl, mix the first six ingredients; give it a good stir. Heat a thin layer of vegetable oil in a nonstick skillet that is placed over a moderate flame. Form the mixture into patties; fry until they're browned on all sides, or about 12 minutes. Arrange the potatoes at the bottom of a baking dish. Sprinkle with the rosemary and thyme; add a drizzle of olive oil. Top with the turkey. Roast for 32 minutes at 365 degrees F, turning once halfway through. Eat warm.

748. Red Currant Cupcakes

Servings: 3   Cooking Time: 20 Minutes

Ingredients:

1 cup all-purpose flour	1 egg
1/2 cup sugar	1/4 cup full-fat coconut milk
1 teaspoon baking powder	1/4 teaspoon ground cardamom
A pinch of kosher salt	1/4 teaspoon ground cinnamon
A pinch of grated nutmeg	1 teaspoon vanilla extract
1/4 cup coconut, oil melted	6 ounces red currants

Directions:
Mix the flour with the sugar, baking powder, salt, and nutmeg. In a separate bowl, whisk the coconut oil, egg, milk, cardamom, cinnamon, and vanilla. Add the egg mixture to the dry ingredients; mix to combine well. Now, fold in the red currants; gently stir to combine. Scrape the batter into lightly greased 6 standard-size muffin cups. Bake your cupcakes at 360 degrees F for 12 minutes or until the tops are golden brown. Sprinkle some extra icing sugar over the top of each muffin if desired. Enjoy!

749. Sweet Corn And Kernel Fritters

Servings: 4   Cooking Time: 20 Minutes

Ingredients:

1 medium-sized carrot, grated	1 medium-sized egg, whisked
1 yellow onion, finely chopped	2 tablespoons plain milk
4 ounces canned sweet corn kernels, drained	1 cup of Parmesan cheese, grated
1 teaspoon sea salt flakes	1/4 cup of self-rising flour
1 heaping tablespoon fresh cilantro, chopped	1/3 teaspoon baking powder
	1/3 teaspoon brown sugar

Directions:
Press down the grated carrot in the colander to remove excess liquid. Then, spread the grated carrot between several sheets of kitchen towels and pat it dry. Then, mix the carrots with the remaining ingredients in the order listed above. Roll 1 tablespoon of the mixture into a ball; gently flatten it using the back of a spoon or your hand. Now,

repeat with the remaining ingredients. Spitz the balls with a nonstick cooking oil. Cook in a single layer at 350 degrees for 8 to 11 minutes or until they're firm to touch in the center. Serve warm and enjoy!

750. Italian Sausage And Veggie Bake

Servings: 4   Cooking Time: 20 Minutes

Ingredients:

1 pound Italian sausage	4 cloves garlic
2 red peppers, seeded and sliced	1 teaspoon dried oregano
2 green peppers, seeded and sliced	1/4 teaspoon black pepper
1 cup mushrooms, sliced	1/4 teaspoon cayenne pepper
1 shallot, sliced	Sea salt, to taste
1 teaspoon dried basil	2 tablespoons Dijon mustard
	1 cup chicken broth

Directions:
Toss all ingredients in a lightly greased baking pan. Make sure the sausages and vegetables are coated with the oil and seasonings. Bake in the preheated Air Fryer at 380 degrees F for 15 minutes. Divide between individual bowls and serve warm. Bon appétit!

751. Easy Frittata With Chicken Sausage

Servings: 2   Cooking Time: 15 Minutes

Ingredients:

1 tablespoon olive oil	Sea salt and ground black pepper, to taste
2 chicken sausages, sliced	4 tablespoons Monterey-Jack cheese
4 eggs	
1 garlic clove, minced	1 tablespoon fresh parsley leaves, chopped
1/2 yellow onion, chopped	

Directions:
Grease the sides and bottom of a baking pan with olive oil. Add the sausages and cook in the preheated Air Fryer at 360 degrees F for 4 to 5 minutes. In a mixing dish, whisk the eggs with garlic and onion. Season with salt and black pepper. Pour the mixture over sausages. Top with cheese. Cook in the preheated Air Fryer at 360 degrees F for another 6 minutes. Serve immediately with fresh parsley leaves. Bon appétit!

752. Bourbon Glazed Mango With Walnuts

Servings: 4   Cooking Time: 20 Minutes

Ingredients:

2 ripe mangos, peeled and diced	2 tablespoons sugar
2 tablespoons	1 teaspoon vanilla essence

bourbon whiskey
2 tablespoons
coconut oil, melted
1/4 teaspoon ground
cardamom

1/4 teaspoon pure
coconut extract
1/2 cup walnuts,
coarsely chopped

Directions:
Start by preheating your Air Fryer to 400 degrees F. Toss all ingredients in a baking dish and transfer to the Air fryer basket.   Now, bake for 10 minutes, or until browned on top. Serve with whipped cream if desired. Bon appétit!

753.   Onion Rings With Mayo Dip

Servings: 3   Cooking Time: 25 Minutes
Ingredients:

1 large onion
1/2 cup almond flour
1 teaspoon salt
1/2 teaspoon ground
black pepper
1 teaspoon cayenne
pepper
1/2 teaspoon dried
thyme
1/2 teaspoon dried
oregano
1/2 teaspoon ground
cumin

2 eggs
4 tablespoons milk
Mayo Dip:
3 tablespoons
mayonnaise
3 tablespoons sour
cream
1 tablespoon
horseradish, drained
Kosher salt and
freshly ground black
pepper, to taste

Directions:
Cut off the top 1/2 inch of the Vidalia onion; peel your onion and place it cut-side down. Starting 1/2 inch from the root, cut the onion in half. Make a second cut that splits each half in two. You will have 4 quarters held together by the root.   Repeat these cuts, splitting the 4 quarters to yield eighths; then, you should split them again until you have 16 evenly spaced cuts. Turn the onion over and gently separate the outer pieces using your fingers.   In a mixing bowl, thoroughly combine the almond flour and spices. In a separate bowl, whisk the eggs and milk. Dip the onion into the egg mixture, followed by the almond flour mixture.   Spritz the onion with cooking spray and transfer to the lightly greased cooking basket. Cook for 370 degrees F for 12 to 15 minutes.   Meanwhile, make the mayo dip by whisking the remaining ingredients. Serve and enjoy!

754.   Chive, Feta And Chicken Frittata

Servings: 4   Cooking Time: 10 Minutes
Ingredients:

1/3 cup Feta cheese,
crumbled
1 teaspoon dried
rosemary
½ teaspoon brown
sugar
2 tablespoons fish
sauce
1 ½ cup cooked

1/2 teaspoon
coriander sprig, finely
chopped
1/3 teaspoon ground
white pepper
1 cup fresh chives,
chopped
1/2 teaspoon garlic
paste

chicken breasts,
boneless and
shredded
3 medium-sized
whisked eggs

Fine sea salt, to taste
Nonstick cooking
spray

Directions:
Grab a baking dish that fit in your air fryer. Lightly coat the inside of the baking dish with a nonstick cooking spray of choice. Stir in all ingredients, minus Feta cheese. Stir to combine well. Set your machine to cook at 335 degrees for 8 minutes; check for doneness. Scatter crumbled Feta over the top and eat immediately!

755.   Crispy Wontons With Asian Dipping Sauce

Servings: 4   Cooking Time: 20 Minutes
Ingredients:

1 teaspoon sesame oil
3/4 pound ground
beef
Sea salt, to taste
1/4 teaspoon Sichuan
pepper
20 wonton wrappers
2 tablespoons low-
sodium soy sauce

Dipping Sauce:
1 tablespoon honey
1 teaspoon Gochujang
1 teaspoon rice wine
vinegar
1/2 teaspoon sesame
oil

Directions:
Heat 1 teaspoon of sesame oil in a wok over medium-high heat. Cook the ground beef until no longer pink. Season with salt and Sichuan pepper.   Lay a piece of the wonton wrapper on your palm; add the beef mixture in the middle of the wrapper. Then, fold it up to form a triangle; pinch the edges to seal tightly. Place your wontons in the lightly greased Air Fryer basket. Cook in the preheated Air Fryer at 360 degrees F for 10 minutes. Work in batches. Meanwhile, mix all ingredients for the sauce. Serve warm.

756.   Roasted Green Bean Salad With Goat Cheese

Servings: 4   Cooking Time: 10 Minutes + Chilling Time
Ingredients:

1 pound trimmed
green beans, cut into
bite-sized pieces
Salt and freshly
cracked mixed
pepper, to taste
1 shallot, thinly sliced
1 tablespoon lime
juice
1 tablespoon
champagne vinegar

1/4 cup extra-virgin
olive oil
1/2 teaspoon mustard
seeds
1/2 teaspoon celery
seeds
1 tablespoon fresh
basil leaves, chopped
1 tablespoon fresh
parsley leaves
1 cup goat cheese,
crumbled

Directions:
Toss the green beans with salt and pepper in a lightly greased Air Fryer basket.   Cook in the preheated

Air Fryer at 400 degrees F for 5 minutes or until tender.   Add the shallots and gently stir to combine.   In a mixing bowl, whisk the lime juice, vinegar, olive oil, and spices. Dress the salad and top with the goat cheese. Serve at room temperature or chilled. Enjoy!

---

757.   Creamy Lemon Turkey

Servings: 4   Cooking Time: 2 Hours 25 Minutes

Ingredients:

1/3 cup sour cream	1 teaspoon fresh
2 cloves garlic, finely minced	marjoram, chopped
	Salt and freshly
1/3 teaspoon lemon zest	cracked mixed peppercorns, to taste
2 small-sized turkey breasts, skinless and cubed	1/2 cup scallion, chopped
1/3 cup thickened cream	1/2 can tomatoes, diced
2 tablespoons lemon juice	1 ½ tablespoons canola oil

Directions:

Firstly, pat dry the turkey breast. Mix the remaining items; marinate the turkey for 2 hours.   Set the air fryer to cook at 355 degrees F. Brush the turkey with a nonstick spray; cook for 23 minutes, turning once. Serve with naan and enjoy!

---

758.   Easy Cheesy Broccoli

Servings: 4   Cooking Time: 25 Minutes

Ingredients:

1/3 cup grated yellow cheese	2 teaspoons dried rosemary
1 large-sized head broccoli, stemmed and cut small florets	2 teaspoons dried basil
	Salt and ground black pepper, to taste
2 1/2 tablespoons canola oil	

Directions:

Bring a medium pan filled with a lightly salted water to a boil. Then, boil the broccoli florets for about 3 minutes.   Then, drain the broccoli florets well; toss them with the canola oil, rosemary, basil, salt and black pepper.   Set your air fryer to 390 degrees F; arrange the seasoned broccoli in the cooking basket; set the timer for 17 minutes. Toss the broccoli halfway through the cooking process. Serve warm topped with grated cheese and enjoy!

---

759.   Greek-style Roasted Figs

Servings: 4   Cooking Time: 20 Minutes

Ingredients:

2 teaspoons butter, melted	1/2 teaspoon cinnamon
8 figs, halved	1 teaspoon lemon zest
2 tablespoons brown sugar	1 cup Greek yogurt
	4 tablespoons honey

Directions:

Drizzle the melted butter all over the fig halves. Sprinkle brown sugar, cinnamon, and lemon zest on the fig slices. Meanwhile, mix the Greek yogurt with the honey.   Roast in the preheated Air Fryer at 330 degrees F for 16 minutes.   To serve, divide the figs among 4 bowls and serve with a dollop of the yogurt sauce. Enjoy!

---

760.   Celery And Bacon Cakes

Servings: 4   Cooking Time: 25 Minutes

Ingredients:

2 eggs, lightly beaten	1/2 tablespoon garlic paste
1/3 teaspoon freshly cracked black pepper	1/3 cup onion, finely chopped
1 cup Colby cheese, grated	1/3 cup bacon, chopped
1/2 tablespoon fresh dill, finely chopped	2 teaspoons fine sea salt
2 medium-sized celery stalks, trimmed and grated	1/3 teaspoon baking powder

Directions:

Place the celery on a paper towel and squeeze them to remove the excess liquid.   Combine the vegetables with the other ingredients in the order listed above. Shape the balls using 1 tablespoon of the vegetable mixture.   Then, gently flatten each ball with your palm or a wide spatula. Spritz the croquettes with a nonstick cooking oil.   Bake the vegetable cakes in a single layer for 17 minutes at 318 degrees F. Serve warm with sour cream.

---

761. Cheesy Pasilla Turkey

Servings: 2   Cooking Time: 30 Minutes

Ingredients:

1/3 cup Parmesan cheese, shredded	1/3 cup mayonnaise
2 turkey breasts, cut into four pieces	1 dried Pasilla peppers
	1 teaspoon onion salt
1 ½ tablespoons sour cream	1/3 teaspoon mixed peppercorns, freshly cracked
1/2 cup crushed crackers	

Directions:

In a shallow bowl, mix the crushed crackers, Parmesan cheese, onion salt, and the cracked mixed peppercorns together.   In a food processor, blitz the mayonnaise, along with the cream and dried Pasilla peppers until there are no lumps.   Coat the turkey breasts with this mixture, ensuring that all sides are covered.   Then, coat each piece of turkey in the Parmesan/cracker mix.   Now, preheat the air fryer to 365 degrees F; cook for 28 minutes until thoroughly cooked.

---

762.   Cheesy Cauliflower Balls

Servings: 4   Cooking Time: 26 Minutes

Ingredients:

4 ounces cauliflower florets	1 egg, beaten
	1/3 teaspoon ground

1/2 cup roasted vegetable stock
1 cup white mushrooms, finely chopped
1/2 cup parmesan cheese, grated
3 garlic cloves, peeled and minced
1/2 yellow onion, finely chopped
black pepper, or more to taste
1 ½ bell peppers, seeded minced
1/2 chipotle pepper, seeded and minced
1/2 cup Colby cheese, grated
1 ½ tablespoons canola oil
Sea salt, to savor

Directions:
Blitz the cauliflower florets in your food processor until they're crumbled (it is the size of rice). Heat a saucepan over a moderate heat; now, heat the oil and sweat the garlic, onions, bell pepper, cauli rice, and chipotle pepper until tender. Throw in the mushrooms and fry until they are fragrant and the liquid has almost evaporated. Add in the stock; boil for 18 minutes. Now, add the cheese and spices; mix to combine. Allow the mixture to cool completely. Shape the mixture into balls. Dip the balls in the beaten egg; then, roll them over the grated parmesan. Air-fry these balls for 6 minutes at 400 degrees F. Serve with marinara sauce and enjoy!

763. Cheese Balls With Spinach

Servings: 4   Cooking Time: 15 Minutes
Ingredients:
1/4 cup milk
2 eggs
1 cup cheese
2 cups spinach, torn into pieces
1/3 cup flaxseed meal
1/2 teaspoon baking powder
2 tablespoons canola oil
Salt and ground black pepper, to taste

Directions:
Add all the ingredients to a food processor or blender; then, puree the ingredients until it becomes dough. Next, roll the dough into small balls. Preheat your air fryer to 310 degrees F. Cook the balls in your Air Fryer for about 12 minutes or until they are crispy. Bon appétit!

764. Grilled Chicken Tikka Masala

Servings: 4   Cooking Time: 35 Minutes + Marinating Time
Ingredients:
1 teaspoon Tikka Masala
1 teaspoon fine sea salt
2 heaping teaspoons whole grain mustard
2 teaspoons coriander, ground
2 large-sized chicken breasts, skinless and halved lengthwise
2 tablespoon olive oil
2 teaspoons onion powder
1 ½ tablespoons cider vinegar
Basmati rice, steamed
1/3 teaspoon red pepper flakes, crushed

Directions:
Preheat the air fryer to 335 degrees for 4 minutes. Toss your chicken together with the other ingredients, minus basmati rice. Let it stand at least 3 hours. Cook for 25 minutes in your air fryer; check for doneness because the time depending on the size of the piece of chicken. Serve immediately over warm basmati rice. Enjoy!

765. Stuffed Mushrooms With Cheese

Servings: 5   Cooking Time: 15 Minutes
Ingredients:
1/2 cup parmesan cheese, grated
2 cloves garlic, pressed
2 tablespoons fresh coriander, chopped
1/3 teaspoon kosher salt
1/2 teaspoon crushed red pepper flakes
20 medium-sized mushrooms, cut off the stems
1 ½ tablespoons olive oil
1/2 cup Gorgonzola cheese, grated
1/4 cup low-fat mayonnaise
1 teaspoon prepared horseradish, well-drained
1 tablespoon fresh parsley, finely chopped

Directions:
Mix the parmesan cheese together with the garlic, coriander, salt, red pepper, and the olive oil; mix to combine well. Stuff the mushroom caps with the parmesan filling. Top with grated Gorgonzola. Place the mushrooms in the Air Fryer grill pan and slide them into the machine. Grill them at 380 degrees F for 8 to 12 minutes or until the stuffing is warmed through. Meanwhile, prepare the horseradish mayo by mixing the mayonnaise, horseradish and parsley. Serve with the warm fried mushrooms. Enjoy!

766. Easy Frittata With Mozzarella And Kale

Servings: 3   Cooking Time: 20 Minutes
Ingredients:
1 yellow onion, finely chopped
6 ounces wild mushrooms, sliced
6 eggs
1/2 teaspoon cayenne pepper
Sea salt and ground black pepper, to taste
1/4 cup double cream
1 tablespoon butter, melted
2 tablespoons fresh Italian parsley, chopped
2 cups kale, chopped
1/2 cup mozzarella, shredded

Directions:
Begin by preheating the Air Fryer to 360 degrees F. Spritz the sides and bottom of a baking pan with cooking oil. Add the onions and wild mushrooms, and cook in the preheated Air Fryer at 360 degrees F for 4 to 5 minutes. In a mixing dish, whisk the eggs and double cream until pale. Add the spices, butter, parsley, and kale; stir until everything is well

incorporated. Pour the mixture into the baking pan with the mushrooms. Top with the cheese. Cook in the preheated Air Fryer for 10 minutes. Serve immediately and enjoy!

767. Cheese And Chive Stuffed Chicken Rolls

Servings: 6   Cooking Time: 20 Minutes
Ingredients:

2 eggs, well-whisked Tortilla chips, crushed	1 ½ cup soft cheese
1 1/2 tablespoons extra-virgin olive oil	1/2 teaspoon whole grain mustard
1 ½ tablespoons fresh chives, chopped	1/2 teaspoon cumin powder
3 chicken breasts, halved lengthwise	1/3 teaspoon fine sea salt
2 teaspoons sweet paprika	1/3 cup fresh cilantro, chopped
	1/3 teaspoon freshly ground black pepper, or more to taste

Directions:
Flatten out each piece of the chicken breast using a rolling pin. Then, grab three mixing dishes. In the first one, combine the soft cheese with the cilantro, fresh chives, cumin, and mustard. In another mixing dish, whisk the eggs together with the sweet paprika. In the third dish, combine the salt, black pepper, and crushed tortilla chips. Spread the cheese mixture over each piece of chicken. Repeat with the remaining pieces of the chicken breasts; now, roll them up. Coat each chicken roll with the whisked egg; dredge each chicken roll into the tortilla chips mixture. Lower the rolls onto the air fryer cooking basket. Drizzle extra-virgin olive oil over all rolls. Air fry at 345 degrees F for 28 minutes, working in batches. Serve warm, garnished with sour cream if desired.

768. Two Cheese And Shrimp Dip

Servings: 8   Cooking Time: 25 Minutes
Ingredients:

2 teaspoons butter, melted	1/2 teaspoon red pepper flakes
8 ounces shrimp, peeled and deveined	4 ounces cream cheese, at room temperature
2 garlic cloves, minced	1/2 cup sour cream
1/4 cup chicken stock	4 tablespoons mayonnaise
2 tablespoons fresh lemon juice	1/4 cup mozzarella cheese, shredded
Salt and ground black pepper, to taste	

Directions:
Start by preheating the Air Fryer to 395 degrees F. Grease the sides and bottom of a baking dish with the melted butter. Place the shrimp, garlic, chicken stock, lemon juice, salt, black pepper, and red pepper flakes in the baking dish. Transfer the baking dish to the cooking basket and bake for 10

minutes. Add the mixture to your food processor; pulse until the coarsely is chopped. Add the cream cheese, sour cream, and mayonnaise. Top with the mozzarella cheese and bake in the preheated Air Fryer at 360 degrees F for 6 to 7 minutes or until the cheese is bubbling. Serve immediately with breadsticks if desired. Bon appétit!

769. Peanut Butter And Chicken Bites

Servings: 8   Cooking Time: 10 Minutes
Ingredients:

1 ½ tablespoons soy sauce	1 teaspoon sea salt
1/2 teaspoon smoked cayenne pepper	32 wonton wrappers
8 ounces soft cheese	1/3 teaspoon freshly cracked mixed peppercorns
1 1/2 tablespoons peanut butter	1/2 tablespoon pear cider vinegar
1/3 leftover chicken	

Directions:
Combine all of the above ingredients, minus the wonton wrappers, in a mixing dish. Lay out the wrappers on a clean surface. Now, spread the wonton wrappers with the prepared chicken filling. Fold the outside corners to the center over the filling; after that, roll up the wrappers tightly; you can moisten the edges with a little water. Set the air fryer to cook at 360 degrees F. Air fry the rolls for 6 minutes, working in batches. Serve with marinara sauce. Bon appétit!

770. Easiest Pork Chops Ever

Servings: 6   Cooking Time: 22 Minutes
Ingredients:

1/3 cup Italian breadcrumbs	3 tablespoons white flour
Roughly chopped fresh cilantro, to taste	1 teaspoon seasoned salt
2 teaspoons Cajun seasonings	Garlic & onion spice blend, to taste
Nonstick cooking spray	6 pork chops
2 eggs, beaten	1/3 teaspoon freshly cracked black pepper

Directions:
Coat the pork chops with Cajun seasonings, salt, pepper, and the spice blend on all sides. Then, add the flour to a plate. In a shallow dish, whisk the egg until pale and smooth. Place the Italian breadcrumbs in the third bowl. Dredge each pork piece in the flour; then, coat them with the egg; finally, coat them with the breadcrumbs. Spritz them with cooking spray on both sides. Now, air-fry pork chops for about 18 minutes at 345 degrees F; make sure to taste for doneness after first 12 minutes of cooking. Lastly, garnish with fresh cilantro. Bon appétit!

771. Keto Brioche With Caciocavallo

Servings: 6   Cooking Time: 15 Minutes

Ingredients:

1/2 cup ricotta cheese, crumbled
1 cup part skim mozzarella cheese, shredded
1 egg
1/2 cup coconut flour
1/2 cup almond flour
1 teaspoon baking soda
2 tablespoons plain whey protein isolate
3 tablespoons sesame oil

2 teaspoons dried thyme
1 ½ cups Caciocavallo, grated
1 cup leftover chicken, shredded
3 eggs
1 teaspoon kosher salt
1 teaspoon freshly cracked black pepper, or more to taste
1/3 teaspoon gremolata

Directions:

To make the keto brioche, microwave the cheese for 1 minute 30 seconds, stirring twice. Add the cheese to the bowl of a food processor and blend well. Fold in the egg and mix again.   Add in the flour, baking soda, and plain whey protein isolate; blend again. Scrape the batter onto the center of a lightly greased cling film.   Form the dough into a disk and transfer to your freezer to cool; cut into 6 pieces and transfer to a parchment-lined baking pan (make sure to grease your hands).   Firstly, slice off the top of each brioche; then, scoop out the insides. Brush each brioche with sesame oil. Add the remaining ingredients in the order listed above. Place the prepared brioche onto the bottom of the cooking basket. Bake for 7 minutes at 345 degrees F. Bon appétit!

772.	Creamed Cajun Chicken

Servings: 6   Cooking Time: 10 Minutes

Ingredients:

3 green onions, thinly sliced
½ tablespoon Cajun seasoning
2 large-sized chicken breasts, cut into strips
1/2 teaspoon garlic powder

1 ½ cup buttermilk
1 teaspoon salt
1 cup cornmeal mix
1 teaspoon shallot powder
1 ½ cup flour
1 teaspoon ground black pepper, or to taste

Directions:

Prepare three mixing bowls. Combine 1/2 cup of the plain flour together with the cornmeal and Cajun seasoning in your bowl. In another bowl, place the buttermilk.   Pour the remaining 1 cup of flour into the third bowl.   Sprinkle the chicken strips with all the seasonings. Then, dip each chicken strip in the 1 cup of flour, then in the buttermilk; finally, dredge them in the cornmeal mixture.   Cook the chicken strips in the air fryer baking pan for 16 minutes at 365 degrees F. Serve garnished with green onions. Bon appétit!

773.	Double Cheese Crêpes

Servings: 3   Cooking Time: 35 Minutes

Ingredients:

1/4 cup coconut flour
1 tablespoon psyllium husk
2 eggs, beaten
3 egg whites, beaten
1/4 teaspoon allspice
1/2 teaspoon salt
1 teaspoon cream of tartar

3/4 cup milk
1/2 cup ricotta cheese
1/2 cup Parmigiano-Reggiano cheese, preferably freshly grated
1 cup marinara sauce

Directions:

Mix the coconut flour, psyllium husk, eggs, allspice, salt, and cream of tartar in a large bowl. Gradually add the milk and ricotta cheese, whisking continuously, until well combined.   Let it stand for 20 minutes.   Spritz the Air Fryer baking pan with cooking spray. Pour the batter into the prepared pan.   Cook at 230 degrees F for 3 minutes. Flip and cook until browned in spots, 2 to 3 minutes longer.   Repeat with the remaining batter. Serve with Parmigiano-Reggiano cheese and marinara sauce. Bon appétit!

774.	Tangy Paprika Chicken

Servings: 4   Cooking Time: 30 Minutes

Ingredients:

1 ½ tablespoons freshly squeezed lemon juice
2 small-sized chicken breasts, boneless
1/2 teaspoon ground cumin
1 teaspoon dry mustard powder
1 teaspoon paprika

2 teaspoons cup pear cider vinegar
1 tablespoon olive oil
2 garlic cloves, minced
Kosher salt and freshly ground mixed peppercorns, to savor

Directions:

Warm the olive oil in a nonstick pan over a moderate flame. Sauté the garlic for just 1 minutes.   Remove your pan from the heat; add cider vinegar, lemon juice, paprika, cumin, mustard powder, kosher salt, and black pepper. Pour this paprika sauce into a baking dish.   Pat the chicken breasts dry; transfer them to the prepared sauce. Bake in the preheated air fryer for about 28 minutes at 335 degrees F; check for doneness using a thermometer or a fork. Allow to rest for 8 to 9 minutes before slicing and serving. Serve with dressing.

775.	Parmesan Broccoli Fritters

Servings: 6   Cooking Time: 30 Minutes

Ingredients:

1 1/2 cups Monterey Jack cheese
1 teaspoon dried dill weed
1/3 teaspoon ground black pepper

3 eggs, whisked
1/2 teaspoon kosher salt
2 ½ cups broccoli florets

1 teaspoon cayenne pepper

1/2 cup Parmesan cheese

Directions:
Blitz the broccoli florets in a food processor until finely crumbed. Then, combine the broccoli with the rest of the above ingredients.   Roll the mixture into small balls; place the balls in the fridge for approximately half an hour.   Preheat your Air Fryer to 335 degrees F and set the timer to 14 minutes; cook until broccoli croquettes are browned and serve warm.

776.   Baked Eggs With Beef And Tomato

Servings: 4   Cooking Time: 20 Minutes

Ingredients:

Non-stick cooking spray	4 eggs, beaten
1/2 pound leftover beef, coarsely chopped	4 tablespoons heavy cream
2 garlic cloves, pressed	1/2 teaspoon turmeric powder
1 cup kale, torn into pieces and wilted	Salt and ground black pepper, to your liking
1 tomato, chopped	1/8 teaspoon ground allspice

Directions:
Spritz the inside of four ramekins with a cooking spray.   Divide all of the above ingredients among the prepared ramekins. Stir until everything is well combined.   Air-fry at 360 degrees F for 16 minutes; check with a wooden stick and return the eggs to the Air Fryer for a few more minutes as needed. Serve immediately.

777. Award Winning Breaded Chicken

Servings: 4   Cooking Time: 10 Minutes + Marinating Time

Ingredients:

1 1/2 teaspoons olive oil	For the Marinade:
1 teaspoon red pepper flakes, crushed	1 ½ tablespoons mayo
1/3 teaspoon chicken bouillon granules	1 teaspoon kosher salt
	For the chicken:
1/3 teaspoon shallot powder	2 beaten eggs
	Breadcrumbs
1 1/2 tablespoons tamari soy sauce	1 ½ chicken breasts, boneless and skinless
1/3 teaspoon cumin powder	1 ½ tablespoons plain flour

Directions:
Butterfly the chicken breasts, and then, marinate them for at least 55 minutes.   Coat the chicken with plain flour; then, coat with the beaten eggs; finally, roll them in the breadcrumbs.   Lightly grease the cooking basket. Air-fry the breaded chicken at 345 degrees F for 12 minutes, flipping them halfway.

778.   Baked Eggs With Cheese And Cauli Rice

Servings: 4   Cooking Time: 30 Minutes

Ingredients:

1 pound cauliflower rice	Sea salt and ground black pepper, to taste
1 onion, diced	6 eggs
6 slices bacon, precooked	1 cup cheddar cheese, shredded
1 tablespoon butter, melted	

Directions:
Place the cauliflower rice and onion in a lightly greased casserole dish. Add the bacon and the reserved quinoa. Drizzle the melted butter over cauliflower rice and sprinkle with salt and pepper. Bake in the preheated Air Fryer at 390 degrees F for 10 minutes.   Turn the temperature down to 350 degrees F.   Make six indents for the eggs; crack one egg into each indent. Bake for 10 minutes, rotating the pan once or twice to ensure even cooking.   Top with cheese and bake for a further 5 minutes. Enjoy!

779.   Scrambled Eggs With Spinach And Tomato

Servings: 2   Cooking Time: 15 Minutes

Ingredients:

2 tablespoons olive oil, melted	4 eggs, whisked
5 ounces fresh spinach, chopped	1/2 teaspoon coarse salt
1 medium-sized tomato, chopped	1/2 teaspoon ground black pepper
1 teaspoon fresh lemon juice	1/2 cup of fresh basil, roughly chopped

Directions:
Add the olive oil to an Air Fryer baking pan. Make sure to tilt the pan to spread the oil evenly. Simply combine the remaining ingredients, except for the basil leaves; whisk well until everything is well incorporated.   Cook in the preheated Air Fryer for 8 to 12 minutes at 280 degrees F. Garnish with fresh basil leaves. Serve warm with a dollop of sour cream if desired.

780.   Dinner Turkey Sandwiches

Servings: 4   Cooking Time: 4 Hours 30 Minutes

Ingredients:

1/2 pound turkey breast	7 ounces condensed cream of onion soup
1 teaspoon garlic powder	1/3 teaspoon ground allspice
BBQ sauce, to savor	

Directions:
Simply dump the cream of onion soup and turkey breast into your crock-pot. Cook on HIGH heat setting for 3 hours.   Then, shred the meat and transfer to a lightly greased baking dish.   Pour in

your favorite BBQ sauce. Sprinkle with ground allspice and garlic powder. Air-fry an additional 28 minutes. To finish, assemble the sandwiches; add toppings such as pickled or fresh salad, mustard, etc.

781. Parmesan-crusted Fish Fingers

Servings: 4   Cooking Time: 20 Minutes

Ingredients:

1 ½ pounds tilapia pieces (fingers)	1 teaspoon onion powder
1/2 cup coconut flour	Sea salt and ground black pepper, to taste
2 eggs	
1 tablespoon yellow mustard	1/2 teaspoon celery powder
1 cup parmesan cheese, grated	2 tablespoons peanut oil
1 teaspoon garlic powder	

Directions:
Pat dry the fish fingers with a kitchen towel. To make a breading station, place the coconut flour in a shallow dish. In a separate dish, whisk the eggs with mustard. In a third bowl, mix parmesan cheese with the remaining ingredients. Dredge the fish fingers in the flour, shaking the excess into the bowl; dip in the egg mixture and turn to coat evenly; then, dredge in the parmesan mixture, turning a couple of times to coat evenly. Cook in the preheated Air Fryer at 390 degrees F for 5 minutes; turn them over and cook another 5 minutes. Enjoy!

782. Philadelphia Mushroom Omelet

Servings: 2   Cooking Time: 20 Minutes

Ingredients:

1 tablespoon olive oil	1 bell pepper, seeded and thinly sliced
1/2 cup scallions, chopped	
6 ounces button mushrooms, thinly sliced	2 tablespoons milk
	Sea salt and freshly ground black pepper, to taste
4 eggs	1 tablespoon fresh chives, for serving

Directions:
Heat the olive oil in a skillet over medium-high heat. Now, sauté the scallions and peppers until aromatic. Add the mushrooms and continue to cook an additional 3 minutes or until tender. Reserve. Generously grease a baking pan with nonstick cooking spray. Then, whisk the eggs, milk, salt, and black pepper. Spoon into the prepared baking pan. Cook in the preheated Air Fryer at 360 F for 4 minutes. Flip and cook for a further 3 minutes. Place the reserved mushroom filling on one side of the omelet. Fold your omelet in half and slide onto a serving plate. Serve immediately garnished with fresh chives. Bon appétit!

783. Turkey With Cheese And Pasilla Peppers

Servings: 2   Cooking Time: 30 Minutes

Ingredients:

1/2 cup Parmesan cheese, shredded	1/3 cup mayonnaise
	1 dried Pasilla peppers
1/2 pound turkey breasts, cut into four pieces	1 teaspoon onion salt
	1/3 teaspoon mixed peppercorns, freshly cracked
1 ½ tablespoons sour cream	

Directions:
In a shallow bowl, mix Parmesan cheese, onion salt, and the cracked mixed peppercorns together. In a food processor, blitz the mayonnaise, along with the cream and dried Pasilla peppers until there are no lumps. Coat the turkey breasts with this mixture, ensuring that all sides are covered. Then, coat each piece of turkey in the Parmesan mixture. Now, preheat the Air Fryer to 365 degrees F; cook for 28 minutes until thoroughly cooked.

784. Muffins With Brown Mushrooms

Servings: 6   Cooking Time: 25 Minutes

Ingredients:

2 tablespoons butter, melted	1 cup brown mushrooms, sliced
1 yellow onion, chopped	1 teaspoon fresh basil
2 garlic cloves, minced	8 eggs, lightly whisked
Sea salt and ground black pepper, to taste	6 ounces goat cheese, crumbled

Directions:
Start by preheating your Air Fryer to 330 degrees F. Now, spritz a 6-tin muffin tin with cooking spray. Melt the butter in a heavy-bottomed skillet over medium-high heat. Sauté the onions, garlic, and mushrooms until just tender and fragrant. Add the salt, black pepper, and basil and remove from heat. Divide out the sautéed mixture into the muffin tin. Pour the whisked eggs on top and top with the goat cheese. Bake for 20 minutes rotating the pan halfway through the cooking time. Bon appétit!

785. Easy Greek Revithokeftedes

Servings: 3   Cooking Time: 30 Minutes

Ingredients:

12 ounces canned chickpeas, drained	1 chili pepper
	1/2 teaspoon cayenne pepper
1 red onion, sliced	Sea salt and freshly ground pepper, to taste
2 cloves garlic	
1 tablespoon fresh coriander	
2 tablespoons all-purpose flour	3 large (6 ½ -inch pita bread

Directions:

Pulse the chickpeas, onion, garlic, chili pepper and coriander in your food processor until the chickpeas are ground. Add the all-purpose flour, cayenne pepper, salt, and black pepper; stir to combine well. Form the chickpea mixture into balls and place them in the lightly greased Air Fryer basket. Cook at 380 degrees F for about 15 minutes, shaking the basket occasionally to ensure even cooking. Warm the pita bread in your Air Fryer at 390 degrees F for around 6 minutes. Serve the revithokeftedes in pita bread with tzatziki or your favorite Greek topping. Enjoy!

786.   Chicken Drumsticks With Ketchup-lemon Sauce

Servings: 6   Cooking Time: 20 Minutes + Marinating Time

Ingredients:

3 tablespoons lemon juice	1/2 teaspoon ground black pepper
1 cup tomato ketchup	2 teaspoons lemon zest, grated
1 ½ tablespoons fresh rosemary, chopped	1/3 cup honey
6 skin-on chicken drumsticks, boneless	3 cloves garlic, minced

Directions:
Dump the chicken drumsticks into a mixing dish. Now, add the other items and give it a good stir; let it marinate overnight in your refrigerator. Discard the marinade; roast the chicken legs in your air fryer at 375 degrees F for 22 minutes, turning once. Now, add the marinade and cook an additional 6 minutes or until everything is warmed through.

787.   Western Eggs With Ham And Cheese

Servings: 4   Cooking Time: 20 Minutes

Ingredients:

6 eggs	1/2 cup milk
2 ounces cream cheese, softened	1/4 teaspoon paprika
Sea salt, to your liking	6 ounces cooked ham, diced
1/4 teaspoon ground black pepper	1 onion, chopped
	1/2 cup cheddar cheese, shredded

Directions:
Begin by preheating the Air Fryer to 360 degrees F. Spritz the sides and bottom of a baking pan with cooking oil. In a mixing dish, whisk the eggs, milk, and cream cheese until pale. Add the spices, ham, and onion; stir until everything is well incorporated. Pour the mixture into the baking pan; top with the cheddar cheese. Bake in the preheated Air Fryer for 12 minutes. Serve warm and enjoy!

788.   Greek Omelet With Halloumi Cheese

Servings: 2   Cooking Time: 17 Minutes

Ingredients:

1/2 cup Halloumi cheese, sliced	4 well-whisked eggs
2 teaspoons garlic paste	1 ½ tablespoons fresh basil, chopped
2 teaspoons fresh chopped rosemary	3 tablespoons onions, chopped
2 bell peppers, seeded and chopped	Fine sea salt and ground black pepper, to taste

Directions:
Spritz your baking dish with a canola cooking spray. Throw in all ingredients and stir until everything is well incorporated. Bake for about 15 minutes at 325 degrees F. Eat warm.

789.   Winter Baked Eggs With Italian Sausage

Servings: 4   Cooking Time: 30 Minutes

Ingredients:

1 pound Italian sausage	2 sprigs thyme
2 sprigs rosemary	2 tablespoons extra-virgin olive oil
1 celery, sliced	1 leek, cut into halves lengthwise
1/2 pound broccoli, cut into small florets	A pinch of grated nutmeg
1 bell pepper, trimmed and cut into matchsticks	Salt and black pepper, to taste
2 garlic cloves, smashed	4 whole eggs

Directions:
Arrange vegetables on the bottom of the Air Fryer baking dish. Sprinkle with the seasonings and top with the sausage. Roast approximately 20 minutes at 375 degrees F, stirring occasionally. Top with eggs and reduce the temperature to 330 degrees F. Bake an additional 5 to 6 minutes. Bon appétit!

790.   Spicy Eggs With Sausage And Swiss Cheese

Servings: 6   Cooking Time: 25 Minutes

Ingredients:

1 teaspoon lard	1 scallion, chopped
1/2 pound turkey sausage	1 chili pepper, seeded and chopped
6 eggs	Sea salt and ground black pepper, to taste
1 garlic clove, minced	1/2 cup Swiss cheese, shredded
1 bell pepper, seeded and chopped	

Directions:
Start by preheating your Air Fryer to 330 degrees F. Now, spritz 4 silicone molds with cooking spray. Melt the lard in a saucepan over medium-high heat. Now, cook the sausage for 5 minutes or until no longer pink. Coarsely chop the sausage; add the

eggs, scallions, garlic, peppers, salt, and black pepper. Divide the egg mixture between the silicone molds. Top with the shredded cheese. Bake in the preheated Air Fryer at 340 degrees F for 15 minutes, checking halfway through the cooking time to ensure even cooking. Enjoy!

791. Masala-style Baked Eggs

Servings: 6   Cooking Time: 25 Minutes

Ingredients:

6 medium-sized eggs, beaten	2 tablespoons sesame oil
1 teaspoon garam masala	Hot sauce, for drizzling
1 cup scallions, finely chopped	1 teaspoon mixed peppercorns, freshly cracked
3 cloves garlic, finely minced	1 teaspoon kosher salt
2 cups leftover chicken, shredded	1/3 teaspoon smoked paprika
1 teaspoon turmeric	

Directions:

Warm sesame oil in a sauté pan over a moderate flame; then, sauté the scallions together with garlic until just fragrant; it takes about 5 minutes. Now, throw in leftover chicken and stir until thoroughly warmed.   In a medium-sized bowl or a measuring cup, thoroughly combine the eggs with all seasonings.   Then, coat the inside of six oven safe ramekins with a nonstick cooking spray. Divide the egg/chicken mixture among your ramekins.   Air-fry approximately 18 minutes at 355 degrees F. Drizzle with hot sauce and eat warm.

792. Super-easy Chicken With Tomato Sauce

Servings: 4   Cooking Time: 20 Minutes + Marinating Time

Ingredients:

1 tablespoon balsamic vinegar	4 Roma tomatoes, diced
½ teaspoon red pepper flakes, crushed	1 ½ tablespoons butter
1 fresh garlic, roughly chopped	1/3 handful fresh basil, loosely packed, sniped
2 ½ large-sized chicken breasts, cut into halves	1 teaspoon kosher salt
1/3 handful fresh cilantro, roughly chopped	2 cloves garlic, minced
2 tablespoons olive oil	Cooked bucatini, to serve

Directions:

Place the first seven ingredients in a medium-sized bowl; let it marinate for a couple of hours. Preheat the air fryer to 325 degrees F. Air-fry your chicken for 32 minutes and serve warm.   In the meantime, prepare the tomato sauce by preheating a deep saucepan. Simmer the tomatoes until you make a chunky mixture. Throw in the garlic, basil, and butter; give it a good stir.   Serve the cooked chicken breasts with the tomato sauce and the cooked bucatini. Bon appétit!

793. Cheddar Cheese And Pastrami Casserole

Servings: 2   Cooking Time: 20 Minutes

Ingredients:

4 eggs	1/4 cup Greek-style yogurt
1 bell pepper, chopped	1/2 cup Cheddar cheese, grated
2 spring onions, chopped	Sea salt, to taste
1 cup pastrami, sliced	1/4 teaspoon ground black pepper

Directions:

Start by preheating your Air Fryer to 330 degrees F. Spritz the baking pan with cooking oil.   Then, thoroughly combine all ingredients and pour the mixture into the prepared baking pan.   Cook for 7 to 9 minutes or until the eggs have set. Place on a cooling rack and let it sit for 10 minutes before slicing and serving.

794. Dinner Avocado Chicken Sliders

Servings: 4   Cooking Time: 10 Minutes

Ingredients:

½ pounds ground chicken meat	1 teaspoon garlic powder
4 burger buns	1 ½ tablespoon extra-virgin olive oil
1/2 cup Romaine lettuce, loosely packed	1 cloves garlic, minced
½ teaspoon dried parsley flakes	Nonstick cooking spray
1/3 teaspoon mustard seeds	Salt and cracked black pepper (peppercorns, to taste)
1 teaspoon onion powder	
1 ripe fresh avocado, mashed	

Directions:

Firstly, spritz an air fryer cooking basket with a nonstick cooking spray.   Mix ground chicken meat, mustard seeds, garlic powder, onion powder, parsley, salt, and black pepper until everything is thoroughly combined. Make sure not to overwork the meat to avoid tough chicken burgers.   Shape the meat mixture into patties and roll them in breadcrumbs; transfer your burgers to the prepared cooking basket. Brush the patties with the cooking spray.   Air-fry at 355 F for 9 minutes, working in batches. Slice burger buns into halves. In the meantime, combine olive oil with mashed avocado and pressed garlic.   To finish, lay Romaine lettuce and avocado spread on bun bottoms; now, add burgers and bun tops. Bon appétit!

795. Easy Zucchini Chips

Servings: 4   Cooking Time: 20 Minutes

Ingredients:

3/4 pound zucchini, peeled and sliced	1 egg, lightly beaten
1/2 cup seasoned breadcrumbs	1/2 cup parmesan cheese, preferably freshly grated

Directions:

Pat the zucchini dry with a kitchen towel. In a mixing dish, thoroughly combine the egg, breadcrumbs, and cheese. Then, coat the zucchini slices with the breadcrumb mixture. Cook in the preheated Air Fryer at 400 degrees F for 9 minutes, shaking the basket halfway through the cooking time. Work in batches until the chips is golden brown. Bon appétit!

---

796. Double Cheese Asparagus Casserole

Servings: 2   Cooking Time: 27 Minutes

Ingredients:

1 cup cauliflower rice	1/3 cup milk
1/3 cup Colby cheese, grated	2 well-beaten eggs
1 1/2 cups white mushrooms, sliced	1/3 teaspoon smoked cayenne pepper
2 asparagus spears, chopped	1 teaspoon ground black pepper, or to taste
1 teaspoon table salt, or to taste	1/3 teaspoon dried rosemary, crushed

Directions:
Throw the cauliflower rice into the baking dish. In a mixing dish, thoroughly combine the eggs and milk. Stir in 1/2 of cheese; add the seasonings. Pour 3/4 of egg/cheese mixture over the bread cubes in the baking dish; press gently using a wide spatula. Now, top with the mushrooms and chopped asparagus. Pour the remaining egg/cheese mixture over the top; make sure to spread it evenly. Top with the remaining Colby cheese and bake for 20 minutes at 325 degrees F.

---

797. Baked Eggs Florentine

Servings: 2   Cooking Time: 20 Minutes

Ingredients:

1 tablespoon ghee, melted	1/4 teaspoon red pepper flakes
2 cups baby spinach, torn into small pieces	Salt, to taste
2 tablespoons shallots, chopped	1 tablespoon fresh thyme leaves, roughly chopped
	4 eggs

Directions:
Start by preheating your Air Fryer to 350 degrees F. Brush the sides and bottom of a gratin dish with the melted ghee. Put the spinach and shallots into the bottom of the gratin dish. Season with red pepper, salt, and fresh thyme. Make four indents for the eggs; crack one egg into each indent. Bake for 12 minutes, rotating the pan once or twice to ensure even cooking. Enjoy!

---

798. Omelet With Mushrooms And Peppers

Servings: 2   Cooking Time: 20 Minutes

Ingredients:

1 tablespoon olive oil	1 bell pepper, seeded and thinly sliced
1/2 cup scallions, chopped	2 tablespoons milk
6 ounces button mushrooms, thinly	Sea salt and freshly ground black pepper, to taste
sliced	1 tablespoon fresh
4 eggs	chives, for serving

Directions:
Heat the olive oil in a skillet over medium-high heat. Now, sauté the scallions and peppers until aromatic. Add the mushrooms and continue to cook an additional 3 minutes or until tender. Reserve. Generously grease a baking pan with nonstick cooking spray. Then, whisk the eggs, milk, salt, and black pepper. Spoon into the prepared baking pan. Cook in the preheated Air Fryer at 360 F for 4 minutes. Flip and cook for a further 3 minutes. Place the reserved mushroom filling on one side of the omelet. Fold your omelet in half and slide onto a serving plate. Serve immediately garnished with fresh chives. Bon appétit!

---

799. Italian-style Broccoli Balls With Cheese

Servings: 4   Cooking Time: 25 Minutes

Ingredients:

1/2 pound broccoli	4 eggs, beaten
1/2 pound Romano cheese, grated	1/2 teaspoon paprika
2 garlic cloves, minced	1/4 teaspoon dried basil
1 shallot, chopped	Sea salt and ground black pepper, to taste
2 tablespoons butter, at room temperature	

Directions:
Add the broccoli to your food processor and pulse until the consistency resembles rice. Stir in the remaining ingredients; mix until everything is well combined. Shape the mixture into bite-sized balls and transfer them to the lightly greased cooking basket. Cook in the preheated Air Fryer at 375 degrees F for 16 minutes, shaking halfway through the cooking time. Serve with cocktail sticks and tomato ketchup on the side.

---

800. Za'atar Eggs With Chicken And Provolone Cheese

Servings: 2   Cooking Time: 20 Minutes

Ingredients:

1/3 cup milk	1 teaspoon Za'atar
1 1/2 Roma tomato, chopped	1/2 chicken breast, cooked
1/3 cup Provolone cheese, grated	1 teaspoon fine sea salt
1 teaspoon freshly cracked pink peppercorns	1 teaspoon freshly cracked pink peppercorns
3 eggs	

Directions:
Preheat your air fryer to cook at 365 degrees F. In a medium-sized mixing dish, whisk the eggs together with the milk, Za'atar, sea salt, and cracked pink peppercorns. Spritz the ramekins with cooking oil; divide the prepared egg mixture among the greased ramekins. Shred the chicken with two forks or a stand mixer. Add the shredded chicken to the ramekins, followed by the tomato and the cheese. To finish, air-fry for 18 minutes or until it is done. Bon appétit!

CPSIA information can be obtained
at www.ICGtesting.com
Printed in the USA
LVHW101539050121
675790LV00010B/356